Health Promotion

Global Principles and Practice

Second Edition

Health Promotion

Global Principles and Practice

2nd Edition

Ruth Cross

Sally Foster

Ivy O'Neil

Simon Rowlands

Louise Warwick-Booth

James Woodall

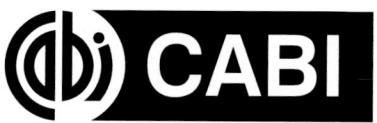

CABI is a trading name of CAB International

CABI
Nosworthy Way
Wallingford
Oxfordshire OX10 8DE
UK

Tel: +44 (0)1491 832111
Fax: +44 (0)1491 833508
E-mail: info@cabi.org
Website: www.cabi.org

CABI
WeWork
One Lincoln St
24th Floor
Boston, MA 02111
USA

Tel: +1 (617)682-9015
E-mail: cabi-nao@cabi.org

© Ruth Cross, Sally Foster, Ivy O'Neil, Simon Rowlands, Louise Warwick-Booth, and James Woodall 2021. All rights reserved. No part of this publication may be reproduced in any form or by any means, electronically, mechanically, by photocopying, recording or otherwise, without the prior permission of the copyright owners.

A catalogue record for this book is available from the British Library, London, UK.

Library of Congress Cataloging-in-Publication Data

Names: Cross, Ruth, author. | C.A.B. International, issuing body.
Title: Health promotion : global principles and practice / Ruth Cross, Sally Foster, Ivy O'Neil, Simon Rowlands, Louise Warwick-Booth, James Woodall.
Description: 2nd edition. | Wallingford, Oxfordshire, UK ; Boston, MA : CABI, [2021] | Preceded by Health promotion / Rahael Dixey ... [et al.]. Wallingford, Oxfordshire : CABI, c2013. | Includes bibliographical references and index. | Summary: "This new edition covers key concepts, theory and practical aspects of health promotion practice worldwide. It reviews social determinants, equality and equity, policy and health, working in partnerships, sustainability, evaluation and evidence-based practice, drawing upon international settings and teaching experience in the global North and South"-- Provided by publisher.
Identifiers: LCCN 2020029725 (print) | LCCN 2020029726 (ebook) | ISBN 9781789245332 (paperback) | ISBN 9781789246148 (ePDF) | ISBN 9781789246155 (epub)
Subjects: MESH: Health Promotion--methods | Community Health Planning | Global Health | Health Communication | Health Policy | Socioeconomic Factors
Classification: LCC RA425 (print) | LCC RA425 (ebook) | NLM WA 530.1 | DDC 362.1--dc23
LC record available at https://lccn.loc.gov/2020029725
LC ebook record available at https://lccn.loc.gov/2020029726

References to Internet websites (URLs) were accurate at the time of writing.

ISBN-13: 9781789245332 (paperback)
          9781789246148 (ePDF)
          9781789246155 (ePub)

Commissioning Editor: Alexandra Lainsbury
Editorial Assistant: Lauren Davies
Production Editor: James Bishop

Typeset by SPI, Pondicherry, India
Printed and bound in the UK by Severn, Gloucester

Contents

The Authors		vii
Introduction *Ruth Cross*		ix
1	The Foundations of Health Promotion *Ruth Cross, Simon Rowlands and Sally Foster*	1
2	People, Power and Communities *Louise Warwick-Booth and Sally Foster*	41
3	Policies for Health in the 21st Century *Louise Warwick-Booth and Simon Rowlands*	75
4	Health Communication *Ruth Cross and Ivy O'Neil*	106
5	Professional Practice *James Woodall and Simon Rowlands*	148
6	Towards the Future of Health Promotion *Ruth Cross, Louise Warwick-Booth and Sally Foster*	186
Index		233

The Authors

Ruth Cross

Ruth is Course Director in Health Promotion and has oversight of the suite of health promotion and public health courses delivered at Leeds Beckett University. She has wide experience in health, health care services and health promotion both in the UK and in sub-Saharan Africa. Ruth is Course Leader for the MSc Public Health Promotion in Ghana. She contributes to all the programmes at Leeds Beckett University facilitating learning about the foundations of health promotion, health communication, health behaviour and research methods. Ruth has co-authored several books and book chapters on health promotion, health communication, global health and health studies.

Sally Foster

Sally is a former Senior Lecturer at Leeds Beckett University. As well as teaching for many years on the Masters courses in Health Promotion in the UK and several countries in Africa, she was also more recently Course Leader for the BSc (Hons) Public Health, which is a 'top-up' degree, delivered in Zambia. A sociologist by background, Sally's interests are in women's health, community involvement in health, and the politics of health and development, particularly in relation to Africa, where she has lived and worked. Sally has also done research on solid waste management in Africa, and is currently researching the benefits of allotments and urban food growing for health and wellbeing.

Ivy O'Neil

Ivy is former Principal Lecturer and Professional Lead for the Health Promotion team at Leeds Beckett University. Her background is in nursing. She is also a Registered General Nurse, a Registered Midwife, a Registered Sick Children's Nurse and a Registered Health Visitor. Ivy's MSc was in research, undertaking primary research into the health needs of ethnic minority families. She was the Course Leader for the MSc Public Health – Health Promotion course and led the development of the distance learning version of the course. Ivy's research interests are in health needs assessment, promoting child, young person and family health. Ivy also has an interest in the education of public health practitioners and public health workforce development. She is the co-author with Dr Ruth Cross and Dr Sam Davis of the book *Health Communication – Theoretical and Critical Perspectives* (2017) and the author of *Digital Health Promotion – A Critical Introduction* (2019).

Simon Rowlands

Simon is a Senior Lecturer and Course Leader in Health Promotion at Leeds Beckett University and teaches a wide range of subjects from Foundations in Health Promotion and Public Health to Policy and Research Methods. Simon has 15 years of experience as a practicing Health Promotion Specialist working for the National Health Service in Bradford, West Yorkshire, as well as various non-governmental organization secondments primarily in the Balkans. Simon's work is largely focused around physical activity and nutrition. His PhD explored the role of gender, and masculinities in particular, in how men manage their bodies.

Louise Warwick-Booth

Louise is a Reader in Health Promotion and a sociologist with specific interests in health policy, social inequalities and vulnerable populations. She teaches modules on sociology, health policy, global health and research methods. Her current research interests focus upon the evaluation of interventions to improve the health of marginalized groups, particularly at-risk women.

James Woodall

James is a Reader and Head of Subject in Health Promotion at Leeds Beckett University. James teaches both postgraduate and undergraduate students and has contributed to several textbooks to support student and practitioner understanding. James is an active researcher in the field of public health and health promotion. His research interests are diverse, but with a common theme of understanding how to reduce health inequalities and improve individual and community health. James has particular interest in prison and offender health and has published several articles in this area.

Introduction

RUTH CROSS

Welcome to the second edition of *Health Promotion: Global Principles and Practice*. We have been updating this book during a time of global pandemic, a time when health and health promotion is at the forefront of many agendas and has become even more central to our everyday lived experiences. The Covid-19 pandemic is occurring against the backdrop of urgent issues such as climate change, threats to planetary health, struggles for racial equality and other matters of social (in)justice. Health promotion has a vital part to play in addressing all of these. As such this book aims to set out some key principles and ideas about health promotion in the 21st century, drawing on contemporary issues, debates and discourse. It is intended as a vehicle to open up the critical conversations required at a postgraduate level; a means to explore what health promotion *is*, what it is *about*, and how it might be *achieved* in order to create a fairer, more equal world.

This book originally came about as a companion text to the Master's level courses on health promotion that we deliver at Leeds Beckett University in Leeds, UK. The first edition of Health Promotion: Global Principles and Practice published in 2013 was edited by Professor Rachael Dixey who played a pivotal role in shaping the book and wrote a substantial amount of the original content alongside contributions from many of the teaching team in post at that time. The writings from the original authors are acknowledged chapter by chapter in this second edition. This second edition retains many of the original writing team members and also welcomes contributions from a newer member of staff, Simon Rowlands. Leeds Beckett University has been facilitating health promotion education for over 40 years and has played a leading role in the academic development of the field. Leeds Beckett staff have made key contributions to the academic health promotion literature including, more recently, Green *et al.* (2019), Cross *et al.* (2017), Warwick-Booth and Cross (2018), Warwick-Booth (2019), O'Neil (2019), and Woodall and Cross (forthcoming). Those familiar with the first edition of *Health Promotion: Global Principles and Practice* will notice that some of the chapter titles have changed slightly. This is to reflect the changes to module titles that have occurred since 2013 through course development and review. However, the core principles and theory of health promotion presented in the first edition remain central. This second edition picks up on many of the arguments presented in the first and takes forward the critical debates therein. It has been refreshed throughout drawing on more recent research and thinking in the field.

The author team, whilst situated in the global North, have experience of working in the global South (particularly in sub-Saharan Africa), and of working with students from around the world. Whilst we do not claim to be the experts on health promotion, nor to (re)present the only worldview on the subject, we do attempt to provide a platform by which health promotion can be critically appraised and to challenge some of the issues that we are all facing. We lay bare and discuss difficult issues for which there are no easy answers – Why do health inequalities persist? How can people be empowered to take control of their health? How do we address social injustice? In doing so we recognize our position of relative privilege, as academics situated in the global North. As such we own that this book presents a specific perspective – the Leeds Beckett view, a culmination of our teaching and thinking about health promotion. The book aims, however, to be useful for a global audience. Not everyone will concur with what we have to say, nor is it possible to include all there is to say about health promotion in a book of this size. We recommend that this book is read alongside other key health promotion texts, for example more practical texts that provide guidance about how to *do* health promotion (such as Naidoo and Wills, 2016; Scriven, 2017; Hubley *et al.*, 2021).

In the words of Professor Rachael Dixey who wrote the introduction to the first edition of *Health Promotion: Global Principles and Practice*:

> Our view of health promotion is that it is a social movement with the central aim of tackling the social determinants of health and so bringing about greater social justice in terms of health. Throughout, we assert that the way societies

are organized has consequences for health: fairer societies lead to healthier lives. As so many aspects of the way societies are organized impact upon health, this gives us a mandate to consider a very wide range of issues – from spending on armaments, to migration, multiculturalism, climate change, women's rights, crime rates, the 'banking crisis', freedom of speech, tourism, land rights and many more. In short, health promoters do not start with blank sheets – we have to start with the messy, true-life realities of our complex world. We present a view of health promotion that has as its central aim the empowerment of communities and we emphasize the importance of working with people, not 'on' them or through them. We thus implicitly criticize top-down, behaviour-change and lifestyle approaches that attempt to manipulate people into healthier behaviours; not that we do not believe that (some) behaviours need to change – the point is the process by which these are made, and the political processes that underpin them. Health promoters often talk of 'interventions', whereas we prefer the idea of 'implementation with people' (2013, pp. xi-xii).

In summary, this book aims to do the following:

- Explore what health promotion is and be critical of it.
- Set out key ideas in health promotion and explore the discourse surrounding it.
- Introduce key thinkers in the field and discuss the relevance and application of their ideas.
- Provide a theoretical basis for health promotion practice.
- Ask some challenging questions and encourage our readers to do the same.
- Comment on the state of academic health promotion.

The Structure of the Book

This second edition is once again organized in step with the curricula of the Leeds Beckett postgraduate courses currently taught in Leeds, Ghana and online (Distant Learning), and formerly in Zambia and The Gambia. It will, however, be highly relevant and appropriate for students on other postgraduate courses in health promotion. This edition builds on the content of the first, which has been refreshed and revived in order to reflect how health promotion theory, practice and research have changed and developed since the publication of the first edition in 2013. It also takes into account how our world has changed in the few years since then.

The first chapter, *The Foundations of Health Promotion*, includes more recent debates and evidence on health, and picks up the discussion of social determinants of health, threshold concepts in health promotion, values in health promotion, empowerment, and developments in the global health agenda. The chapter outlines the key principles and approaches to health promotion as we see them and introduces the disciplinary basis of health promotion.

The next three chapters expand on some of the key ideas introduced in the first one. Chapter 2, *People, Power and Communities*, explores the importance of community for health. It has been updated and refreshed to include more recent debates about healthy communities drawing on developments in evidence associated with community wellbeing (What Works Wellbeing) and new understandings of community engagement (community-centred approaches). Recent work from the World Health Organization on measuring community resilience, linked to asset-based approaches, is also discussed.

Chapter 3, *Policies for Health in the 21st Century*, focuses on health in all policies forefronting the importance of policy for the promotion of health. It has been updated to reflect changes in the global policy context including new content on the Sustainable Development Goals. More recent examples of policy approaches in relation to inequalities are discussed alongside examples of policy as a social determinant of health.

Chapter 4, *Health Communication*, considers communication for health. It has been updated and refreshed to include discussion about the nature of communication, critique of existing approaches, and more recent development in the socio-psychological theories of behaviour change. There has been a substantial rewrite of the digital communication section that includes a more in-depth consideration of social media, digital health technology and Big Data.

Chapter 5, *Professional Practice*, considers the professional context of health promotion. It has been revised to consider developments in relation to the core skills and competencies needs for those working in health promotion. 'Settings' is a major theme of this chapter, as are evaluation and evidence-based practice.

The final chapter, *Towards the Future of Health Promotion*, continues to consider the role of the academic health promotion community and question where health promotion is going, and its potential as a social movement to effect global health and to bring about a fairer, more just world in which everyone has good health and can achieve their potential. The content has been refreshed in relation to new and emerging public health issues, changing health promotion discourse, and more contemporary understandings of wellbeing. The importance of lay knowledge is reinforced, and the value base of health promotion is revisited reflecting on future challenges in the field.

We hope you enjoy reading this book. We hope that it challenges and inspires you. We hope that the critical discussion herein causes you to not only question what health promotion is about but also encourage you to make a difference in order to promote health wherever you are and whatever your role.

This book is dedicated to all our students – past, present and future.

References

Cross, R., Davis, S. and O'Neil, I. (2017) *Health Communication: Theoretical and Critical Perspectives.* Polity, Cambridge.
Green, J., Cross, R., Woodall, J. and Tones, K. (2019) *Health Promotion: Planning and Strategies*, 4th edn. Sage, London.
Hubley, J., Copeman, J. and Woodall, J. (2021) *Practical Health Promotion*, 3rd edn. Polity, Cambridge.
O'Neil, I. (2019) *Digital Health Promotion: A Critical Introduction.* Polity, Cambridge.
Naidoo, J. and Wills, J. (2016) *Foundations for Health Promotion*, 4th edn. Elsevier, London.
Scriven, A. (2017) *Promoting Health: A Practical Guide*, 7th edn. Elsevier, London.
Warwick-Booth, L. (2019) *Social Inequality: A Student Guide*, 2nd edn. Sage, London.
Warwick-Booth, L. and Cross, R. (2018) *Global Health Studies: A Social Determinants Perspective.* Polity, Cambridge.
Woodall, J. and Cross, R. (forthcoming) *Essentials of Health Promotion.* Sage, London.

1 The Foundations of Health Promotion

Ruth Cross, Simon Rowlands and Sally Foster[1]

This chapter aims to:
- explore concepts of 'health' held by lay people and health promoters;
- introduce recent work on the social determinants of health;
- introduce certain threshold concepts including salutogenesis, social models of health and upstream thinking;
- establish the value base of health promotion;
- introduce the disciplinary foundations of health promotion
- outline in more detail 'empowerment' as a key value in health promotion; and
- describe the key WHO conferences, which provide the milestones in the development of health promotion.

The aim of this chapter is to provide an orientation to current thinking in health promotion and offer some of the material that would be covered in an introductory module, laying the foundations for a course of study. It is essential to understand that health promotion is a political and ethical activity, with a sound value base providing the platform for practice and setting its direction.

Our view of health promotion is that it is a social movement with the central aim of tackling the social determinants of health and so bringing about greater social and health justice. By the 'social determinants of health' we mean those factors that enable people to live healthy and productive lives – these factors include the obvious ones of decent housing, access to education, employment opportunities, nourishing food, well-functioning and accessible health care, cohesive communities, good systems of government and peaceful, safe nation-states. The social determinants of health can either enable people and communities to flourish and do well, or not, depending on whether (or how) they create opportunities for better health. Social justice is harder to define, and is often used interchangeably with related concepts such as 'fairness', 'equality' and 'equity'. Aristotle's *Ethics* suggest that equity is where like but different individuals are both regarded and treated justly because they are equally valued. Thus, regardless of ability/ disability, gender, sexual orientation, ethnicity, age or any other variable that differentiates people, *all* individuals have equal value. Treating individuals with equal value is *just* and therefore contributes to social justice. Logically, following from this is the idea that 'social goods' such as health should be distributed fairly. Harvey (1973, p. 98), in his attempt to outline the 'skeleton concept' of social justice, says that it starts with a 'just distribution justly arrived at'. We can argue that where access to a good, decent and productive life is not available to some, where some live in abject poverty and others in excessive wealth, then there is clearly not 'a just distribution'. This raises the question of whether people have the *right* to good health, and we would assert that people do indeed have the right to those determinants that produce good health. This is enshrined in the Universal Declaration of Human Rights: that people have the right to the conditions necessary to achieve the highest possible standard of health (United Nations, 1948; Marks, 2004). This rights-based approach to health was strongly reiterated in the 2030 Agenda for Sustainable Development and Universal Health Coverage (WHO, 2017). Health promotion has, at its heart, the drive to eliminate health inequities, if inequity means the failure to regard and treat 'like but different' individuals and groups justly because they are not equally valued.

Individual readers might pause at this point and think that they do indeed see all individuals as having equal worth. However, we can clearly see that at a global scale we do not treat individuals as having equal worth – otherwise children would not be dying in the 'developing' world due to preventable diseases such as diarrhoea, respiratory infections or measles, whilst others live in unimaginable luxury. There would not be the less dramatic differences between individuals within the same country, such as in England, with children growing up in situations described as below the poverty line (for a 'developed' country) and those living in very comfortable wealth. Inequities in health experience and outcomes are being highlighted at the time of updating this chapter amid the Covid-19 pandemic (April 2020). Ratcliffe (2020) points out how the pandemic is emphasizing existing inequality and disproportionately affecting certain groups of people, despite the rhetoric that 'we are all in this together' – see Box 1.1 for further elaboration.

This central concern with health equity has been present since the Ottawa Charter, and was present in the World Health Organization (WHO) from 1946. According to Whitehead and Dahlgren (2007, p. 5), health equity

> ... implies that ideally everyone could attain their full health potential and that no one should be disadvantaged from achieving this potential because of their social position or other socially determined circumstance. This refers to everyone and not just to a particularly disadvantaged segment of the population. Efforts to promote social equity in health are therefore aimed at creating opportunities and removing barriers to achieving the health potential of all people. It involves the fair distribution of resources needed for health, fair access to the opportunities available, and fairness in the support offered to people when ill.

The outcome of these efforts would be a gradual reduction of all systematic differences in health between different socioeconomic groups. The ultimate vision is the elimination of such inequities, by levelling up to the health of the most advantaged.

The concern with health inequities culminated in the global health promotion community cohering behind the work of the Commission on Social Determinants of Health (CSDH). The Commission was established by the WHO in 2005 and chaired by Sir Michael Marmot. It was essentially an independent enquiry into the social and environmental issues affecting health and planned to investigate actions with the potential to promote greater health equity that has been referred to as a 'global blue-print for the health promotion community and the stakeholders we work with' (Smith et al., 2018. p. 3). The work of the CSDH preceded other work led by Sir Michael Marmot including the Strategic Review of Health Inequalities in England post-2010 (Fair Society, Healthy Lives) (Marmot, 2010) and a 53-nation European Review (Marmot, 2013). The primary outcome of the CSDH work was a set of recommendations to reduce health inequity focusing on upstream influences including improving the conditions of daily living, tackling the inequitable distribution of power, money and resources, and measuring and understanding the problem and

---

Box 1.1. Health inequity and Covid-19 in England (April, 2020).

'What is interesting about the risk of death (from Covid-19) is that it almost perfectly tracks your current risk of death. So, if you are already sick, from a BAME background, grew up in poverty or are already older you are more likely to develop serious symptoms and/or die. The economic impacts will be most acutely felt by those with the fewest resources: people in low paid jobs, people who have chronic mental of physical illness, people on temporary or "zero hours" contracts and those who are living from pay check to pay check. It is also likely that those in low paid manual jobs (e.g. [working in] supermarkets, social care, construction etc.) will be less able to socially distance by working from home and, hence, less able to minimise the risk of infection. Those who are confined to home in poor quality or cramped housing will have the most miserable experience and those living in the least affluent, vibrant and green surroundings will suffer the biggest fall in wellbeing. These individuals are all part of the same group: the poorest in society. [...] Covid-19 has taken the social determinants of health, which have been insidiously working away behind the scenes, slowly eroding peoples' health and wellbeing, and exploded their impact into full view' (Ratcliffe, 2020, www.fairhealth.org.uk).

assessing the impact of action (WHO, 2008; Schrecker, 2019). Ten years after the report was published there have been some reflections on the progress that has been made; however, the extent to which we have made headway is open to question (Smith *et al.*, 2018). Schrecker (2019) has argued that 'in some respects the report has sunk like a stone' causing some ripples 'but not the erosion of the pond's shoreline that [was] hoped for' (p. 610). The ripples referred to include a greater appreciation (in theory at least) of the social determinants of health; for example, advances in understanding the impact of stress, environmental pollution and climate change on health inequity. In many countries, however, income inequality (which is directly linked to health inequality) has been increasing, hence the lack of erosion of the shoreline referred to by Schrecker. On the other hand, there is also greater understanding of the social determinants of health (Smith *et al.*, 2018), and the adoption of the Sustainable Development Goals (SDGs) gives rise to some optimism, Schrecker (2019) argues. The achievement of the SDGs will, however, require significant political will in order to effect change. Friel *et al.* (2009) noted that money can be found to tackle anything if the political will to do so is in place. They called for social solidarity in terms of public sector leadership – to enable redistributive justice such as in tackling poverty through fairer redistribution of taxes, for example. The current economic climate in the majority of the world further hampers health equity (Farrer *et al.*, 2015). In fact, it mitigates against it because a capitalist system perpetuates differences in wealth that then manifest in differences in health outcomes. This has caused many to advocate for radical redistributive economic policies (Schrecker, 2019). Likewise, Elwell-Sutton *et al.* (2019), among others, call for cross-governmental action and investment to create the right conditions for healthier lives. In addition, they stress the need for greater accountability and argue that 'stronger measures are needed' in this regard (p. 2). Friel *et al.* (2009) also called for social solidarity in terms of the power of communities. In the Australian context, for example, Smith *et al.* (2018) note that action on the social determinants of health has been limited 'particularly for those priority populations that would benefit most' (p. 7). Social groups and communities could be empowered to engage in decision making and agenda setting, and to form the grassroots organizations that would lead to the 'nutcracker effect' described by Baum (2007), who has called for 'combining top down political commitment and policy action with bottom up action from communities and civil society groups' (Baum, 2007, p. 192). She questions the assumption that economic growth can bring about improvements to the lives of the poor and she calls for a challenge to the 'basic tenets of neoliberalism'. (This will be returned to in Chapter 6.) Outlining a vision for 2040, she quotes the Charter of the People's Health Movement:

> Equity, ecologically-sustainable development and peace are at the heart of our vision of a better world – a world in which a healthy life for all is a reality; a world that respects, appreciates and celebrates all life and diversity; a world that enables the flowering of people's talents and abilities to enrich each other; a world in which people's voices guide the decisions that shape our lives.
>
> (Baum, 2009, p. 73)

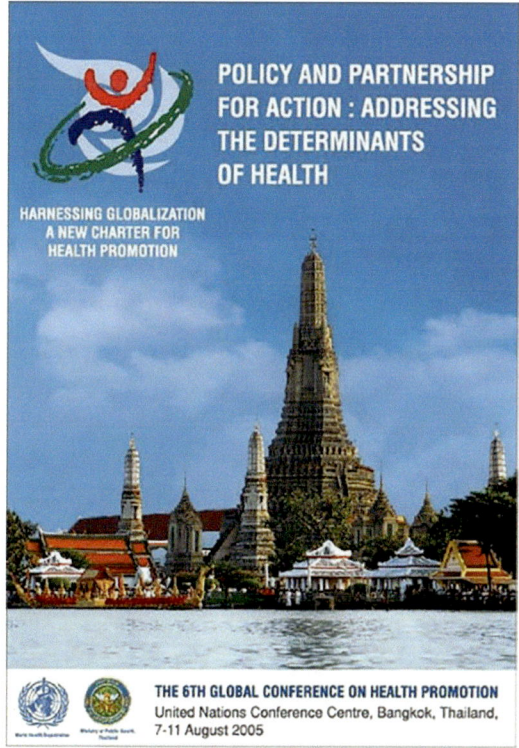

Addressing the social determinants of health.

This captures part of what health promotion is all about – that is, the wish to envision what kind of world we want to create – for ourselves and for future generations. Envisioning the future has been a central activity of health promotion since its inception at the Ottawa conference in 1986. The Ottawa Charter, coming up to its 35th anniversary, remains a central document for anyone studying health promotion. It is the cornerstone of the modern health promotion movement. Its value lies in its outline of strategies and activities to achieve health for all. Whereas 'Health for All by the Year 2000' was a call to mobilize governments, the Ottawa Charter is more of a guide to how to go about putting the vision into practice.

The central concern with the social determinants of health is what distinguishes health promotion from public health. Health promotion takes a different approach from 'mainstream' public health, and we suggest that health promotion is more a form of politics than a part of the medical enterprise – that it is more allied to social policy than it is a profession allied to medicine. The politicized nature of health promotion is captured nicely by Larsen and Manderson (2009) when they write that health promotion is about:

> … representing marginalized populations, advocating equity, giving voice to the powerless and educating people in civic rights, democracy and politics, that is, in citizenship. In this respect, health promotion represents a humanist discourse aimed at creating a more equal and just society.
> (Larsen and Manderson, 2009, p. 608)

More will be said on citizenship in subsequent chapters.

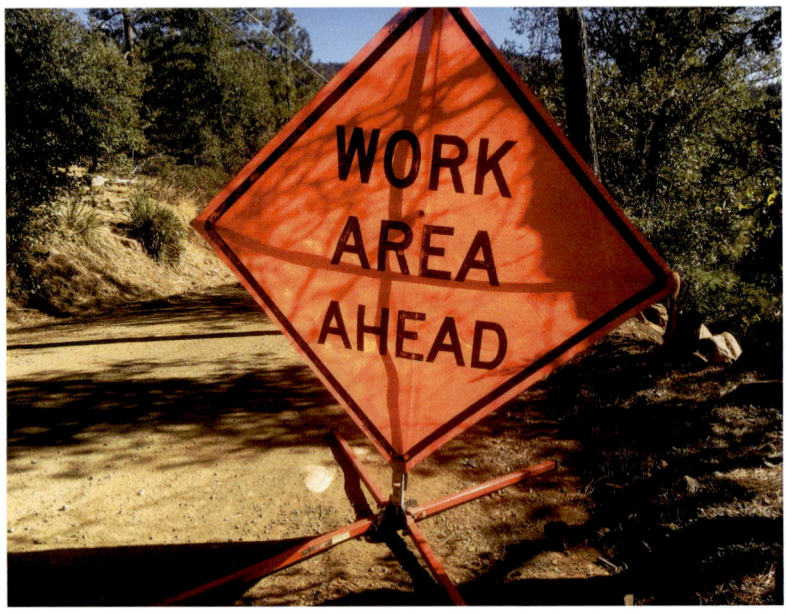

Employment – a social determinant of health (from Creative Commons source: Work is Going on by cogdogblog is licensed under CC0 1.0).

That we do not live in an equal and just society is easy to demonstrate. Data on inequalities in health abound, whether this is within rich countries such as the UK, between richer countries, such as the USA and Japan, or in poorer countries of the global South. The reasons for the existence of these inequalities are more contentious. Wilkinson and Pickett (2009) claim to have produced an undeniable argument that inequalities in health within countries are explained by inequalities in wealth, not by the absolute wealth of that country, and that the more unequal a society, the more inequalities in health there are in that society. As epidemiologists who have worked on health inequalities, they show the socially corrosive impacts of inequality, and how 'almost everything – from life expectancy to mental illness, violence to illiteracy – is affected not by how healthy a society is, but how equal it is' (2009, back cover). *The Spirit Level* (Wilkinson and Pickett, 2009) received a great deal of attention and also criticism; however, since its publication the evidence of a causal relationship between inequalities and health outcomes is actually more robust than ever (see, for example, Pickett and Wilkinson, 2015; Bambra, 2016). The Black Report of 1980 was the first major report in the UK to highlight how health is systematically related to social class, and it put forward a number of reasons for this. Later work has refined analysis of health inequalities, and most notably the Marmot review of the social determinants of health highlights the role of psychosocial factors in explaining the fine gradients in health between social groups. Early 2020 saw the publication of *Health Equity in England: The Marmot Review 10 Years on* (Marmot et al., 2020), in which Sir Michael Marmot and his team examined the decade that had passed since the publication of the original Marmot Review in 2010 (Marmot, 2010). Despite the set of recommendations that were made to government in the original review, the period of time since 2010 has seen a dramatic slowing in improvements in life expectancy, and in some areas it even went down (Marmot et al., 2020). This is contrary to what we have previously seen in England where life expectancy had been following an upward trend. Marmot et al. (2020) argue that such worrying health trends are indicative of a broader problem in society as a whole – 'when a society is flourishing health tends to flourish' (p. 5). *Healthy Equity in England* (Marmot et al., 2020) highlights a number of markers of worsening outcomes including, for example, rising child poverty, rising homelessness, and declines in education and early years funding. Marmot et al. (2020) hold the government responsible for not having put into place the recommendations of the original review that, it is argued, would have mitigated against increased health inequalities.

Whilst this body of work shows that inequalities in health *do* exist, why should we be concerned? Could we not simply agree that some people will 'naturally' experience better health, and also that it is inevitable that the better off, whether in 'developed' or 'developing' countries, in 'good' jobs and living in nicer neighbourhoods, with no major stresses, will be healthier? If we accept that inequality is an inevitable feature of capitalist societies, then surely so are inequalities in health? This *is* the position adopted by many, and can be seen in the discourse that describes 'differences in health' rather than inequalities. Although there may be disagreements on this point among all those working in public health and health promotion, we would argue that these inequalities are *not* inevitable, thus providing a political justification for action. Whitehead (1992) has argued that a health difference becomes a health inequity when it is avoidable, unnecessary and unjust. If these three criteria are met, she argues that a response is needed, in the cause of social justice. Meanwhile, 'health inequalities are systematic differences in health among social groups that are caused by unequal exposure to – and distributions of – the social determinants of health. They are persistent between and within countries despite action taken to reduce them' (Farrer et al., 2015, p. 392).

Ethical justification for intervention to tackle inequalities, or to improve anyone's health, needs to be mentioned here too. It would not, at first sight, appear to be contentious that we ought to 'help' those less fortunate than ourselves, whether this is in terms of richer countries giving foreign aid, directing resources to poorer areas and communities within rich countries, or aiding individuals living in deprived circumstances. The parable of the good Samaritan is a powerful motif in Western cultures, Islam and other cultures and religions, i.e. of providing charity to the less fortunate; it informs our moral codes whilst appealing to a human sense of 'natural justice'. Thomas Pogge (Jaggar, 2010) is perhaps the most outspoken of those arguing the moral case for intervention. He suggests that citizens commit a monumental crime against humanity when they collude with their governments in wealthy countries in maintaining the injustices of the world order.

We are entering a series of debates, however, which could turn into a minefield. It is also possible to stray into condescension, paternalism and unwanted interference. The Zambian economist, Dambisa Moyo (2009), in her critique of overseas aid to Africa, argued that aid is part of the problem, not part of the solution, that the aid-based development model will not generate sustained economic growth in Africa, and that it can lead to corruption. Angus Deaton, the winner of the Nobel Prize in economics, argues that foreign aid is often actually detrimental to poorer countries which should be allowed to develop in their own ways (Swanson, 2015). Riddell (2008) also provides an in-depth analysis of the failures of aid to promote development, and although he tentatively suggests that aid is necessary, he makes persuasive arguments for radical changes in the way that aid is administered. The entry of wealthy philanthropists such as Bill Gates, in the form of the Bill & Melinda Gates Foundation, provides huge quantities of money for health projects, but there is also the danger of distorting priorities (as these are seen through a particular lens of the benefactors), and secondly, those funds can be withdrawn at any time, which is the weakness of a 'charitable' as opposed to a rights-based approach. In addition, as Park (2019) argues, aid in itself cannot lead to development – other factors must come into play.

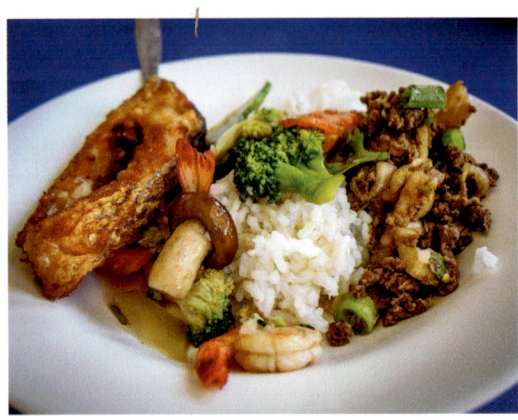

Nutrition – a social determinant of health. ('Monk celebration food' by maxim303 is licensed under CC BY-SA 2.0).

David Sanders (Sanders with Carver, 1985), who was one of the most influential practitioners to highlight the 'struggle for health' in much of the developing world, and particularly in Africa, writes that the 'concerned health worker' will have to think carefully about their role, given that 'health in the underdeveloped world can only come by the actions of the people themselves – it will not come from outside' (Sanders with Carver, 1985, p. 218). He continues:

> The concerned health worker may arrive in a village, overflowing with brilliant, progressive ideas for preventive or promotive schemes, only to discover that the inhabitants are obstinately uninterested in them … And the visiting health worker must accept that more often than not, the villagers are right.
> (Sanders with Carver, 1985, p. 218)

Sanders' views have since become mainstreamed and so may seem less radical than they were in the 1980s, the so-called lost decade of development. This questioning of how communities can be 'helped' continues to be a vexed one, even in situations of dire emergency, such as after a tsunami or earthquake, where help from 'outside' may not always be welcome or may not actually help. The world today is a more complex and polarized place than ever before and the past few decades have seen increasing ecological crisis alongside increasing health, social and economic inequality (Labonté, 2016; Marmot et al., 2020). The idea that health can only be achieved by people taking action for themselves will be returned to later, particularly in discussing empowerment.

At the level of the individual or of communities, what right do we have to intervene in order to improve health and at what point do we have the right to constrain people's behaviour if it is felt that it is damaging to health? It is possible to see health promotion being hijacked by governments who wish to propagandize and manipulate, to even force people to live in 'healthier ways'. Thus Larsen and Manderson (2009, p. 608) suggest that

> another way of seeing health promotion is as an 'extended arm' of the neo-liberal discourse … health promotion is one way of 'governing the masses' and health education is explicit in this task: people are directed to eat healthy foods, not to smoke cigarettes or use drugs, consume alcohol moderately, exercise regularly, participate in community life, and be responsible for their own life.

At best, this can be seen as part of the 'nanny state' and at worse, could be seen as a form of 'health fascism'. However, if governments do not take responsibility for ensuring the health rights of their populations, they could be accused of negligence. It is not a 'nanny state' that provides decent housing, employment opportunities, and good education and health systems, though it might be a 'nanny state' if it forbids people to smoke. A key question therefore is: what is the proper role of the state in ensuring that citizens enjoy the best possible health and what are the responsibilities of individuals for their own health? This debate is a key one in health promotion and it returns to the whole question of the determinants of health – to what extent is my health determined by factors external to me, such as the country I live in, the levels of pollution, level of development, the opportunities in my neighbourhood for good schooling, a satisfying job, good parenting ... and so on, and to what extent is my health determined by those factors under my control – by the choices I freely make, my lifestyle and so on? Of course, in reality these two – the external and internal – are intertwined. Social policies that support equality in health include things such as a universal basic income (UBI Lab Leeds, 2020), free education, free and accessible healthcare, good infrastructure, opportunities for employment and a good public transport system.

The focus on lifestyles and the need to adopt healthier behaviours is a recurring theme in public policy and is propagated in the mass media. A recent example from the UK (as of April 2020) is the reporting of findings from the Cancer Research Report UK 2019, which proposed that more than 135,000 cancers per year in the UK are caused by lifestyle factors including smoking, unhealthy diets, alcohol and obesity. The report estimated that up to four in ten cancer cases in the UK are preventable and cited smoking and excess body weight as the two largest preventable causes of cancer. The report was based on research carried out by Brown *et al.* (2018), which examined 13 lifestyle and environmental risk factors in an attempt to estimate what proportion of cancers were avoidable. Interestingly, only two of the 13 factors could really be labelled 'environmental' (exposure to occupational hazards and air pollution). Attention was not paid to the wider socio-environmental factors, which we, in health promotion, would pay heed to. We need to be critical of information that solely focuses on poor health outcomes as being down to issues of behaviour and personal choice.

The focus on lifestyle factors and individual behaviours is not peculiar to industrialized countries now that we are witnessing the rise of non-communicable diseases (NCDs) within less wealthy countries. It is estimated that a total of 41 million people die each year from NCDs globally and that 85% of these deaths occur in people aged 30–69 years (i.e. prematurely) in low- and middle-income countries (WHO, 2018). NCDs are cited as the major challenge to development in the 21st century and are predicted, by 2030, to be the leading cause of mortality in the sub-Saharan African region (Bigna and Noubiap, 2019). The modifiable risk factors are identified as being tobacco use, unhealthy diets, physical activity and harmful use of alcohol. However, poverty is closely linked with NCDs along with many other social determinants of health. We therefore need to move beyond policy that focuses on individual behaviour, choice and responsibility towards policy that addresses the causal mechanisms of health inequalities (Kriznik *et al.*, 2019).

So far, we have established that health promotion is both a political and ethical activity. Broader ethical questions are taken up again in Chapter 5. Health promotion is both political and ethical because it asks the question: what sort of society do we want to live in? This implicitly asks questions about who has power and who does not, and about how societies can be re-organized so that they are fairer.

Before offering a short history of the development of health promotion, noting the key milestones in its development, we suggest that there are a number of concepts that require understanding. In our teaching, we have found it useful to think in terms of threshold concepts, where, as the name suggests, the learner steps over into another realm of understanding. The point about a threshold is that once it is crossed, there is no going back. In educational terms, they are important, as they are concepts that have to be understood before being able to proceed to the next idea. They have proved useful, for example, in mathematics education, where one block of knowledge has to be mastered before being able to progress. Meyer and Land (2005) suggest that crossing a threshold can transform a person's worldview and additionally cause fundamental shifts in that person's sense of identity and reconstruction of who they are (Meyer and Land, 2005; Meyer *et al.*, 2010). Thus, crossing a threshold can lead to a fundamental questioning of, for example, one's career to date. We introduce three threshold concepts early on in our courses – 'upstream thinking', salutogenesis and the social model of health.

Threshold Concepts

Upstream thinking

Zola (1970, in McKinlay, 1979) is credited with developing the river analogy, which has become such a potent image within health promotion (Box 1.2).

> **Box 1.2. The 'upstream' approach (McKinlay, 1979).**
>
> There I am standing by the shore of a swiftly flowing river and I hear the cry of a drowning man. So I jump into the river, put my arms around him, pull him to shore and apply artificial respiration, and then, just when he begins to breathe, there is a cry for help. So I jump back into the river, reach him, pull him to shore, apply artificial respiration, and then just as he begins to breathe, another cry for help. So back in the river again, without end, goes the sequence. You know, I am so busy jumping in, pulling them to shore, applying artificial respiration, that I have no time to see who is upstream pushing them all in.
>
> (This is also cited in Hubley *et al.* (2013, p. 16) and in Tones and Tilford (2001, p. 27).)

It refers to the medical enterprise of rescuing people once they have got into difficulties. Whilst this is essential for those who have become ill or contracted a disease, it would be better to have stopped them becoming so in the first place. Whilst we would assert that health promotion is the profession that walks up the river bank to find out what is pushing all the people into the river (i.e. health promotion is *the* profession dedicated to tackling the determinants of health), it remains the case that many who work within health promotion are actually working downstream. This is perhaps one of the gaps identified above – that although much of the international, epistemic health promotion community talks about upstream working, many or even most, frontline workers in health promotion are not in positions where they *can* affect change upstream. Furthermore, they may be located in arenas that are strictly *not* political organizations, such as the UK's NHS. Many health promoters are civil servants with explicit contracts not to engage in political activity, and, as we saw above, health promotion is inherently political – hence a contradiction!

A further issue is that the further upstream one looks, the harder it is to be sure of the chain of causality. A death downstream will have a series of causes: a child who dies of diarrhoea in a poor country will most likely also have an infection, be malnourished and live in a poor household. Whilst intervention that is most close to the diarrhoea and infection would be effective, those conditions are likely to reoccur; a health worker could treat those conditions but malnutrition is not likely to be within their remit or expertise. Tackling undernutrition and food security would require a strategic intervention, as would tackling the causes of poverty, and would require politicians and policy makers both nationally and globally to take action. Similarly, we can consider the challenge of obesity using an upstream 'lens'. Whilst certain behavioural risk factors (such as eating more than we need or not doing enough exercise) can lead to obesity there are many upstream influences that increase the likelihood of putting on weight, the majority of which can be linked to our wider environment (Lakerveld and Mackenbach, 2017). Creating a 'problem tree' of causes enables us to identify factors contributing to an obesogenic environment (an environment that 'creates' obesity or enables it to flourish) – lack of green spaces for leisure and physical activity, the number of fast food outlets in a neighbourhood, the availability of cheap high-sugar, high-fat food, market forces, and socio-economic inequality, for example. As Lakerfeld and Machenbach (2017, p. 219) assert, 'the types of environments in which upstream determinants of obesity appear can be divided into physical (what is available?), socio-cultural (what are the attitudes and beliefs?), economic (what are the costs) and political (what are the 'rules'?)'. Thus, the causal pathways have both technical and political dimensions, and the further up the chain, the less likely are those with 'health' in their job title to be able to tackle the issue.

Medical and social models of health

Health promotion holds a 'social' model of health. The central ideas about the social model of health are that understandings of health are broad and complex. The social model of health encompasses 'lay' perspectives about health, taking into account subjective experience and understandings. Crucially, it also takes into account the wider determinants of health (Dahlgren and Whitehead, 1991, 2006, 2007; Commission on the Social Determinants of Health, 2008; Marmot, 2010; Marmot *et al.*, 2020) regarding health as holistic and multidimensional and emphasizing *social* responsibility for health. These ideas are in direct contrast to more biomedical perspectives, which view health rather more narrowly, focusing on disease and disability at the individual level, elevating objective, scientific and expert ideas and emphasizing *personal* responsibility for health.

A social model of health views the 'health service' as a sickness service, essential when people become ill and are in need of medical help, but not the key player in terms of *creating* health, except where services are preventive, such as in immunization and screening. A social model tends to see the health service as treating symptoms and not causes – the causes of ill health are rooted in society, in poor housing, food insecurity, lack of employment, lack of money, poor education and so on. In short, the causes are 'upstream' and the medical model 'saves' people in a downstream fashion. Whereas the medical model sees ill health as caused by disease, the social model sees ill health as caused by social conditions (Table 1.1).

A social model of health naturally begins to question the 'illness', or negative view of health, and moves towards asking what a positive view of health would look like. If we are not measuring health in terms of mortality, morbidity, years of life lost, or years of life compromised by poor health, how should we measure health? We can begin to realize that most of our measures or indices of 'health' are actually measures of ill health. It is clearly important to have these facts about negative health – (life expectancy *is* a matter of life and death!) – but we also need to develop positive concepts of health and the means to measure this. Several writers are attempting to do this, based on Antonovsky's idea of salutogenesis.

Salutogenesis

Salutogenesis will be discussed later in this chapter in some depth as part of an attempt to define health. It is mentioned here as a threshold concept, as it represents a real attempt to move towards seeing health differently. Often when we talk of 'health', we are actually talking about 'ill health', and it is easier to describe what illness and sickness, or sanity, are, compared with health, wellbeing, wellness or sanity. It can be very difficult to re-conceptualize health away

Table 1.1. Comparing and contrasting the medical and social models of health (adapted from: Lyons and Chamberlain, 2006; Earle, 2007; Warwick-Booth *et al.*, 2021).

Negative view of health	Positive view of health
Narrow or simplistic understanding of health	Broad or complex understanding of health
Explanations of disease and illness are rooted in biological science	Explanations for ill health are rooted in a range of social factors. Ill health is caused by structural factors such as poverty and inequalities
Medically biased definitions focusing on the absence of disease or disability; the focus on pathology emphasizes individual risk factors	More holistic definition of health taking a wide range of factors into account such as mental and social dimensions of health
Wider influences on health not taken into account (outside of the physical body)	Takes into account wider influences on health such as the impact of the environment and inequalities
Health is located within the individual body; the physical body is seen as separate to social and/or psychological processes	Health is socially constructed and subjectively experienced
Influenced by scientific and expert knowledge, a high value is put on this and it is privileged over other types of knowledge	Takes into account lay knowledge and understandings
Emphasizes personal, individual responsibility for health	Emphasizes collective, social responsibility for health
Focuses on health education to change knowledge, attitudes and behaviour	Focuses on empowerment; working *with* people to facilitate change
Quantitative scientific evidence and the positivist paradigm is more highly valued	Qualitative scientific evidence and the interpretative paradigm is more highly valued
Forms the basis of 'Western' health care systems	Forms the basis of traditional and 'alternative' health care systems
Reductionist	**Inclusive**
Ill health requires expert intervention	Ill health requires collective intervention

from illness and the negative, towards a positive notion of health – from the pathogenic to the salutogenic. The concept of salutogenesis has been wholeheartedly adopted in the epistemic health promotion community (Bauer *et al.*, 2019) as indicated by Mittelmark *et al.*'s international *Handbook of Salutogenesis* (Mittelmark *et al.*, 2017). Antonovsky (1996) attempted to show how the model can be used to guide health promotion. More will be said in this chapter about salutogenesis when we start to discuss in detail what we mean by 'health'.

A Short History of the Development of Health Promotion

A history of health promotion usually starts in 1974 with the publication of the Lalonde Report in Canada, and then proceeds to the Ottawa Charter in 1986, which was followed by a series of conferences that further explicated the WHO agenda for health promotion. The Ottawa conference was aimed at 'industrialized countries' and, from a global perspective, the Alma-Ata conference on primary health care in 1978 is an equally, if not more, important milestone.

The Lalonde report (Lalonde, 1974) was the first attempt by a Western democracy to assert that the approach to health was misguided, and it called for a radically new approach to tackling the issues of 'lifestyle' in a rich country. It started the trend to thinking that health was not merely the responsibility of the health service, but needed a broader approach, first to stem human misery caused by illness, but also to reduce the runaway costs of health care. It focused more attention than hitherto on the role of the environment and on lifestyle, thus calling for a shift towards prevention. Much of this thinking subsequently found its way into the Ottawa Charter, and Canada has remained a powerhouse for health promotion ideas ever since (Pederson *et al.*, 2005).

The Ottawa Charter provided a definition of health promotion: 'Health promotion is the process of enabling people to increase control over, and to improve, their health' (WHO, 1986a, p. 1).

The Charter provided a list of the prerequisites for health (Box 1.3).

It suggested three processes through which to work: Advocate, Enable and Mediate (Box 1.4).

And it proposed five areas of action:

- Build healthy public policy.
- Create supportive environments.
- Strengthen community actions.
- Develop personal skills.
- Reorient health services.

These five areas should be seen as having equal worth, not as being ranked. The Charter made the powerful statement, 'health promotion goes beyond health care', to assert the fact that health care is but a minor part in creating health. It called for all policy makers to consider the health consequences of their decisions and made the point that many government sectors contain the key to health creation – especially employment, trade and industry, education, transport, housing and so on – 'It is coordinated action that leads to health …' (WHO, 2009, p. 3). Thus healthy public policy requires joint action and is a foundation for tackling the social determinants of health.

Creating supportive environments explicitly recognizes the importance of the natural environment and sustainability of ecosystems, calling for a socio-ecological approach to health. That people live their lives inextricably bound up with the environments in which they live is obvious but tends to be overlooked by a medical model of health. Health promotion 'generates living and working conditions that are safe, stimulating, satisfying and enjoyable' (p. 3) – and clearly not everyone enjoys this in the world today.

Box 1.3. Prerequisites for health.

The fundamental conditions and resources for health are:

- peace;
- shelter;
- education;
- food;
- income;
- a stable eco-system;
- sustainable resources; and
- social justice and equity.

Improvement in health requires a secure foundation in these basic prerequisites.

(WHO, 2009, p. 1)

> **Box 1.4. Three processes of health promotion.**
>
> ADVOCATE
> Good health is a major resource for social, economic and personal development and an important dimension of quality of life. Political, economic, social, cultural, environmental, behavioural and biological factors can all favour health or be harmful to it. Health promotion action aims at making these conditions favourable through advocacy for health.
>
> ENABLE
> Health promotion focuses on achieving equity in health. Health promotion action aims at reducing differences in current health status and ensuring equal opportunities and resources to enable all people to achieve their fullest health potential. This includes a secure foundation in a supportive environment, access to information, life skills and opportunities for making healthy choices. People cannot achieve their fullest health potential unless they are able to take control of those things that determine their health. This must apply equally to women and men.
>
> MEDIATE
> The prerequisites for health cannot be ensured by the health sector alone. More importantly, health promotion demands coordinated action by all concerned: by governments, by health and other social and economic sectors, by non-governmental and voluntary organizations, by local authorities, by industry and by the media. People in all walks of life are involved as individuals, families and communities. Professional and social groups and health personnel have a major responsibility to mediate between differing interests in society for the pursuit of health.
>
> Health promotion strategies and programmes should be adapted to the local needs and possibilities of individual countries and regions to take into account differing social, cultural and economic systems.
>
> (WHO, 2009, p. 2)

Strong communities are the third central plank of the infrastructure for health promotion:

> Health promotion works through concrete and effective community action in setting priorities, making decisions, planning strategies, and implementing them to achieve better health. At the heart of this process is the empowerment of communities, their ownerships and control of their own destinies (p. 3).

The fourth area concerns helping people to develop personal skills, and is centred on the need to support personal development, provide information and education for health, and to enhance life skills. If people really are to take control of the factors influencing their health, they need to be equipped to learn throughout their lives, but action is also required by educational institutions, workplaces and the voluntary sector to enable and provide such learning opportunities.

Finally, health services need to be reoriented, 'embrace an expanded mandate' and move beyond their curative focus, but must also be more sensitive to the needs of individuals and communities and respect diverse cultural needs.

Two subsequent conferences, in Adelaide and Sundsvall, took up the first two action areas, expanding on what these might mean in practice. The Adelaide conference took up the theme of building healthy public policy, reasserting that 'inequalities in health are rooted in inequities in society' (WHO, 2009, p. 7). Healthy public policy explicitly places at the forefront the importance of health and equity in all areas of policy and requires all policies to consider their health impacts. In terms of immediate action, the Adelaide conference suggested four areas:

- Supporting the health of women: ensuring that countries develop healthy public policy around equal sharing of caring work, birthing practice based on women's preferences, and supportive mechanisms for the caring that women do in terms of childcare and other caring. It emphasized the rights of all women 'especially those from ethnic, indigenous and minority groups, to have the right to self-determination of their health and should be full partners in the formation of healthy public policy to ensure its cultural relevance'.
- Food and nutrition: the elimination of hunger and malnutrition must be a fundamental objective, incorporating agricultural, economic and environmental policy. Taxations and subsidies should be used to enable better access to healthier diets.

- Tobacco and alcohol: these are 'two major health hazards that deserve immediate action'. It was noted that tobacco, not only as a direct cause of ill health and premature death, but as a cash crop in impoverished countries, has serious ecological consequences and can be linked to crises in food production and distribution. It called upon all governments to reduce tobacco growing and alcohol production, marketing and consumption.
- Creating supportive environments: as so many people live and work in hazardous environments, coordinated inter-sectoral efforts are needed to protect health across national borders. It argues: 'Policies promoting health can only be achieved in an environment that conserves resources through global, regional, and ecological strategies' (WHO, 2009, pp. 8–9).

The Sundsvall conference took up the theme of supportive environments, suggesting that they comprise four aspects:

- The social dimension, including the way that norms, customs and social processes affect health; changes to traditional ways of life are not always health-enhancing.
- The political dimension, requiring governments to guarantee democratic participation in decision making and decentralization of responsibilities and resources, and to make a commitment to peace, human rights and a shift of resources away from armaments.
- The economic dimension, requiring a re-channelling of resources to achieve better health.
- A gender dimension, whereby women's skills and knowledge are recognized in all sectors, including policy making and the economy in order to develop a more positive infrastructure for supportive environments (WHO, 2009, p. 14).

It could have been expected that subsequent conferences might have taken up the other key planks of health promotion, after Adelaide and Sundsvall tackled the first two. However, Jakarta took a different tack, and although it built very much on Ottawa, it was the first to be held in a so-called 'developing country' (the Ottawa conference was aimed at 'industrialized countries'), and was the first to include what it called the 'private sector'. It wished to reflect on what had been learnt about effective health promotion and to re-examine the social determinants of health. It asserted that there were new challenges, including greater integration of the global economy, financial markets and trade, changed access to the media and communications technology, greater environmental degradation, new and re-emerging infectious diseases. Demographic trends such as increases in older people, greater urbanization, more sedentary behaviour and a host

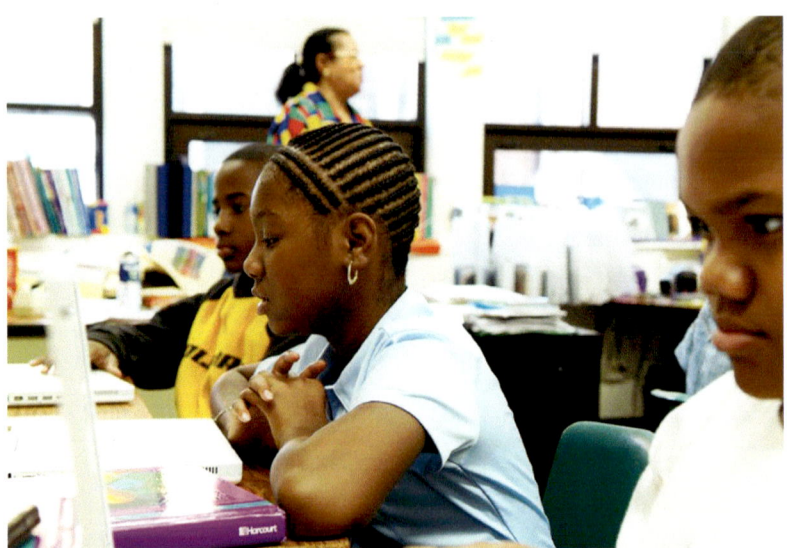

Education – a key determinant of health (from Creative Commons source – 50847569.Kellman30 by torres21 licensed under CC BY-SA 2.0).

of other emerging issues led the conference to call for new responses, greater investment in health, and more capacity in health promotion by developing its infrastructure and maximizing its impact. It called for emphasis on 'settings for health' (taken up in Chapter 5 of this book). It also called for new kinds of partnerships and a more robust documentation of experiences in health promotion so as to develop the evidence base.

Mexico, in 2000, took up the last point, asserting that there was 'ample evidence that good health promotion strategies of promoting health are effective' (WHO, 2009, p. 22). The Mexico conference had the subtitle of 'Bridging the Equity Gap', and in the spirit of 'From Ideas to Action', 88 countries signed up to support country-wide plans of action for promoting health, to take a lead role in ensuring the active participation of all sectors and civil society, to expand partnerships for health and to support national and international networks to promote health.

The Bangkok conference (2005) reiterated many of the key aspects of the previous conferences and noted that action had not always followed the signing of the resolutions by national governments. It therefore offered a series of actions and called for four commitments, to make the promotion of health:

- central to the global development agenda;
- a core responsibility for all of government;
- a key focus of communities and civil society; and
- a requirement for good corporate practice (WHO, 2009, p. 26).

Notably, after the Bangkok conference, the WHO added to its definition of health promotion to include an emphasis on the determinants of health – 'health promotion is the process of enabling people to increase control over their health *and its determinants*, and thereby to improve their health' (WHO, 2005, italics ours). The Nairobi conference was the first to be held in Africa, in 2009. It wished to mainstream health promotion into priority programmes such as HIV/AIDS, malaria, tuberculosis, mental health, maternal and child health, violence and injury, neglected tropical diseases, and NCDs such as diabetes (WHO, 2009). The Nairobi Call to Action put great emphasis on countries to strengthen leadership and workforces, empower communities and individuals, enhance participatory processes, and apply knowledge for the effective implementation of health promotion. According to the call to action, countries are to build capacity in health promotion, to strengthen health systems, to ensure community empowerment, to develop partnerships and inter-sectoral actions relevant to addressing the determinants of health, and to help improve health literacy and healthy lifestyles (Petersen and Kwan, 2010).

The Helsinki conference (2013) returned to a focus on policy, highlighting the importance of healthy public policy and emphasizing the need for 'health in all policies' and intersectoral action and collaboration. The resulting conference statement promoted the 'Health in All Policies' agenda calling for political will and cross-governmental action (WHO, 2013). The most recent international conference (at the time of writing) took place in Shanghai, China, in 2016 and resulted in the Shanghai Declaration (WHO, 2016). This included the following call to action:

> We recognize that health is a political choice and we will counteract interests detrimental to health and remove barriers to empowerment – especially for women and girls. We urge political leaders from different sectors and from different levels of governance, from the private sector and from civil society to join us in our determination to promote health and wellbeing in all the Sustainable Development Goals. Promoting health demands coordinated action by all concerned, it is a shared responsibility. With this Shanghai Declaration, we, the participants, pledge to accelerate the implementation of the SDGs through increased political commitment and financial investment in health promotion.

The declaration forefronted health promotion in the global sustainable development agenda (Kickbusch and Nutbeam, 2017) recognizing that 'health and wellbeing are essential to achieving the United Nations Development Agenda and its Sustainable Development Goals [reinforcing] the importance of structural factors and of the wider determinants of health' (WHO 2016, p. 2). The declaration reflects how the world has changed since the Ottawa Charter was written, emphasizing commitments to harnessing digital technologies, creating supportive consumer environments, and reiterating the significance of good governance. However, as Fleming (2020) points out, the legacy of the Ottawa Charter in the Shanghai Declaration is clear; the heritage of the strategies outlined within the latter declaration can be traced back to the earlier charter.

It can be seen that, whereas Ottawa, Adelaide and Sundsvall explored and expanded on key principles of health promotion, the subsequent conferences have been aimed at developing high-level political commitment for health promotion. They thus involved ministers and others in powerful governmental roles in signing up to the actions required to tackle health inequalities. Whilst this is necessary, it has meant that the two action areas – building healthy public policy and creating supportive environments – have been more fully developed compared with the other three. The Shanghai conference likewise developed these two areas further as discussed; however, some attention was also paid to the third priority of the Ottawa Charter – strengthen community action. The declaration reiterates the role of communities as crucial settings for health, the importance of strong community engagement, and the necessity to put people and communities at the heart of health promotion. The vital role community plays in health promotion is discussed in more detail in Chapter 2.

The whole ethos of the Ottawa Charter was, to a large extent, a reaction against the individualistic approach of health education where individuals were exhorted to adopt new behaviours in the face of personal risks to their health. The charter represented a paradigm shift focusing, instead, on policy and environmental solutions (Nutbeam, 2019). This shift has been reinforced in the subsequent WHO agenda for health promotion. At the same time, activities in many countries are called 'health promotion' but do not appear to be touched by the Ottawa vision. Rather, health promotion is seen as health education, behaviour change approaches and lifestyle advice. 'In the UK, [currently] there remains an over emphasis on personal responsibility and behaviour change, rather than tackling the fundamental societal-wide issues' (Thompson et al., 2018). Thus, the entire political point of the need for radical structural change is missed, and these reductionist activities persist in what some would regard as 'victim-blaming'. More than 40 years have now passed since the Alma Ata declaration and, whilst we are living in a very different world in many ways, the thrust of it remains as important as ever and still resonates strongly in health promotion – strong health systems, underpinned by comprehensive primary healthcare and multisectoral approaches to reduce inequalities and ill health (Bhutta et al., 2018).

Of course, health promotion has a history that is wider than this series of conferences, but they do provide a backbone for our movement. A number of writers consider whether the radical intention of Ottawa has been diluted in subsequent years (Baum and Sanders, 1995; Potter, 1997; Thompson et al., 2018), providing commentaries on what has happened in the intervening years, and these are covered in Chapter 6, where we discuss where health promotion is going next.

An overview of the key conferences is presented in Table 1.2.

What Are the Inequalities that Health Promotion Is Attempting to Address?

Many different types of health inequalities exist between and within countries that are unfair, unjust and, most importantly, avoidable (Williams et al., 2020). Williams et al. (2020) usefully point out that health inequalities can involve differences in health status, access to care, quality and experience of care, behavioural risks to health, and/or the wider determinants of health; differences also exist between groups of people based on a range of factors such as socio-economic aspects, geographical location, and specific characteristics (such as gender and ethnicity). One of health promotion's central remits is to tackle inequality in order to promote social justice. The problem is huge, however, and it is sometimes hard to fully appreciate the number of deaths from preventable diseases that run into literally millions of people. Labonté (2016) refers to this as 'rampant inequality' fuelled by ecological crisis and economic disparities (p. 675). However, numbers and statistics can help us to understand some of the issues faced and provide a stark illustration of health inequalities. For example, in the UK 'long-term improvement in life expectancy and mortality […] have stalled and are falling behind other high-income countries. At the same time the difference between the health of the people living in the best- and worst-off communities is widening' (Elwell-Sutton et al., 2019, p. 2) – healthy life expectancy is 70 years in the most affluent areas as compared with 52 years in the most deprived. So, whilst people are living longer, in general inequalities persist and are getting worse. In a further example, the world's richest country, the USA, has lower life expectancy (78.5) than countries with less income (such as Sweden, 82.3, and Japan, 84.1). There are also middle-income countries that have higher life expectancy than might be expected. Sri Lanka is one such example, with average life expectancy of 76.6 (World Bank,

Table 1.2. Summary of the key global conferences on health promotion.

Meeting of the World Health Organization at the 30th World Health Assembly (1977)	• 'Health for All by the year 2000' launched
Alma-Ata Declaration (1978) – seen as the means to achieve 'Health for All'	• Focus on primary health care Key issues: • Social justice • Addressing inequalities • Government responsibility
First International Conference on Health Promotion in Ottawa, Canada (1986), resulted in the **Ottawa Charter**	Five key areas: • Building healthy public policy • Creating supportive environments • Strengthening community action • Developing personal skills • Reorienting health services To be achieved through: • Advocacy • Enabling • Mediation
Second International Conference on Health Promotion in **Adelaide**, Australia (1988)	• Focus on healthy public policy • Alliances for health
Third International Conference on Health Promotion in Sundsvall, Sweden (1991), resulted in the **Sundsvall Statement on Supportive Environments for Health**	• Focus on supportive environments for health • Reinforced health as a basic human right • Identified *settings* as key to promoting health

Fourth International Conference on Health Promotion in Jakarta, Indonesia (1997), resulted in the **Jakarta Declaration on Leading Health Promotion into the 21st Century**	• Set out the following priorities:
	  ◦ Promote social responsibility for health
	  ◦ Increase investments for health development
	  ◦ Consolidate and expand partnerships for health
	  ◦ Increase community capacity and empower the individual
	  ◦ Secure an infrastructure for health promotion
	• Highlighted the need to invest in health

Fifth International Conference on Health Promotion in Mexico City, Mexico (2000)	• Create an infrastructure for health promotion • Reduce inequity
Sixth International Conference on Health Promotion in Bangkok, Thailand (2005), resulted in the **Bangkok Charter for Health Promotion in a Globalized World**	• Emphasized policy and partnership • The need to address determinants of health
Seventh International Conference on Health Promotion in Nairobi, Kenya (2009), resulted in **The Nairobi Call to Action**	Five sub-themes: • Build capacity for health promotion • Strengthen health systems, partnerships and inter-sectoral action • Community empowerment • Health literacy • Health behaviours
Eighth International Conference on Health Promotion in Helsinki, Finland (2013)	Reinforced the importance of intersectoral action, healthy public policy and political will. Emphasized the 'Health in All Policies' approach
Ninth International Conference on Health Promotion in Shanghai, China (2016), resulted in the **Shanghai Declaration**	Reaffirmed health as a universal right, an essential resource for everyday living, a shared social goal and a political priority for all countries 'We are determined to leave no one behind' (WHO, 2016)

2019a). Sri Lanka and Cuba are both examples of high health-achieving countries as a result of national-level policies that created access to basic social services (Mehrotra, 2000).

Infectious diseases are a major global burden of disease that disproportionately affect poorer regions, contributing to health inequalities between and within countries (Wang *et al.*, 2017), yet these are often highly preventable. For example, it is estimated that in 2018, 19.4 million infants did not receive routine immunizations against diseases such as measles and polio (WHO, 2019). The overwhelming majority of these infants were in the global South. Those in weak social, economic and political positions, such as women, are much more at risk of certain conditions such as malnutrition, violence, sexually transmitted infections and respiratory conditions. Women and children bear the main burden of global health inequalities. For example, in sub-Saharan Africa young women aged 15–24 years represent 10% of the population, yet this age group accounted for 80% of new HIV infections in 2017 (cited in Karim and Baxter, 2019). In Europe, Roma communities experience poorer health outcomes than majority populations (Orton and Anderson de Cuevas, 2019). Put simply, within all societies death rates are typically highest amongst the poorest and marginalized. Data on many sources of inequalities go uncollected – information on the health of refugees, asylum seekers, prisoners, indigenous peoples, uncontacted tribes, gypsies and travellers, the homeless, and a range of other marginalized groups is not available, often for obvious reasons. Data are often aggregated too, disguising inequalities within regions and groups. Infant mortality is often used as a rough guide to the scale of inequalities (see Box 1.5).

Box 1.5. Infant mortality as an indicator of health inequalities.

Using the example of infant mortality as a crude indicator of health we can map clear health inequalities at local, regional and global levels. If we start with Leeds, which is where we are based at Leeds Beckett University, we can see differences within the city itself:

- In 2016 in Leeds there were 4.8 infant deaths for every 1000 live births compared with 3.9 for the rest of the country. The most deprived parts of the city had a higher rate (above 5) and the least deprived had a lower rate (below 4).

Moving to the regional level, we can see differences between Yorkshire and Humber (the region where Leeds is located) and the rest of England:

- In 2014–2016, the average infant mortality rate (IMR) for the whole of England was 3.9 deaths per 1000 live births and 4.1 deaths per 1000 for Yorkshire and Humber. Within the Yorkshire and Humber region, there were variations from 2 (East Riding) to 5.7 (City of Bradford) (PHE, 2018). Within the whole of North-East England, observed infant mortality for the same period was 3.2 deaths per 1000 live births (IHME, 2019).

There are differences between England and the rest of Europe:

- In 2014–2016, the average infant mortality rate was 3.9 in England per 1000 live births; however, this varied across the country from the lowest rate of 1.6 to the highest at 7.9 (PHE, 2018). Compare this with, for example, the highest rates – 6.7 in Malta and Romania, and the lowest – 1.3 in Cyprus or 2 in Finland whilst the average in Europe in 2017 was 3.6 deaths per 1000 live births (Eurostat, 2019).

There are differences between Europe and the rest of the world:

- In 2018, the average infant mortality rate in the countries comprising Latin America and the Caribbean was 14 per 1000 live births compared with the average infant mortality rate in the countries of the European Union, which was 3 per 1000 live births. There is a clear difference here between 'developed' and 'developing' countries. For 'fragile and conflict affected situations', the IMR was 51 for the same year whilst high income countries averaged 3. The average global IMR rate for 2018 was 29 deaths per 1000 live births (World Bank, 2019b).

There are also differences within continents:

- Within the continent of Asia, for example, in 2018, the infant mortality rate was 48 per 1000 live births in Afghanistan, compared with 2 per 1000 live births in Japan in the same year. In Africa for the same year, South Sudan's IMR was 62 whilst South Africa's was 29 (World Bank, 2019b).

(Note that, in most regions of the world, IMRs have reduced significantly in the past decade.)

What is Health?

Thus far, we have seen health as a common-sense concept and assumed that we have a working definition of it. We need to consider in some detail what we really *do* mean by health – if we are trying to promote it, we need at least to be clear that health is a complex, multifaceted and contested concept (Green *et al.*, 2019), a consensual definition of which is virtually impossible. The examples given above of inequalities in health are from literature, which is disease orientated. Health is usually measured in disease terms – mortality, morbidity, life expectancy are the key features. These are not to be minimized, but they only give a partial picture. Definitions of health also fall short and are criticized. For example, some have suggested that the WHO's definition of health should include spiritual wellbeing (Chirico, 2016). Health means different things to different people (Green *et al.*, 2019). When asked what makes them well and happy, however, people will usually produce a list (assuming that they have had their basic needs satisfied, such as for shelter, food, clothing and so on, and are living free from terror, war or violence) that includes all or some of the following: feeling loved and wanted, being close to family and friends; doing something useful and with purpose, such as paid or unpaid work; being part of a community; having leisure time, being able to relax and rest, sleeping well, feeling alive, being in touch with nature, enjoying a cultural life; being free from violence, feeling safe, being able to access health care when needed; having hope for the future … This list could continue, but what is clear is that the items on it do not feature on indices of 'health'. Derived from the UN's SDGs, Raworth (2017) sets out a minimum set of requirements for a 'good life' including food and clean water, housing, sanitation, energy, education, health care, gender equality, income and political voice. At the time of writing (April 2020), many countries around the world are experiencing some level of lockdown as we experience the impact of Covid-19 on families, communities and nations. This is bringing into sharp relief what people feel is important for health and wellbeing. We do not know how many people in the world, for example, feel safe most of the time, how many feel loved or how many enjoy reasonable leisure time. In other words, we know little about those things that most cause us to be at ease, happy and healthy, in terms of official statistics. There are international attempts to develop 'happiness' indices, but these remain to be inserted into the debates about how to address the social determinants of health. These issues will be taken up in Chapter 6.

The professional view

The health promotion community necessarily puts a high value on health – as something worth trying to promote. Duncan (2007) offers a critical discussion about the nature of health, emphasizing the importance of examining what 'health' is in order to determine how we might create or improve it. He concludes that continuous dialogue is needed 'as part of a strategy for examining and understanding perspectives on health' (2007, p. 214) as well as the constant awareness that alternative (and perhaps equally valid) positions exist. Different discourses on health hold different views about ideas such as where health is located (whether it is at the individual, community, societal or even global level), how health is defined, how health is experienced and how health is valued. If people do not hold health in high regard then there is little impetus to try to promote it.

The nature of health and how it is defined have been extensively discussed and debated in the wider literature. In summary, health is conceptualized in many ways – as abstract (Earle, 2007), as contested, as subjective, as difficult to define (Chronin de Chavez *et al.*, 2005) and as dichotomous (Green *et al.*, 2019). Differing theoretical, ideological and philosophical perspectives influence the way in which health is viewed (Warwick-Booth *et al.*, 2021). In addition, we know that concepts of health are influenced by a range of different factors including our culture (Chirico, 2016), our socio-economic position (Duncan, 2007; Blaxter, 2010; Bopp *et al.*, 2012), our individual experiences across the lifespan (Brannen and Storey, 1996; Chapman *et al.*, 2000; Lawton, 2003) and our gender (Emslie and Hunt, 2008; Yang *et al.*, 2018). Many people have examined lay perspectives on health and offer interesting accounts and understandings, for example Calnan (1987), Seedhouse (2001), Stainton-Rogers (1991), Murray *et al.* (2003), Blaxter (2010) and Svalastog *et al.* (2017). Lay perspectives are discussed in more detail later in this chapter and in Chapter 2.

Salutogenic perspectives

One of the key critiques of research that has claimed to have investigated perspectives on health is that relatively few of them have actually examined concepts of health and instead have focused on aspects of illness (Hughner and Kleine, 2004; Green *et al.*, 2019). Clearly, health can be viewed in negative or positive ways, and the classic WHO definition of 1946 (cited in WHO, 1986b) highlights how health should be seen as much more than the absence of illness, disease and disability. But if it is not simply the absence of these things, what is health? It is somewhat easier to frame health in negative rather than positive ways, and easier to talk about those things that create ill health rather than those that create health. Biomedical accounts of health remain the most influential within Western contexts (Sidell, 2010) but salutogenic ways of thinking about health are more positive and focus on what creates health and wellbeing rather than on what causes ill health (Antonovsky, 1996). As Becker *et al.* (2010) put it:

> Pathogenesis works retrospectively from disease to determine how individuals can avoid, manage, and/or eliminate that disease. Salutogenesis provides a framework for researchers and practitioners to help individuals, organizations, and society move towards optimal well-being (p. 25).

Logically, health promotion should align itself with more salutogenic ways of understanding and conceptualizing health – focusing on what causes, creates or supports health (Svalastog *et al.*, 2017). The concept has therefore been adopted in health promotion research and practice with a burgeoning literature on salutogenesis and salutogenic approaches (Bauer *et al.*, 2019).

'Salutogenesis' is one attempt to capture a positive view of health and its causes and challenge negative ways of conceptualizing health. It is the opposite of pathogenesis, which is the attempt to understand disease. Antonovsky (1996) coined the term 'salutogenesis' and challenges the 'pathogenic' nature of the medical model of health by arguing that we should be focusing on wellness not illness. Rather than emphasizing the biomedical dichotomy of health versus illness and disease, Antonovsky argues that we are all on a continuum that he calls the 'health-ease-dis-ease' continuum and that we move up and down this continuum all of the time – no-one ever really achieving 'full' health. He argues that the achievement of full health is impossible, given that we are all biological beings subject to the pathogenic forces of disease and decay. He also called for a move away from focus on the unwell and those deemed 'at risk' (a key tenet of public health approaches; Green *et al.*, 2019). Whilst pathogenic approaches might be described as 'retrospective', salutogenic approaches are 'prospective' (Becker *et al.*, 2010).

Antonovsky further developed his ideas of what health is composed of with what he calls a Sense of Coherence. This encompasses three key elements – comprehensibility, meaningfulness and manageability. These relate, in turn, to our understanding of our world and making sense of our experiences, how we feel about these and to what extent we can cope with the demands that we face (Sidell, 2010). This idea becomes crucial in terms of understanding and accounting for our 'place' on the 'health-ease-dis-ease continuum' – those with a stronger Sense of Coherence, Antonovsky argues, are more likely to be able to move towards the 'health' end of the continuum. Research consistently demonstrates that a stronger sense of coherence is related to reported better health and higher levels of wellbeing (Eriksson, 2017). The emphasis in salutogenesis is much more on adaptation and the mobilization of available resources to create health (Bhattacharya *et al.*, 2020). Work undertaken by the Global Working Group on Salutogenesis of the International Union of Health Promotion and Education has expanded on Antonovsky's original ideas resulting in the 'salutogenic orientation', which includes the need to foster resources and capacities to increase health (Bauer *et al.*, 2019).

Health as happiness and wellbeing

Intuitively, it makes sense that happiness is fundamentally related to health. Many governments have introduced measures of wellbeing and quality of life in order to determine people's experience and obtain indicators of 'progress' above and beyond economic ones. The World Economic Forum (2015) has recognized that it is important to find better measures of lived experience aside from simply looking at how much money a person (or country) has. Measuring 'happiness' and 'wellbeing' is not an exact science, although many people, when asked, will equate happiness with health (Cloninger and Zohar, 2011). Wellbeing is another term that is well used yet not well defined. Grant *et al.* (2007) offer a useful way of conceptualizing 'wellbeing'. They draw on the WHO's 'holistic' definition of health as a starting point for discussion then go on to bring together ideas about wellbeing from the wider literature, drawing on psychological, philosophical and sociological definitions. Their summary is presented in Box 1.6. Wellbeing includes having one's basic psychological needs met and is linked with mental health (experiencing positive emotions) and social health (engaging with others and having meaningful relationships), as well as achieving things (Gu *et al.*, 2015; Johnson *et al.*, 2016).

Another useful model of health is offered by Labonté, in Fig. 1.1. This places wellbeing in the centre, which is the point of reference for many people when thinking about their health. (In the UK for example, a common greeting is 'Are you well?' We do not say 'Are you healthy?') The model also centralizes the notion of 'control', a notion that is central to definitions of health promotion. Kobasa *et al.* (1979) assert that control, the idea that an individual is able to influence the course of events, is one of three common factors in salutogenesis. The other two factors are commitment – having a sense of curiosity for life and a sense of meaningfulness in life – and challenge – the expectation that life will change and that change is beneficial. Helping people to make appropriate changes, as individuals, families, communities and organizations, is a key task of health promotion. The model captures the importance of meaningfulness and a sense of purpose – to be meaningfully occupied is almost a definition of health (Dixey, 2010).

Box 1.6. Capturing 'wellbeing' – core elements.

Grant *et al.* (2007) identify three dimensions of 'wellbeing': the psychological dimension, the physical dimension and the social dimension. Each dimension contains several core elements as follows:

- *Psychological*: includes agency, satisfaction, self-respect and capabilities.
- *Physical*: includes nourishment, shelter, health care, clothing and mobility.
- *Social*: includes participating in community, being accepted in public and helping others.

(Adapted from Grant *et al.*, 2007, p. 52)

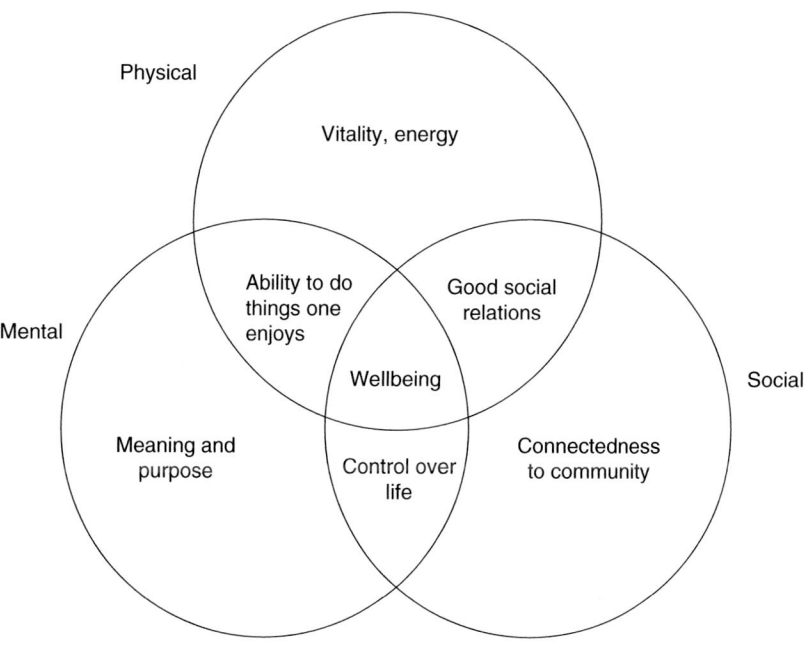

Fig. 1.1. Labonté's model (1998, cited in Orme *et al.*, 2003, p. 287).

The material presented so far is from the viewpoint of professionals – thinkers, academics, health workers – and not from lay people's perspective. We use the term 'lay' to mean the ideas of those who are not professionally trained in health – people in communities and in cultures who have developed their own ideas about health. It is important that we explore these beliefs in some detail, as, in keeping with our philosophical standpoint, we start with where people are, regarding their views on health and illness as a form of knowledge that needs to be recognized and respected.

Lay health knowledge

What do we know of lay people's ideas about health and how these relate to their health-related behaviours? Anthropology, in its attempt to 'make the strange comprehensible' (Lambert and McKevitt, 2002, p. 212), has long studied lay ideas about health in non-Western cultures and, in particular, medical anthropology 'generates in-depth knowledge about the ways people understand health and frame health-related decisions' (Panter-Brick and Eggerman, 2018, p. 237). Sociology has come more recently to the study of lay beliefs, although in their comprehensive review of the literature on views of health in the lay sector, Hughner and Kleine (2004) point out that much of this research has focused on illness, and linking lay beliefs about particular conditions to people's behaviours in relation to these, rather than their views on health more generally. However, from the late 1970s, there have been a number of studies on lay ideas about health and health-relevant behaviours, and what follows is an account of some of the main findings, followed by a discussion of the ways in which lay people feel that health can be promoted, or illness prevented. Important to this discussion is recognition of the importance of culture, ethnicity, social class, gender and age, as well as place, in relation to ideas about health.

As in the biomedical model, a common lay conception of health is as the absence of disease; indeed Kleinman (1980) points out that professional, folk and popular ideas about health co-exist, and are not distinct. In the classic Health and Lifestyle study in the UK reported on by Blaxter (1990), 'absence of illness' was one of the main definitions of health. However, she also noted that illness and health were not always conceived as dichotomous states, and that respondents talked about being healthy in spite of illness. A study by Abbott et al. (2006) of post-soviet citizens in Russia and Ukraine also found that the 'most frequently cited indicator of health included in people's accounts was absence of illness (or in some cases serious illness), mentioned by nearly half our informants' (p. 231). In contrast, in a study of Polynesian ideas about health, Capstick et al. (2009) point out that 'for Samoans, it is inaccurate to conceptualize health as absence of illness and illness as absence of health – instead illness is seen as an inevitable though potent disruption to life and social systems' (p. 1342). They also say that the Polynesian languages have no equivalent to the biomedical constructs of 'health' and 'disease' (p. 1342).

'Health as instrumental' is another conception of health, which is outlined in Blaxter's (1990) study, where she describes responses that linked health with ability to function. In Abbott et al.'s post-soviet study, they note that a quarter of their informants talked about health as a resource: 'A healthy man should be able to easily walk 20 km and be able to lift with one hand a 50 kg sack of potatoes' (2006, p. 231). This quote also suggests elements of 'health as fitness', which was another category in Blaxter's typology (1990) and Abbott et al. (2006) report that a third of their respondents mentioned physical appearance as part of a definition of health, with sporty appearance also mentioned. Physical appearance and fitness relate to more positive concepts of health, but in such positive concepts social and psychological wellbeing feature the most. Indeed, Blaxter (1990) found that health was described as wellbeing and Abbott et al. (2006) found that many of their respondents saw healthy people as happy and positive about life, with one respondent combining several concepts and noting: 'A healthy person is rarely ill, does not have any chronic diseases – is always in a good mood, has a healthy complexion, good hair and shinning [sic] eyes and allocates time for work and rest' (Abbott et al., 2006, p. 232).

This links with the way that many of these ideas about health are also underpinned by important notions of balance or equilibrium. In another classic study by Herzlich (1973), 'health as equilibrium' was one of three main conceptualizations of health. Interestingly, according to Stacey (1986, cited in Pierret, 1993, p. 17), 'this positive conception of health as an equilibrium is more frequently found in French than British studies'. Harmony was also a feature of Polynesian ideas about health (Capstick et al., 2009), as were notions of balance and harmony in Kwok and Sullivan's (2007) study of Chinese Australians; this same study highlighted the emphasis on 'everything in moderation' in Chinese culture. And what needs to be kept in equilibrium? For Polynesians, health is about harmony with the environment and the family (Capstick et al., 2009). Omonzejele (2008) in his study of concepts of health in Nigeria also concludes that health is about more than individual stability: 'Good health for the African consists of mental, physical, spiritual, and emotional stability for oneself, family members, and community' (p. 120). A more recent contribution is that of Charlier et al. (2017), who suggest that indigenous peoples could offer us a new definition of health that includes environmental equilibrium, spirituality and an ability to adapt. An example they give is the Mathias Colomb First Nation community (Canada) for whom 'being in good health means having a good relationship with the land, having access to good foods, but also having access to traditional culture' (Charlier et al., 2017, p. 36).

There are other themes that emerge from the studies, which relate more to how much health can be maintained, and where responsibility for this lies. For instance, some studies explore the degree to which people feel health is under their control. Pill and Stott (1982), in an early study of lay health beliefs in Wales, suggested that their respondents' ideas about health and illness could be grouped into those ideas that were 'fatalistic', where health and illness were regarded as states that just happened, and those that emphasized 'lifestyles' where, in contrast, it was felt that an individual's behaviours could affect health and the occurrence of illness. However, in a later paper, Pill and Stott (1987) cautioned against categorizing people as 'fatalists' or 'lifestylists', and observed that rather than seeing these as opposing views, respondents tended to combine elements of each view. Similarly, Davison et al. (1992) argued that 'fatalism' is not a contrast to a lifestyle-orientated viewpoint, but rather tends to arise from people's observations of the limitations of a purely lifestyle-focused discourse; in other words, people are well aware of messages that particular behaviours are linked to health maintenance or to the causes of illness, but if their own experiences do not support this view, they may become more fatalistic. Exploring the relationship between people's ideas and the messages they receive about health is clearly important, as so much of current health promotion discourse focuses on healthy lifestyles. However Abbott et al. (2006) found that amongst post-soviet citizens, few explicitly mentioned healthy lifestyles in their definition of health, and the authors attributed this to a lack of understanding of 'healthy lifestyles' as promoted in the West.

Conceiving of health as something that can be controlled also raises questions about how that control can be achieved. On the theme of control and responsibility, Mullen (1994) gives an account of male Glaswegians' concepts of health in which both activist and fatalist dimensions can be found. He points out, however, that:

... activist thinking was seen to have three strands: personal activism, social activism, and religious activism. Further, fatalistic thinking was not about passive submission but rather the belief that control lay outwith the person in the realm of the social, natural or supernatural worlds.

(Mullen, 1994, p. 414)

Pierret (1993) suggested another dilemma in relation to health; whilst one conception of health was as 'health-product', as an objective to be reached, in this conception there were also tensions, and the need for balance, as health was seen as a product of controlled risk on the one hand, and pleasure on the other. This theme of tension is also pursued in Crawford's (1984) work in the USA, where he discussed health as 'release' and health as 'self-control'. Nowhere is this theme more pronounced than in ideas about eating and health, where the pleasure from food consumption is contrasted with the need for restraint and moderation (Askegaard et al., 2014).

So how much do people accept that they are responsible for their own health? In Abbot et al.'s (2006) study, virtually all their respondents felt that individuals were responsible for their own health, and this is a theme in many studies. For instance, the issue of health as an achieved rather than an ascribed status is evident in the work of Backett (1992). This study of middle-class Scottish respondents also revealed that 'healthiness was defined on moralistic grounds' (p. 261). Crawford (1984) also highlighted the moral dimensions of health, pointing out that as health comes increasingly to be seen as a state to be achieved by effort and self-control, health becomes an issue of morality.

Another conception of health highlighted by Pierret is that of 'health-institution', where health is seen as a matter of public policy and institutions;

Pierret comments on the peculiarly French nature of this construct, which might be a product of French social policy (Pierret, 1993, p.19). Certainly, in Abbot et al.'s (2006) study, few respondents felt the post-soviet state was responsible for their health. As we will see later, however, a growing emphasis on the role of wider social and economic factors in health is reflected in the recognition of the wider policy environment in more recent studies of lay health knowledge.

Throughout this overview of findings about lay concepts of health, there has been evidence of cultural differences in such concepts. This reminds us of the importance of the social context of such ideas, or worldviews. There is also evidence of the importance of social location in terms of social class, gender, age and place. A number of studies have compared and contrasted concepts of health among middle- and working-class respondents. For instance, in d'Houtaud and Field's study (1984) of 4000 French respondents, when socio-economic status was taken into account, clear differences emerged, with those in the higher and middle groups associating health with hedonism, equilibrium, vitality and the body, whereas those in the lower socio-economic groups were more likely to see health as the absence of sickness, and link it with hygiene and psychological wellbeing. d'Houtaud and Field (1984) conclude that the more personalized representation of health in the higher groups contrasts with a more socialized conception of health in the lower groups, where health is instrumental and about performing one's social duties and these differences reflect 'corresponding roles of mastery on the one hand and the execution of social tasks on the other' (p. 47). These findings are echoed in the Welsh study by Pill and Stott (1982), who also found that functional definitions of health were more common among working class women. However, Calnan (1987) cautions against overemphasizing social class differences in defining health, suggesting that seeming differences may relate more to the way people respond in interviews, and also to whether respondents are referring to their own health or that of others.

Another dimension that has received increasing attention in recent years is the role of gender in ideas about health. Blaxter (1990) found women more expansive in their ideas about health than men; she also found that younger women saw health as being about vitality, energy and functioning, whereas younger men were more likely to see health as being about physical fitness. Many of the early studies were purely on women (e.g. Herzlich, 1973; Pill and Stott, 1982); however, recent studies have focused on men and their definitions of health. For instance, Robertson (2006) found that direct questions about defining health were problematic for his male respondents, and he attributed this to cultural notions of masculinity, which made it harder for men to express concern about health: 'It's [health] important to women, innit? But blokes don't really bother about it' (Robertson, 2006, p. 178). He goes on to describe echoes of Crawford's description of health as an outcome of control and release, as shown in this quote from a respondent (p. 179):

> I do keep fit. Um, don't drink too much, don't smoke too much, well I probably do at times [laughs]. Watching what I eat to a certain extent, eating fruit and vegetables. Um, so keeping fit, eating healthily and not living life in too much of an excess.

However, Macintyre et al. (2006) concluded from their Scottish study of both men and women that there were no significant sex differences. They comment: 'This suggests the need for caution in interpreting single sex studies from which implicit comparisons might be drawn with the opposite sex on the assumption that there are always gender differences' (p. 737). Whilst this may indeed be true, a recent study by Alidu and Grunfeld (2017) explored both gender and cultural differences amongst Ghanaian and Indian migrants and White British participants in an urban area of the UK, and concluded that gender differences as well as cultural differences were apparent in health beliefs. Echoing earlier research, they comment that: 'men's beliefs about health are shaped by societal prescription of their role and "being masculine" may involve being able to withstand challenges, conceal emotion and not disclose distress' (p. 6).

Age is also a factor in concepts of health. Blaxter (1990) found definitions of health varied through the life course, with negative concepts and views of health as ability to function perhaps unsurprisingly more common among older people, whereas adolescent boys in a Swedish study took physical health for granted and for them health was more about positive emotions and relationships (Randell et al., 2016). A final important factor in views about health is that of place. Small et al. (2012) stress the importance of place in their account of shared narratives of health in Barnsley, UK, a former mining town. In their study of patients with chronic obstructive pulmonary disease (COPD), they conclude that 'views about health are shaped by collective history', and they link their respondents' views on health to the consequences of working lives spent in the coalmines or in heavy industry, where breathing problems are considered commonplace.

The causes of illness and 'lay epidemiology'

Much of the research on concepts of health and maintenance of health also contains evidence about lay people's ideas about the causes of illness. For instance, if health is seen as a product of harmony and social relationships, then disruption to this balance and problems with relationships might be assumed to be the causes of ill health. However, it is important to realize that causes of health and causes of illness may not be conceptualized as opposites. For instance, in Herzlich's (1973) work, health was seen as something that could be enhanced by individual actions, but illness was seen as something that was beyond control. Broadly, however, causes of illness in lay ideas have been categorized as internal or external, as under control or beyond control. An example of a focus on external factors is the following: 'Illness in the Pacific may be perceived as coming about through conflicts with family members, or because of otherwise unbalanced or unsettled social relations' (Capstick et al., 2009, p. 1343). Similarly, Swami et al. (2009) conclude that among their Malaysian respondents the social world was seen as an important source of both health and illness. In Nigeria, Omonzejele (2008) stresses ideas about disequilibrium with ancestors, or evil spirits as the cause of disease. However, given the emphasis on health promotion and disease prevention through behaviour change in health policies in the last decades, much research focuses on ideas about the relative weighting given to personal behaviour in promoting health or causing disease (i.e. factors under control), as opposed to external factors in the wider social and economic environment. An example is Mackenzie et al.'s (2017) study of working-class discourses about health in two de-industrialized areas in Scotland. In their study, they describe how 'discourses around lifestyles indicate knowledge of the association between behaviours or cultural practices and health' (Mackenzie et al., 2017, p. 244). However, they then note that the majority of their respondents saw these lifestyles and poor health as products of neoliberal policies and austerity measures.

Whilst many lay accounts of illness, and its causes, often recognize those factors that are stressed in professional accounts, these ideas also coexist with other accounts of health and illness, and 'lay epidemiology' is the term applied to this. Frankel et al. (1991, p. 428) define 'lay epidemiology' as the process by which 'individuals interpret health risks through the routine observation and discussion of cases of illness and death in personal networks and in the public arena, as well as from formal and informal evidence arising from other sources, such as television and magazines'. Davison et al.'s (1991) early study of lay ideas about 'candidacy' and coronary heart disease risk shows that lay people are often well aware of risk communication, and factors such as lifestyles are often cited as important in causing disease. However, such awareness does not extend to a wholehearted acceptance of official medical thinking and advice. Indeed, Bury (1994, p. 28) points out that 'people rationally assess official information and apply it to their lived experiences on an ongoing basis'. So, for instance, 'smoking kills' is a message that may well be treated with some scepticism when we see smoking centenarians around us. Or a focus on lifestyle choices whilst people are struggling to cope with poverty may be seen as unrealistic or 'victim blaming'. Such lay ideas about risk and disease have been explored in terms of, for example, gender and heart disease (Emslie et al., 2001), social class, smoking and ill health (Lawlor et al., 2003), ethnicity and heart disease (Grunau et al., 2008), and vaccination of children in Denmark (Pihl et al., 2017) and Zambia (Pugliese-Garcia et al., 2018). A particular recent focus of research has been on the role of the mass media and social media in influencing lay views. For instance, de-Graft Aikins et al. (2014) comment on the role of the mass media in explanatory models of diabetes among the urban poor in Ghana. Another example is the impact of media coverage of the health risks of mobile phone masts on lay understanding (Collins, 2010), and even more recently (2020) we have had the example of links being made on social media between 5G technology and the Covid-19 pandemic. Deborah Lupton has been a key writer on these issues; having highlighted how much people learn about health and illness from the mass media, more recently she has pointed out that digital technologies are having significant effects on both professional and lay 'ideas and practices concerning how human bodies should be understood, experienced and treated' (Lupton, 2016, p. 53). These issues are discussed further in Chapter 4.

The research on lay health beliefs and knowledge outlined here has revealed rich and complex ideas, which have implications for those engaged in promoting health, and it suggests the need, at the very least, for what has been called 'cultural sensitivity' in messages about health (e.g. Krumeich *et al.*, 2001). But it also suggests something more. In the case of many of the studies, the respondents live in a context where they are surrounded by the messages of the past few decades about personal responsibility for health, and the role of individual behaviours in maintaining health and preventing disease. If they do not respond to these, it is surely not a question of a 'knowledge deficit' (Henderson, 2010), but rather one of people's experiences and contexts giving them different opportunities and a different understanding, which may be complex and entirely rational. As Gabe *et al.* (2004, p. 139) point out: 'universities and laboratories are not the only places in which evidence is debated and knowledge generated. Knowledge is found in the home, the street, the pub and the workplace'. How health promotion needs to take account of, and work with, such lay knowledge is a theme of this book.

The Disciplinary Foundations of Health Promotion

Health promotion has been criticized by some for being a 'magpie' profession (Seedhouse, 2004) on the premise that it has collected together many different facets from other disciplines (bodies of knowledge) rather than having developed a distinct scholarship around a single discipline of its own. However, the fact that health promotion draws on a number of different disciplines can also be considered one of its strengths as it brings together various fields of study in a common enterprise. Macdonald and Bunton (2002) distinguish between two different levels of 'feeder' disciplines – referred to as 'primary' and 'secondary'. Primary feeder disciplines make a significant contribution to health promotion theory and include sociology, psychology, education, economics, epidemiology and communication theory. Secondary feeder disciplines include ethics and philosophy, social policy, genetics, and marketing. These also make a contribution but to a lesser extent. That is not to say that Macdonald and Bunton's list of primary and secondary feeder disciplines is exhaustive. For example, more recently Klein *et al.* (2015) have argued the case for the major role that social psychology plays in promoting public health. The breadth and depth of health promotion necessarily requires a multi-disciplinary approach. Enabling people to live healthier lives is a very complex endeavour requiring multisectoral action (Fleming, 2020). Bringing together knowledge from various disciplines is essential to understanding how this might be achieved even whilst, as Cribb (2015) argues, operating from different premises may cause some ethical challenges. All of these disciplines are referred to, and drawn upon, in this book in relation to the different areas that are discussed in each chapter. In that sense they serve as a foundation for exploring what health promotion is about and for establishing the principles and practice that underpin efforts to promote health and wellbeing. We take up this discussion again in Chapter 6; however, in the final part of this chapter, we turn to empowerment, another threshold concept in health promotion and, arguably, the most important.

Empowerment

From what has been said so far, it is becoming apparent that our view of health promotion will favour an approach that puts people at the centre, is empowering and that challenges the social structure. Sen (1993) articulated the idea of capability, meaning all those aspects that enable people to live lives with meaning and value to themselves; capability also contains aspects that constrain individual agency – the ability to act freely. As health promotion is defined as the ability to take control of the determinants of health, it follows that people need a certain amount of power in order for them to do so. Empowerment is essential in terms of becoming the author of one's own life (Baxter Magolda, 2001).

We are thus clear in our view that empowerment is the key to promoting health. This view has been consistent at Leeds Beckett from the work of its first professor of health promotion, Keith Tones, who asserted that 'empowerment is central to the philosophy and practice of health promotion' (Tones, 1997, p. 39), through to our current work trying to assess the effectiveness of empowerment approaches (Woodall *et al.*, 2010, 2012; Green *et al.*, 2019). Empowerment is mentioned in all the key conference documents from Ottawa to

Shanghai. Empowerment fits with humanistic approaches, where we assume that people are competent and capable of making changes in their own lives; that competence is gained through life experiences and not from being told what to do; and that empowerment cannot be 'given', it can only be worked on collaboratively in a process where workers or 'professionals' aim to decrease the powerlessness felt by individuals and communities. It is also clear that power and thus empowerment, like capability, are distributed in massively unfair ways.

Despite the central importance of empowerment, there have been difficulties in articulating exactly what it means. Victoria Grace (1991), for example, highlighted the inconsistencies and contradictions of 'empowerment' within health promotion and our recent review reiterated the ambiguity and confusion surrounding the term, suggesting that 'empowerment' was being deployed somewhat 'casually' in the health promotion literature (Woodall *et al.*, 2010, 2012). Raeburn and Rootman (1998) have been two prominent authors highly disparaging of empowerment and its status as a 'buzz word' in the health promotion discourse. They, like Rissel (1994), argue that the absence of a clear definition leads to misuse and misunderstanding of the term. Its use has thus become problematic (Minkler, 2000; Labonté and Laverack, 2008).

Describing a vicious theory–practice circle, Cattaneo and Chapman (2010, p. 646) assert that '... one might argue that the lack of precise definition has made it amenable to diffuse applications, which have then exacerbated the lack of precision in its definition'.

This semantic slippage may reflect the ubiquitous spread of neoliberal ideas within health promotion, and modern life more generally, that favour the individual over the social. It is in this context that Woodall *et al.* (2012) argue that the word has lost its power and original orientation toward social and political change. Interviews with practising health promoters show that, although empowerment as a concept is highly valued but frequently perceived as idealistic, day-to-day application in the field is all too often stymied by top down organizational hierarchy and target-driven culture with their ever-present issues of time, funding and quantifiable measurement (Berry *et al.*, 2014).

Somewhat compounding this issue is that the discourse of empowerment within health promotion has not evolved consistently throughout the world, so it is little wonder that the term has been misrepresented and inconsistently applied. For example, empowerment has been viewed by some as a 'Eurocentric phenomenon' (MacDonald, 1998, p. 40), perhaps because it was a central tenet in the original WHO European Healthy Cities programme in the late 1980s (Heritage and Dooris, 2009) and because of the burgeoning amount of academic writing on the issue from European authors. However, in Africa, community development and empowerment approaches have been a key strategy for some time (Nyamwaya, 2005), where academic commentary now exists but has been relatively slow to emerge (Moore *et al.*, 2014; Onditi and Odera, 2017). In contrast, Anme and McCall (2011) argue that empowerment is a reasonably new concept in Asian countries. These semantic difficulties should not divert attention from the overwhelming importance of empowerment. Discussion of a working definition can be found in the Altogether Better programme in the UK (Woodall *et al.*, 2010). Related to but going beyond definitional dilemmas is the problem of measurement, which is discussed in some detail by Cross *et al.* (2017) and Cyril *et al.* (2016).

Power and powerlessness

The concept of power is at the heart of empowerment – empowerment can only occur when communities take power (Rappaport, 1985). The radical roots of empowerment can be traced to the Brazilian humanitarian and educator, Paulo Freire (1921–1997), whose key text, the *Pedagogy of the Oppressed* (1972), introduced important ideas such as critical awareness or 'conscientization', which have entered the health promotion discourse. Freire brings in the issue of oppression, necessitating a working definition of this term, too, but as Dalyrymple and Burke (2001) argue, oppression is a complex and emotive term and to explain it simply would be to deny this complexity. Empowerment approaches should inevitably be anti-oppressive, and we would assert that health promotion needs to develop anti-oppressive practice. 'Anti-oppressive practice ... means recognizing power imbalances and working towards the promotion of change to redress the balance of power' (Dalyrymple and Burke, 2001, p. 15). This way of working also requires reflection on the power imbalances between professional health promoters and communities, and challenging oppression wherever it is encountered, a task taken up again in Chapter 6.

Within health promotion, empowerment is generally regarded as a process enabling people who lack power to become more powerful and gain some degree of control over their lives and health (Green et al., 2019). Empowerment is associated with addressing the causes of powerlessness and disempowerment. In its widest and most radical sense, empowerment is concerned with combating oppression and injustice and is a process by which people work together to increase the control they have over events that influence their lives and health (Laverack, 2006). This suggests that empowerment approaches must operate at various levels, from the individual through to organizations and communities. Empowerment in the Freirarian sense only happens when a person makes the links between their personal position and structural inequalities, i.e. when they not only feel a sense of personal power but when they begin to question their position in society. An example of this awakening (or conscientization) is this:

> During the depression years of the 1930s, cookery classes were organised for women in poor communities in an attempt to help them to provide nutritious meals for their families despite low incomes. One particular evening a group of women were being taught how to make cod's head soup – a cheap and nourishing dish. At the end of the lesson the women were asked if they had any questions. 'Just one', said a member of the group, 'whilst we're eating the cod's head soup, who's eating the cod?'
>
> (Quoted in Popay and Dhooge, 1989; a cod is a fish commonly eaten in Europe)

A more recent example of this raising, at a social and international level, of critical awareness of unfair and unjust structural inequalities might be the way in which the death of George Floyd at the hands of the Minneapolis Police Department has brought together a global movement for challenge and change.

Powerlessness, in Solomon's view, comes from three potential sources: first there are systems that systematically deny powerless groups opportunities to take action; secondly there are the negative images that oppressed people have of themselves, a form of self-oppression; and thirdly there are the negative experiences that oppressed people undergo in their everyday interactions with systems, institutions or the media (Solomon, 1976).

Experiencing powerlessness means that people feel further excluded, rejected, treated as inferior and in a downward spiral, then feel that they are inadequate, unworthy and deserving of the role of 'second-class citizen'. Those experiencing powerlessness could occupy a stigmatized role, such as a

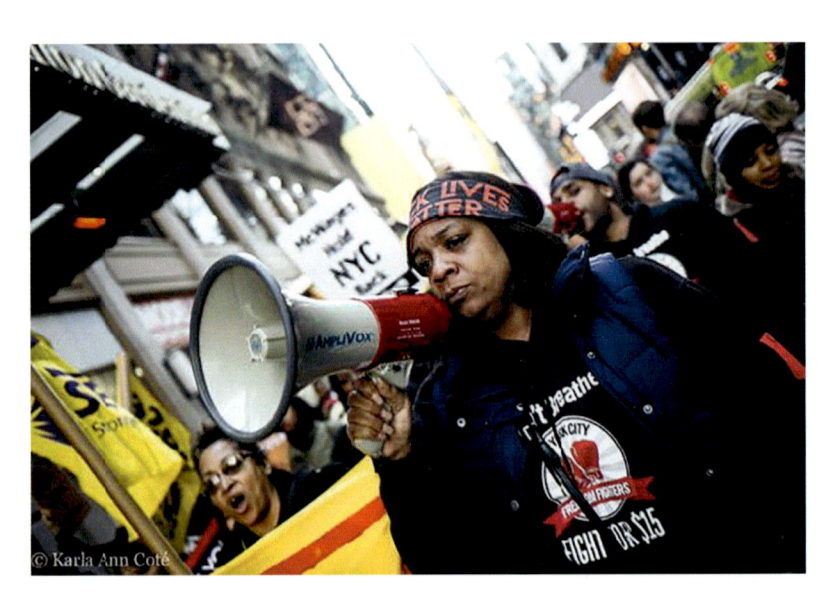

Community empowerment – Black Lives Matter, June 2020, New York ('New York Protest' © KarlaAnnCoté).

'traveller', Gypsy, 'ethnic minority', 'gay', 'asylum seeker', 'ex-convict', 'mentally ill', and/or could be facing insecurity in terms of joblessness, income, housing, education, literacy. Dalyrymple and Burke (2001, p. 15) comment:

> If we consider that people's relations are structured by power then we are less likely to stereotype, make assumptions or misinterpret other people's actions. It is when we do stereotype, make assumptions and misinterpret other people's actions that we start to oppress.

Individual and community empowerment

Empowerment is a necessary stage in the process of transformation. As Freire (1972, p. 34) said:

> In order for the oppressed to be able to wage the struggle for their liberation, they must perceive the reality of oppression, not as a closed world from which there is no exit, but as a limited situation which they can transform.

Empowerment resonates with the important sociological concept of agency: 'agency' suggests that people have 'internal powers and capacities which, through their exercise, make her an active entity constantly intervening in the course of events going on around her' (Barnes, 2000, p. 25). It means that people have the will, power and capacities to act. Agency, however, also requires an understanding of how one stands in relation to others – an appreciation of one's identity and standing in relation to the rest of the community in which one is located. This moves us into considering individual empowerment and its relationship with community empowerment. These two concepts are often presented as being separate but, of course, they are connected, as summed up in the basic tenet of the feminist movement, that 'the personal *is* political'.

A prominent theme within health promotion discourse has been that of fostering individual forms of empowerment. Individual empowerment (also referred to as psychological or self-empowerment) can occur without participation in collective action or political activity and is concerned with developing attributes that are needed for people's personal capacity to be realized – it is associated with people having the genuine potential for making choices (Tones and Tilford, 2001). Choice is an embedded term in the empowerment process, as empowered people often have better health because they are more capable of making informed decisions about their life (Linhorst *et al.*, 2002; Rifkin, 2003; Larsen and Manderson, 2009). Staples (1990) suggests that individual empowerment concerns the way people think about themselves and also the knowledge, capacities, skills and mastery they actually possess. At the individual level, individuals who become more empowered feel better about themselves (Staples, 1990). Indeed, there is good evidence showing that empowerment interventions focusing on the individual increase participants' psychological wellbeing, including self-efficacy, confidence and self-esteem (Gibbon, 2000; Crossley, 2001; Jacobs, 2006; Laverack, 2006; Wallerstein, 2006; Aday and Kehoe, 2008; Fisher and Gosselink, 2008). Two comprehensive reviews, for example, both showed how participation in various groups and programmes had led to increases in these particular health-related outcomes (Laverack, 2006; Wallerstein, 2006). Whereas powerlessness can lead to depression and immobilization, increasing empowerment can enable a shift in the individual's perspective, away from self-blame and towards feeling that change is possible. Greater individual empowerment is not at the expense of others and is thus a non-zero-sum form of power. This type of power is infinite – an increase in one person's individual empowerment is not at the expense of anyone else's – it is a 'win-win situation' (Rissel, 1994, p. 40).

Individual empowerment, however, may not consider or challenge the social determinants of people's health (Wallerstein, 2006) and in our view does not constitute full empowerment in the sense of transforming the relations of power. Individual empowerment alone has a limited impact on addressing health inequalities and may be illusory in that it does not lead to an increase in actual power or resources. In reality, empowerment simply at the individual level does little to influence social change:

> Individual empowerment is not now, and never will be, the salvation of powerless groups. To attain social equality, power relations between 'haves,' 'have-a-littles,' and 'have-nots' must be transformed. This requires a change in the structure of power.
>
> (Staples, 1990, p. 36)

This is not to say that individual empowerment is unimportant, but if it remains at this level, it overlooks change in the political and social context in which people live (Riger, 2002).

Individual and community empowerment should be seen as linked, with the former constituting an early stage of the latter in some cases where individually empowered people come together to create social movement for change (Woodall *et al.*, 2010). Community empowerment (Box 1.7) is a 'synergistic interaction' between the individual and broader social and political action (Laverack, 2007, p. 14). It refers to processes by which individuals join together to make changes to their situation and is tied to principles of social justice. Green *et al.* (2019) suggest that if empowerment consists of facilitating voluntaristic decision making and 'free choice', then it should not only target the individual but also the community and environment. This is encapsulated by Wallerstein (1992, p. 198) who defines community empowerment as:

> ... a social-action process that promotes the participation of people, organizations and communities towards the goals of increased individual and community control, political efficacy, improved quality of life and social justice.

Community empowerment (Boxes 1.8 and 1.9) has a political orientation in which members are made conscious of their powerlessness and actively participate in redistributing resources to challenge social injustice and oppression (Ward and Mullender, 1991; Rissel, 1994). Wise (1995) believes that the

---

Box 1.7. Similarities and differences.

According to Laverack and Wallerstein (2001), community empowerment has been superseded by a plethora of other terms, such as community capacity, community competence, community cohesiveness and social capital.

Community empowerment has similarities with, but is still different from, terms like community capacity and social capital. In summary, community empowerment concerns power relations and intervention strategies which ultimately focus on challenging social injustice through political and social processes (Wallerstein, 2006). The overall aim is to allow people to take control of the decisions that influence their lives and health.

Box 1.8. African-American community health advisors' role in transformational change.

The inclusion of Community Health Advisors (CHAs) in a breast and cervical cancer programme for African-American women in Alabama helped to bridge the gap between professionals and the community by identifying barriers to health for this marginalized group. Experiences of inequity relating to socio-economic status, education and healthcare utilization were recounted through photovoice focus groups and the need for greater cultural awareness and sensitivity was highlighted. The images collected were then used to promote dialogue, critical thinking and to identify causes of powerlessness. Being described as a 'transformational' process, this allowed the women to better advocate for change and resulted in an improvement in the development of more culturally appropriate health services and, more broadly, greater educational opportunities for their peers (Mayfield-Johnson *et al.*, 2014).

Box 1.9. Immigrant Latina survivors of domestic violence: promotora model of community leadership.

A programme designed to enhance leadership of Latina immigrant survivors of domestic violence in the USA utilized peer support and information sharing to facilitate transformational change. Not only did the approach engender individual empowerment with respect to the intrapersonal, interactional and behavioural, but the women also reported a reduction in fear, an increase in knowledge and *'a sense that they could promote change in their community'* (Serrata *et al.*, 2016, page 37).

underlying philosophy involves enabling the oppressed to understand how structural processes (e.g. racial, gender, social inequalities, etc.) impact upon them as individuals and concerns mobilizing people to take community action (Baum, 2003). Community empowerment in this respect is a zero-sum relationship – power in essence is finite. For example, resources being directed at some people can cause the displacement of power (disempowerment) from others due to competition for the same resources (Riger, 2002; Heritage and Dooris, 2009). Consequently, Gutiérrez (1991) suggests that this form of empowerment is based on a conflict model.

'Outcome' or a 'process'

Whether community empowerment is an 'outcome' or a 'process' has been a debated issue. An empowerment outcome could, for instance, be the redistribution of resources to redress health inequalities or a change of policy in favour of community groups that have come together to create change. Laverack (2004) has developed a continuum of community empowerment, which outlines the process of community empowerment. As illustrated in Fig. 1.2, Laverack has proposed a series of actions that progressively contribute to more organized community and social action. Starting with an individual's concerns about a given issue, the process of community empowerment starts with the development of small mutual groups, then community organizations, partnerships and ultimately to groups of people taking political and social action to create social change through the redistribution of resources and power (Wallerstein, 2002; Laverack, 2006). The continuum is useful from a theoretical perspective, as it allows practitioners to identify how they can be involved in empowerment approaches in their everyday work. However, in reality, the process of community empowerment is dynamic, iterative and complex as opposed to linear (Laverack, 2010).

Participation is an important feature of Laverack's continuum (Fig. 1.2). Individuals have a better chance of achieving their health goals if they can share these matters with other people who are faced with similar problems. Through participation, individuals are likely to experience some degree of control as they are better able to define and analyse their concerns and together they are capable of finding joint solutions to act on their issues (Laverack, 2005). Figure 1.3 demonstrates the assumed relationship between levels of participation and degrees of empowerment.

While participation forms 'the backbone of empowering strategies' (Wallerstein, 2006, p. 9), participation alone does not guarantee empowerment, as it can often be manipulative and passive, rather than truly engaging and empowering. It is perhaps also naive to consider empowerment a panacea for improving people's health and wellbeing (Hyung Hur, 2006), as Baistow (1994, p. 40) argues that 'problems' are often complex and interconnected, and a simple 'dose of empowerment' is unlikely to provide the full solution. Indeed, some authors offer more critical perspectives on empowerment. For example, Spencer (2015) highlights the potential for unintended consequences and ethical dilemmas, which may require professional reflexivity. Jacobs (2011) considers the difficulties and dissonances in bringing more abstract concepts of power to the day-to-day work of health promotion on the ground, which may be more task orientated. Notwithstanding this criticism, it is imperative that the relationship between the professional and the community is equal in order to facilitate empowerment-based approaches (Jacobs, 2006). Empowerment cannot be given to people, but comes from individuals and communities empowering themselves. The role of the health promoter here, rather than imposing professional perspectives and solutions, or employing manipulative or persuasive techniques, is to help to create a situation where empowerment may be more likely, through facilitation and support, but only when groups of people gain their own momentum, acquire skills and advocate for their own change will empowerment have been fully realized (Rissel,

Personal action — Small mutual groups — Community organizations — Partnerships — Social and political action

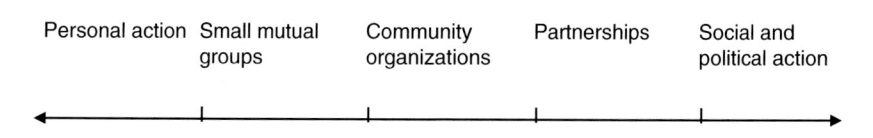

Fig. 1.2. Community empowerment as a continuum (Laverack, 2004, p. 48).

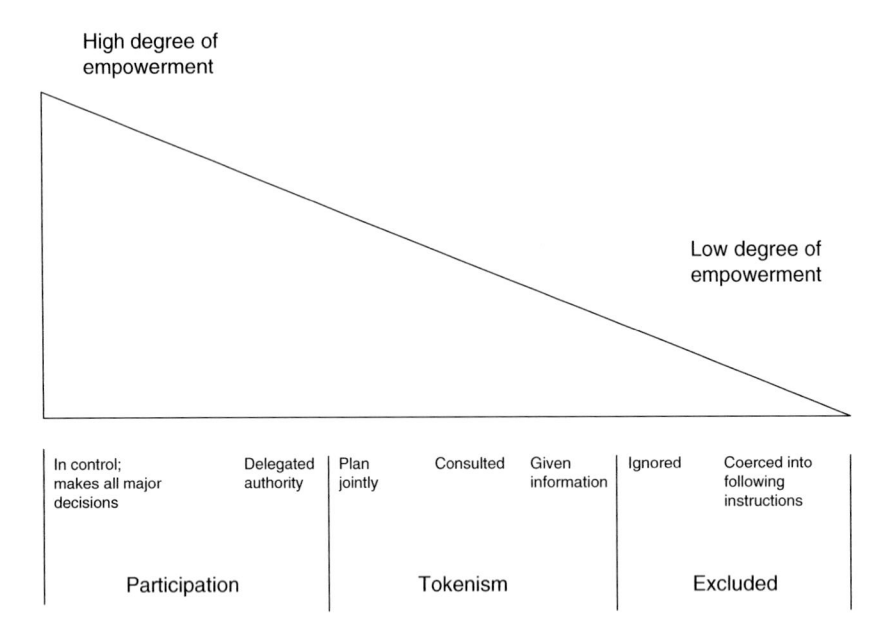

```
High degree of
empowerment



                                                          Low degree of
                                                          empowerment



In control;      Delegated  Plan      Consulted  Given        Ignored   Coerced into
makes all major  authority  jointly              information            following
decisions                                                               instructions

        Participation              Tokenism                    Excluded
```

Fig. 1.3. Participation and empowerment gradient (from Green *et al.*, 2019, p. 54).

1994; Wallerstein, 2006). Yet this does raise some interesting issues, such as how do we know if our intentions and practices to empower really are empowering and can we and should we attempt to facilitate the empowerment of all people? According to Allah Nikkhah and Redzuan (2009), if power cannot change, i.e. if it is inherent in social structures, then empowerment is not possible. The question as to whether health promoters should work toward empowerment with all people returns to our view of health promotion as a moral activity. Riger (2002) argues that there are some groups who should become less empowered, rather than more powerful, but who should decide which groups? Our work on health in prisons presents interesting contradictions between the central tenet of empowerment and the stripping away of power that the prison experience engenders.

Prisons arguably represent an environment where empowerment cannot be fostered. It is a setting where little choice can be sanctioned, where autonomy and personal agency are frowned upon and where prisoners are under surveillance, controlled and forced into subservience and obedience (Maeve, 1999; Smith, 2000; de Viggiani, 2006). The 'power over' individuals can be particularly damaging to health and contribute to a loss of control and disempowerment (Woodall *et al.*, 2010). The empowerment of people in prison is a potentially contentious area, but the WHO (1995) claim that prisons should be concerned with empowerment. This has been reiterated more recently by the UK government in their delivery plan for health and criminal justice (DOH, 2009), where the strategy alluded to the increased participation and empowerment of offenders. The rationale for empowering prisoners is justifiable, given the fact that most people serve short prison sentences and return to the community. However, there are some writers who feel that the empowerment of prisoners is 'morally questionable and politically dangerous' (The Aldridge Foundation and Johnson, 2008, p. 2).

The Value Base of Health Promotion

So far, this chapter has explicated a number of key values held by health promotion, including the importance of listening to lay views, empowerment and participation. We will end this chapter by further outlining the value base, by presenting the views of a number of thinkers. Seedhouse (1997) usefully summarized the debate about whether health promotion is, and should be, driven by values or by evidence. Wills and Woodhead (2004, p. 12) later argued that a 'technical-rational model' of public health with its focus on 'applying expert knowledge objectively to analyse problems and provide the solutions' gives 'little attention to value based questions about what outcomes are desirable, how situations are framed as problems, and what constitutes valid professional knowledge' – a position with which we concur.

We would assert that not only is health promotion driven by values, but also that some sets of values *are* better than others: justice, peace and democracy are all values, and we would say that they are better than their opposites. We (the authors) are thus not value-neutral. Furthermore, we believe that health promotion should be underpinned by a set of values and principles that guide practice. There is general agreement in the health promotion community that health promotion is underpinned by three core values – empowerment, equity and social justice (Green *et al.*, 2019). If health promotion is values-driven, it raises the question of how the evidence base for health promotion should be used, as evidence-based practice not only is part of current professional life, but it is also ethical to work in ways that we believe will work (however 'working' is defined). Evidence-based practice is taken up in Chapter 5, with the obvious caveat that not everything that counts can be counted, and with a scepticism towards the current obsession with not doing anything that cannot be 'evaluated'. A values-based approach should not be seen in opposition to an evidence-based approach – it is not necessarily an 'either/or'. Incorporating evidence-based practice is an ethical value and should be one of the principles of practice *within* a values-based approach. Some attempts at delineating sets of values for health promotion work will be discussed here.

The WHO, in 1986, developed a set of concepts in its Copenhagen discussion paper mentioned above (WHO, 2009). These principles are covered in Box 1.10.

Health promotion focuses on the population as a whole in their everyday life, not just those seen to be 'at risk' of particular disease conditions; it is directed towards action on the determinants or causes of health; it combines diverse but complementary methods and approaches; it aims to obtain effective public participation; it requires professionals to play an enabling role.

In an attempt to detail what a 'people-centred' health promotion might look like, Raeburn and Rootman, in 1998, wrote a book with that title, which provided a set of principles. Health promotion should be concerned with real, living people and focus on positive, life-enhancing factors and not on social problems or disease symptoms; it should focus on people's strengths rather than their weaknesses; it should focus on health outcomes rather than more general (but equally important)

Box 1.10. Health Promotion Principles.

1. Health promotion involves the population as a whole in the context of their everyday life, rather than focusing on people at risk for specific diseases. It enables people to take control over, and responsibility for, their health as an important component of everyday life – both as spontaneous and organized action for health. This requires full and continuing access to information about health and how it might be sought for by all the population, using, therefore, all dissemination methods available.

2. Health promotion is directed towards action on the determinants or causes of health. Health promotion, therefore, requires a close cooperation of sectors beyond health services, reflecting the diversity of conditions that influence health. Government, at both local and national levels, has a unique responsibility to act appropriately and in a timely way to ensure that the 'total' environment, which is beyond the control of individuals and groups, is conductive to health.

3. Health promotion combines diverse, but complementary, methods or approaches, including communication, education, legislation, fiscal measures, organizational change, community development and spontaneous local activities against health hazards.

4. Health promotion aims particularly at effective and concrete public participation. This focus requires the further development of problem-defining and decision-making life skills both individually and collectively.

5. While health promotion is basically an activity in the health and social fields, and not a medical service, health professionals – particularly in primary health care – have an important role in nurturing and enabling health promotion. Health professionals should work towards developing their special contributions in education and health advocacy.

(WHO, 2009, pp. 29–30)

outcomes such as social justice or social equality; empowerment, justice, equity, cultural appropriateness and spirituality are central values to health promotion; health promotion takes time and should not be judged on 'quick results'; health promotion must be efficient, well-organized and systematic.

Those countries – Australia, Canada, the USA and New Zealand – with a large indigenous population that was subsequently overwhelmed by the invading Europeans have attempted to develop ways to make health promotion meaningful for those native populations. Durie (2004), for example, has argued that for health promotion to be useful to indigenous peoples it must be consistent with their values, attitudes and aspirations. (The same could be said of all communities, of course.) An Indigenous model of health promotion has been developed in New Zealand that combines Maori world views and health perspectives. Given the importance of the symbolism of the Southern Cross constellation (Te Pae Mahutonga), the model adopts an Indigenous icon to increase understanding and to make health promotion relevant. The model proposes four key areas for health ('ora'), each representing one of the central Southern Cross stars.

> Waiora refers to the natural environment and environmental protection; Mauri Ora is about cultural identity and access to the Maori world; Toiora includes wellbeing and healthy lifestyles; and Whaiora encompasses full participation in the wider society. The two pointer stars symbolize capacities that are needed to make progress: effective leadership (Nga Manukura) and autonomy (Mana Whakahaere).
>
> (Durie, 2004, p. 181)

Another excellent guide to health promotion using an 'aboriginal lens' is provided by the Mungabareena Aboriginal Corporation and Women's Health Goulburn North East (2008), in a guide that is useful to everyone working in health promotion, wherever they practise, as it presents ideas on how to work in culturally appropriate, participative ways. It considers each stage of a health promotion work cycle through an 'aboriginal lens':

There are 10 components within the framework. Each section describes a health promotion concept, and then presents it through an Aboriginal lens. Following this are examples of practice and useful resources. The 10 components of the framework are:

1. Identifying guiding values and principles
2. Identifying theoretical underpinnings and frameworks
3. Analysing health promotion practice environments
4. Evidence gathering and needs analysis
5. Identifying settings and sectors for health promotion
6. Determining and implementing health promotion strategies and approaches
7. Evaluation design and delivery
8. Partnerships, leadership and management
9. Workforce capacity building for the Aboriginal community and generalist (non-Aboriginal) health and community sector
10. Infrastructure and resources for sustainability

(Mungabareena Aboriginal Corporation and Women's Health Goulburn North East, 2008, p. 3)

These ideas are taken up by Mahoney and Fleming (2020) who emphasis the centrality of self-determination as a value conceptualized as 'determining the health of Aboriginal peoples by them and for them' (p. 100). Health promotion has been influenced by the principles of community development, such as described by Ife (2000), and we assert that these principles provide a suitable basis for health promotion as well:

- social justice principles, which address structural disadvantage, power differentials, institutionalized prejudice;
- local principles, valuing local knowledge, cultures, skills, ways of working, assets;
- process principles, working ethically and with integrity, processes which have appropriate timing and pace, are inclusive and lead to community building, engender cooperation, consensus, peace, non-violence, conflict resolution, and enable vision and outcomes to be realized;
- ecological principles, which consider sustainability, diversity, holism, and the environment;
- global principles, which link the global and local (thinking globally, acting locally), makes connections, using anti-colonial practice.

The principles of working with communities are the focus of the next chapter.

The detailed discussion of the concept of health shows that it is not a simple one, is seen differently by different people, and changes over time; discussion of the social determinants of health show that health is the product of complex processes. Thus promoting 'health' is not a straightforward matter. Health promotion has attempted to distance itself from the reductionist, narrow approaches adopted by the medical and psycho-behavioural models, and ways of working that show a gap between the rhetoric of health promotion and the reality in practice:

> ... a significant proportion of present health promotion practice is underpinned by a conventional biomedical model of health that is concerned primarily with the physical body and its diseases ... many health promoters find themselves focusing primarily or exclusively on the conventional immediate or proximal behavioural risk factors for specific disease conditions, without the opportunity to address the distal or social determinants of health.
>
> (Gregg and O'Hara, 2007a, p. 10)

To address this gap, Gregg and O'Hara (2007b) propose a new model that is explored more fully in Chapter 6, when we offer some ways of thinking suitable for the 21st century. Whether the values and principles are adequate for providing a reliable foundation and whether this foundation is translatable into action remains a moot point, and some of this discussion is taken up again at the very end of the book. For now, distilling the key points from this discussion, we propose (in no particular order) that health promotion therefore should:

1. Resist biomedical models of health and advocate for the broader social model of health to be adopted at policy-making levels.
2. Place empowerment and the redistribution of power at the centre, so as to bring transformation to individuals, communities, organizations and societies with the aim of producing greater health.
3. Involve collaborative working and strong partnerships.
4. Take a salutogenic approach and promote the importance of 'good health'.
5. Take an assets perspective (rather than a deficits one), with a stress on capability.
6. Prioritize the most vulnerable and disadvantaged communities, thus tackling areas facing the worst inequities.
7. Start with where people are, use 'constructionist epistemologies', respect and value local knowledge and lay epidemiologies.
8. Use ethical change processes.
9. Have capable, skilled health promotion workers working alongside communities as allies.
10. Adopt anti-oppressive practices, challenge racism, sexism, disablism and any other practices and institutions that oppress people.
11. Adopt ecological principles, sustainability and a concern for the environment.
12. Invest in the capabilities of the health promotion workforce (both professional and lay), paying attention to life-long learning.
13. Use evidence-based practice, 'real world' evaluation methods.
14. Produce 'big picture' change at the societal level and also 'small picture' change, working with communities and individuals.

Summary

This chapter has provided a foundation upon which to base further study; it has presented the key values and principles of health promotion; emphasized the need to tackle the social determinants of health; presented a history of health promotion's development through the WHO-led conferences; introduced some threshold concepts; introduced the disciplines that contribute to health promotion; outlined professional and lay concepts of health; and suggested that empowerment approaches are the essence of health promotion. The next three chapters provide detail on three central aspects of health promotion, which follow logically from what we have outlined thus far: working with communities, developing healthy public policy and communicating about health. These three areas also, logically, form modules of study on many postgraduate courses.

Note

[1] The previous version of this chapter was written by Rachael Dixey, Ruth Cross, Sally Foster and James Woodall.

Further Reading

Fleming, M. and Baldwin, L. (eds) (2020) *Health Promotion in the 21st Century: New Approaches to Achieving Health for All*. Allen & Unwin, London.

Global Health Watch (2017) *Global Health Watch 5: An Alternative World Health Report*. Zed Books, London.

Green, J., Cross, R., Woodall, J. and Tones, K. (2019) *Health Promotion: Planning and Strategies*, 4th edn. Sage, London, UK.

Mittelmark, M.B., Sagy, S., Eriksson, M., Bauer, G.F., Pelikan, J.M. and Lindström, B. (2017) *The Handbook of Salutogenesis*. Springer, New York.

Warwick-Booth, L. (2019) *Social Inequality*, 2nd edn. Sage, London.

References

Abbott, P.A., Turmov, S. and Wallace, C. (2006) Health world views of post-soviet citizens. *Social Science & Medicine* 62, 228–238.

Aday, R.H. and Kehoe, G. (2008) Working in old age: benefits of participation in the Senior Community Service Employment Program. *Journal of Workplace Behavioral Health* 23, 1–2.

Alidu, L. and Grunfeld, E.A. (2017) Gender differences in beliefs about health: a comparative qualitative study with Ghanaian and Indian migrants living in the United Kingdom. *BMC Psychology* 5(1), 8. https://doi.org/10.1186/s40359-017-0178-z

Allah Nikkhah, H. and Redzuan, M. (2009) Participation as a medium of empowerment in community development. *European Journal of Social Sciences* 11, 170–176.

Anme, T. and McCall, M.E. (2011) Empowerment in health and community settings. In: Muto, T., Nakahara, T. and Woo Nam, E. (eds) *Asian Perspectives and Evidence on Health Promotion and Education*. Springer, London.

Antonovsky, A. (1996) The salutogenic model as a theory to guide health promotion. *Health Promotion International* 11, 11–18.

Askegaard, S., Ordabayeva, N., Chandon, P., Cheung, T., Chytkova, Z., Cornil, Y., Corus, C. Edell, J., Mathras, D., Junghans, A., Kristensen, D., Mikkonen, I., Miller, E., Sayarh, N. and Werle, C. (2014) Moralities in food and health research. *Journal of Marketing Management* 30, 17 –18, 1800–1832.

Backett, K. (1992) Taboos and excesses: lay health moralities in middle class families. *Sociology of Health and Illness* 7, 110–117.

Baistow, K. (1994) Liberation and regulation? Some paradoxes of empowerment. *Critical Social Policy* 14, 34–46.

Bambra, C. (2016) *Health Divides: Where You Live Can Kill You*. Policy Press, Bristol, UK.

Barnes, B. (2000) *Understanding Agency*. Sage, London.

Bauer, G.F., Roy, M., Bakibinga, P., Contu, P., Downe, S., Eriksson, M., Espnes, G.A. *et al.* (2019) Future directions for the concept of salutogenesis: a position article. *Health Promotion International*, 1–9, doi: 10.1093/heapro/daz057

Baum, F. (2003) *The New Public Health*, 2nd edn. OUP, South Australia.

Baum, F. (2007) Cracking the nut of health equity: top down and bottom up pressure for action on the social determinants of health. *Promotion & Education* 14, 90–95.

Baum, F. and Sanders, D. (1995) Can health promotion and primary health care achieve Health for All without a return to their more radical agenda? *Health Promotion International* 10, 149–160.

Baxter Magolda, M. (2001) *Making Their Own Way: Narratives for Transforming Higher Education to Promote Self-development*. Stylus, Sterling, Virginia.

Becker, C., Glascoof, M.A. and Felts, M. (2010) Salutogenesis 30 years later: Where do we go from here? *International Electronic Journal of Health Education*, 13, 25–32.

Berry, N., Murphy, J. and Coser, L. (2014) Empowerment in the field of health promotion: recognizing challenges in working toward equity. *Global Health Promotion* 21(4), pp. 35–43.

Bhattacharya, B., Pradhan, K.B., Bashar, M.A., Tripathi, S., Thiyagarajan, A. Srivastava, A. and Singh, A. (2020) Salutogenesis: a bona fide guide towards health preservation. *Journal of Family Medicine and Primary Care* 9 (1), 16–19.

Bhutta, Z.A., Atun, R., Ladher, N. and Abbasi, K. (2018) Alma Ata and primary healthcare: back to the future. *BMJ* 363, doi: 10.1136/bmj.k4433

Bigna, J.J. and Noubiap, J.J. (2019) The rising burden of non-communicable diseases in sub-Saharan Africa. *The Lancet* 7 (10), E1295–E1296.

Blaxter, M. (1990) *Health and Lifestyles*. Routledge, London.

Blaxter, M. (2010) *Health*, 2nd edn. Polity Press, Cambridge.

Bopp. M., Braun, J., Gutzwiller, F. and Faeh, D. (2012) Health risk or resource? Gradual and independent association between self-rated health and mortality persists over 30 years. *PlOS ONE*, https://doi.org/10.1371/journal.pone.0030795

Brannen, J. and Storey, P. (1996) *Child Health in Social Context: Parental Employment and the Start of Secondary School*. Health Education Authority, London.

Brown, K.F., Rumgay, H., Dunlop, C. *et al.* (2018) The fraction of cancer attributable to modifiable risk factors in England, Wales, Scotland, Northern Ireland and the United Kingdom in 2015. *British Journal of Cancer*, doi: 10.1038/s41416-018-0029-6

Bury, M. (1994) Health promotion and lay epidemiology: a sociological view, *Health Care Analysis* 2, 23–30.

Calnan, M. (1987) *Health and Illness: The Lay Perspective*. Tavistock Publications, London.

Cancer Research (2019) *Cancer in the UK 2019*. Cancer Research, London, UK. Available at: https://www.cancerrearchuk.org (accessed 30 April 2020).

Capstick, S., Norris, P., Sopoaga, F. and Tobata, W. (2009) Relationship between health and culture in Polynesia: a review. *Social Science & Medicine* 68, 1341–1348.

Cattaneo, L. and Chapman, A. (2010) The process of empowerment: a model for use in research and practice. *American Psychologist* 65, 646–659.

Chapman, N., Emerson, S., Gough, J., Mepani, B. and Road, N. (2000) *Views of Health 2000*. Save the Children, London Development Team, London.

Charlier, P., Coppens, Y., Malaurie, J., Brun, L., Kepanga, M., Hoang-Opermann, V., Correa Calfin, J.A., Nuku, G., M., Ushiga, M., Schor, X.E., Deo, S., Hassin, J. and Hervé, C. (2017) A new definition of health? An open letter of autochthonous peoples and medical anthropologists to the WHO. *European Journal of Internal Medicine* 37, 33–37.

Chirico, F. (2016) Spiritual well-being in the 21st century: it is time to review the current WHO's health definition. *Journal of Health and Social Sciences* 1 (1), 11–16.

Chronin de Chavez, A., Backett-Milburn, K., Parry, O. and Platt, S. (2005) Understanding and researching well-being: its usage in different disciplines and potential for health research and health promotion. *Health Education Journal* 64, 70–87.

Cloninger, R.C. and Zohar, A.H. (2011) Personality and the perception of health and happiness. *Journal of Affective Disorders* 128 (1–2), 24–32.

Collins, J.W. (2010) Mobile phone masts, social rationalities and risk: negotiating lay perspectives on technological hazards. *Journal of Risk Research* 13 (5), 621–637.

Commission on the Social Determinants of Health (2008) *Closing the Gap in a Generation: Health Equity through Action on the Social Determinants of Health. Final Report of the Commission on Social Determinants of Health.* WHO, Geneva.

Crawford, R. (1984) A cultural account of health: control, release and the social body. In: McKinlay, J.B. (ed.) *Issues in the Political Economy of Health.* Tavistock, London, pp. 60–103.

Cribb, A. (2015) Operating from different premises: the ethics of inter-disciplinarity in health promotion. *Health Promotion Journal of Australia* 26, 200–204.

Cross, R., Woodall, J. and Warwick-Booth, L. (2017) Empowerment: challenges in measurement. *Global Health Promotion* 26(2), 93–96.

Crossley, M.L. (2001) The 'Armistead' project: an exploration of gay men, sexual practices, community health promotion and issues of empowerment. *Journal of Community & Applied Social Psychology* 11, 111–123.

Cyril, S., Smith, B. and Renzaho, A. (2016) Systematic review of empowerment measures in health promotion. *Health Promotion International* 31(4), 809–826.

D'Houtaud, A. and Field, M.G. (1984) The image of health: variations in perception by social class in a French population. *Sociology of Health and Illness* 6, 30–60.

Dahlgren, G. and Whitehead, M. (1991) *Policies and Strategies to Promote Social Equity in Health.* Institute of Futures Studies, Stockholm.

Dahlgren, G. and Whitehead, M. (2006) *European Strategies for Tackling Social Inequities in Health: Levelling up Part 1.* WHO, Copenhagen.

Dahlgren, G. and Whitehead, M. (2007) *Policies and Strategies to Promote Social Equity in Health.* Background document to WHO – Strategy paper for Europe, Institute for Futures Studies, Stockholm.

Dalyrymple, J. and Burke, B. (2001) *Anti-oppressive Practice: Social Care and the Law.* Open University Press, Buckingham, UK.

Davison, C., Davey-Smith, G. and Frankel, S. (1991) Lay epidemiology and the prevention paradox. *Sociology of Health and Illness* 13, 1–19.

Davison, C., Frankel, S. and Davey Smith, G. (1992) The limits of lifestyle: re-assessing fatalism in the popular culture of illness prevention. *Social Science and Medicine* 34, 675–685.

De-Graft Aikins, A., Awuah, R.B., Pera, T.A., Mendez, M. and Ogedegbe, G. (2014) Explanatory models of diabetes in urban poor communities in Accra, *Ghana, Ethnicity & Health*, doi: 10.1080/13557858.2014.921896

de Viggiani, N. (2006) Surviving prison: exploring prison social life as a determinant of health. *International Journal of Prisoner Health* 2, 71–89.

Dixey, R. (2010) Health promotion and occupational therapy. In: Curtin, M., Molineux, M. and Supyk-Mellson, J. (eds) *Occupational Therapy and Physical Dysfunction: Enabling Occupation*, 6th edn. Churchill-Livingstone/Elsevier, London.

DOH (2009) *Improving Health, Supporting Justice: The National Delivery Plan of the Health and Criminal Justice Programme Board.* DOH, London.

Duncan, P. (2007) *Critical Perspectives on Health.* Palgrave Macmillan, Basingstoke, UK.

Durie, M. (2004) An indigenous model of health promotion. *Health Promotion Journal of Australia* 15, 181–185.

Earle, S. (2007) Promoting public health: exploring the issues. In: Earle, S., Lloyd, C.E., Sidell, M. and Spurr, S. (eds) *Theory and Research in Promoting Public Health.* Sage, London, pp. 1–36.

Elwell-Sutton, T., Finch, D. and Bibby, J. (2019) *The Nation's Health: Priorities for the Next Government.* The Health Foundation, London.

Emslie, C. and Hunt, K. (2008) The weaker sex? Exploring lay understandings of gender differences in life expectancy: a qualitative study. *Social Science & Medicine* 67, 808–816.

Emslie, C., Hunt, K. and Watt, G. (2001) Invisible women? The importance of gender in lay beliefs about heart problems. *Sociology of Health and Illness* 23, 203–233.

Eriksson, M. (2017) The sense of coherence in the salutogenic model of health. In: Mittelmark, M.B., Sagy, S., Eriksson, M., Bauer, G.F., Pelikan, J.M. and Lindström, B. (eds) *The Handbook of Salutogenesis.* Springer, New York.

Eurostat (2019) Infant Mortality Halved between 1997 and 2017. Available at: https://ec.europa.eu/eurostat/web/products-eurostat-news/-/DDN-20190719-1 (accessed 7 April 2020).

Farrer, L., Marinetto, C., Cavaco, Y.K. and Costongs, C. (2015) Advocacy for health equity: a synthesis review. *The Milbank Quarterly* 93 (2), 392–437.

Fisher, B.J. and Gosselink, C.A. (2008) Enhancing the efficacy and empowerment of older adults through group formation. *Journal of Gerontological Social Work* 51, 1–2.

Fleming, M. (2020) The importance of health promotion principles and practices. In: Fleming, M. and Baldwin, L. (eds) *Health Promotion in the 21st Century: New approaches to achieving health for all*. Allen & Unwin, London. pp. 1–12.

Frankel, S., Davison, C. and Davey Smith, G. (1991) Lay epidemiology and the rationality of responses to health education. *British Journal of General Practice* 41, 428–430.

Freire P (1972) *Pedagogy of the Oppressed*. Penguin, London.

Friel, S., Bell, R., Houweling, A.J. and Marmot, M. (2009) Calling all Don Quixotes and Sancho Panzas: achieving the dream of global health equity through practical action on the social determinants of health. *Global Health Promotion Supplement* 1, 9–13.

Gabe, J., Bury, M. and Elston, M.A. (2004) *Key Concepts in Medical Sociology*. Sage, London.

Gibbon, M. (2000) The health analysis and action cycle: an empowering approach to women's health. *Sociological Research Online*, 4.

Grace, V. (1991) The marketing of empowerment and the construction of the health consumer: a critique of health promotion. *International Journal of Health Services* 21, 329–343.

Grant, A.M., Christianson, M.K. and Price, R.H. (2007) Happiness, health, or relationships? Managerial practices and employee well-being tradeoffs. *Academy of Management Perspectives* August, 51–63.

Green, J., Cross, R., Woodall, J. and Tones, K. (2019) *Health Promotion: Planning and Strategies*, 4th edn. Sage, London, UK.

Gregg, J. and O'Hara, L. (2007a) Values and principles evident in current health promotion practice. *Health Promotion Journal of Australia* 18, 7–11.

Gregg, J. and O'Hara, L. (2007b) The Red Lotus Health Promotion Model: a new model for holistic, ecological and salutogenic health promotion practice. *Health Promotion Journal of Australia* 18, 12–19.

Grunau, G.L., Ratner, P. and Hossain, S. (2008) Ethnic and gender differences in perceptions of mortality risk in a Canadian urban centre. *International Journal of General Medicine* 1, 41–50.

Gu, J., Strauss, C., Bond, R. and Cavanagh, K. (2015) How do mindfulness-based cognitive therapy and mindfulness-based reduction improve mental health and wellbeing? A systematic review and meta-analysis of mediation studies. *Clinical Psychology Review* 37, 1–12.

Gutiérrez, L. (1991) Empowering women of color: a feminist model. In: Bricker-Jenkins, M., Hooyman, N.R. and Gottlieb, N. (eds) *Feminist Social Work Practice in Clinical Settings. Sage*, London.

Harvey, D. (1973) *Social Justice and the City*. Arnold, London.

Henderson, J. (2010) Expert and lay knowledge: a sociological perspective. *Nutrition and Dietetics* 67, 4–5.

Heritage, Z. and Dooris, M. (2009) Community participation and empowerment in healthy cities. *Health Promotion International* 24, 45–55.

Herzlich, C. (1973) *Health and Illness*. Academic Press, New York.

Hubley, J., Copeman, J. and Woodall, J. (2013) *Practical Health Promotion*, 2nd Ed. Polity Press, Cambridge, UK.

Hughner, R.S. and Kleine, S.S. (2004) Views of health in the lay sector: a compilation and review of how individuals think about health. *Health* 8, 395–422.

Hyung Hur, M. (2006) Empowerment in terms of theoretical perspectives: exploring a typology of the process and components across disciplines. *Journal of Community Psychology* 34, 523–540.

Ife, J. (2000) *Community Development: Community Based Alternatives in an Age of Globalisation*. Longman, Melbourne, Australia.

IHME (Institute for Health Metrics and Evaluation) (2019) *North East England*. Available at: www.healthdata.org (accessed 7 April 2020).

Jacobs, G. (2006) Imagining the flowers, but working the rich and heavy clay: participation and empowerment in action research for health. *Educational Action Research* 14, 569–581.

Jacobs, G. (2011) Take control or lean back? Barriers to practicing empowerment in health promotion. *Health Promotion Practice* 12, 94–101.

Jaggar, A. (ed.) (2010) *Thomas Pogge and his Critics*. Polity Press, Cambridge, UK.

Johnson, D., Deterding, S., Kuhn, K., Staneva, A., Stoyanov, S. and Hides, S. (2016) Gamification for health and wellbeing: a systematic review of the literature. *Internet Interventions* 6, 89–106.

Karim, S.S.A. and Baxter, C. (2019) HIV incidence rates in adolescent girls and young women in sub-Saharan Africa. *The Lancet* 7 (11), doi: 10.1016/S2214-109X(19)30404-8.

Kickbusch, I. and Nutbeam, D. (2017) Editorial: A watershed for health promotion: The Shanghai Conference. *Health Promotion International* 32 (1), 2–6.

Klein, W.M.P., Sheppard, J.A., Suls, J., Rothman, A.J. and Croyle, R.T. (2015) Realizing the promise of social psychology in improving public health. *Personality and Social Psychology Review* 19 (1), 77–92.

Kleinman, A. (1980) *Patients and Healers in the Context of Culture*. University of California Press, London.

Kobasa, S., Hiker, R. and Maddi, S. (1979) Who stays healthy under stress? *Journal of Occupational Medicine* 21, 595–598.

Kriznik, N.M., Kinmouth, A.L., Ling, T. and Kelly, M. (2019) Moving beyond individual choice in policies to reduce health inequalities: the integration of dynamic with individual explanations. *Journal of Public Health* 40 (4), 764–775.

Krumeich, A., Weitjts, W., Reddy, P. and Meijer-Weitz, A. (2001) The benefits of anthropological approaches for health promotion research and practice. *Health Education Research* 16, 121–130.

Kwok, C. and Sullivan, G. (2007) Health seeking behaviours among Chinese-Australian women: implications for health promotion programmes. *Health* 11, 401–415.

Labonté, R. (2016) Health promotion in an age of normative equity and rampant inequality. *International Journal of Health Policy and Management* 5 (12), 675–682.

Labonté, R. and Laverack, G. (2008) *Health Promotion in Action*. Palgrave Macmillan, Basingstoke, UK.

Lakerfeld, J. and Mackenbach, J. (2017) The upstream determinants of adult obesity. *Obesity Facts: The European Journal of Obesity* 10, 216–222.

Lalonde, M. (1974) *A New Perspective on the Health of Canadians: A Working Document*. Ministry of National Health and Welfare, Ottawa.

Lambert, H. and McKevitt, C. (2002) Anthropology in health research: from qualitative methods to multidisciplinarity. *British Medical Journal* 325, 210–213.

Larsen, E.L. and Manderson, L. (2009) 'A good spot': health promotion discourse, healthy cities and heterogeneity in contemporary Denmark. *Health and Place* 15, 606–613.

Laverack, G. (2004) *Health Promotion Practice: Power and Empowerment*. Sage, London.

Laverack, G. (2005) *Public Health. Power, Empowerment and Professional Practice*. Palgrave, Basingstoke, UK.

Laverack, G. (2006) Improving health outcomes through community empowerment: a review of the literature. *Journal of Health, Population and Nutrition* 24, 113–120.

Laverack, G. (2007) *Health Promotion Practice*. Open University Press, Maidenhead, UK.

Laverack, G. (2010) Influencing public health policy: to what extent can public action defining the policy concerns of government? *Journal of Public Health* 18, 21–28.

Laverack, G. and Wallerstein, N. (2001) Measuring community empowerment: a fresh look at organizational domains. *Health Promotion International* 16, 179–185.

Lawlor, D.A., Frankel, S., Shaw, M., Ebrahim, S. and Smith, G.D. (2003) Smoking and ill-health: does lay epidemiology explain the failure of smoking cessation programs among deprived populations? *American Journal of Public Health* 93, 266–270.

Lawton, J. (2003) Lay experiences of health and illness: past research and future agendas. *Sociology of Health and Illness* 25, 23–40.

Linhorst, D.M., Hamilton, G., Young, E. and Eckert, A. (2002) Opportunities and barriers to empowering people with severe mental illness through participation in treatment planning. *Social Work* 47, 425–434.

Lupton, D. (2016) Towards critical digital health studies: reflections on two decades of research in health and the way forward. *Health* 20(1), 49–61.

Lyons, A.C. and Chamberlain, K. (2006) *Health Psychology*. Cambridge University Press, Cambridge, UK.

MacDonald, T.H. (1998) *Rethinking Health Promotion: A Global Approach*. Routledge, London.

Macdonald, G. and Bunton, R. (2002) Health promotion: disciplinary developments. In: Bunton, R. *Health Promotion: Disciplines, Diversity and Developments*, 2nd edn. Taylor & Francis Ltd, Abingdon, UK, pp. 9–27.

Maeve, M.K. (1999) Adjudicated health: incarcerated women and the social construction of health. *Crime, Law and Social Change* 31, 49–71.

Mahoney, R. and Fleming, M. (2020) Promoting health in Aboriginal and Torres Strait Islander communities. In: Fleming, M. and Baldwin, L. (eds) *Health Promotion in the 21st Century: New approaches to achieving health for all*. Allen & Unwin, London, pp. 88–116.

Marks, D. (2004) Rights to health, freedom from illness: a life and death matter. In: Murray, M. (ed.) *Critical Health Psychology*. Palgrave Macmillan, Basingstoke, UK.

Marmot M. (2010) *Fair Society, Healthy Lives: Strategic Review of Health Inequalities in England Post-2010*. London.

Marmot, M. (2013) *Review of Social Determinants and the Health Divide in the WHO European Region: Final Report*. WHO European Region, Copenhagen, Denmark.

Marmot, M., Allen, J., Boyce, T., Goldblatt, P. and Morrison, J. (2020) *Health Equity in England: The Marmot Review 10 Years on*. Institute of Health Equity, London.

Macintyre, S., McKay, L. and Ellaway, A. (2006) Lay concepts of the relative importance of different influences on health: are there major socio-demographic variations? *Health Education Research* 21, 731–739.

Mackenzie, M., Collins, C., Connolly, J., Doyle, M. and McCartney, G. (2017) Working class discourses of politics, policy and health: 'I don't smoke; I don't drink. The only thing wrong with me is my health'. *Policy & Politics* 45 (2), 231–249.

Mayfield-Johnson, S., Rachal, J. and Butler, J. (2014) When we learn better, we do better? describing changes in empowerment through photovoice among community health advisors in a breast and cervical cancer health promotion program in Mississippi and Alabama. *Adult Education Quarterly* 64, 91–109.

McKinlay, J.B. (1979) A case for refocusing upstream: the political economy of illness. In: Jaco, E.G. (ed.) *Patients, Physicians and Illness*. The Free Press, New York.

Mehrotra, S. (2000) *Integrating Economic and Social Policy: Good Practices from High Achieving Countries*. Innocenti Working Paper No. 80. UNICEF, Florence, Italy.

Meyer, J. and Land, R. (2005) Threshold concepts and troublesome knowledge (2): epistemological considerations and a conceptual framework for teaching and learning. *Higher Education* 49, 373–388.

Meyer, J., Land, R. and Baille, C. (eds) (2010) *Threshold Concepts and Transformational Learning*. Sense Publishers, Boston, Massachusetts.

Minkler, M. (2000) Health promotion at the dawn of the 21st century: challenges and dilemmas. In: Schneider Jamer, M. and Stokols, D. (eds) *Promoting Human Wellness. New Frontiers for Research, Practice, and Policy*. University of California Press, London.

Mittelmark, M.B., Sagy, S., Eriksson, M., Bauer, G.F., Pelikan, J.M. and Lindström, B. (2017) *The Handbook of Salutogenesis*. Springer, New York.

Moore, L., Chersich, M., Steen, R., Reza-Paul, S., Dhana, A., Vuylsteke, B., Lafort, Y. and Scorgie, F. (2014), Community empowerment and involvement of female sex workers in targeted sexual and reproductive health interventions in Africa: a systematic review. *Globalization & Health* (1) 1–35.

Moyo, D. (2009) *Dead Aid: Why Aid Is Not Working and How there Is Another Way for Africa*. Penguin, London.

Mullen, L. (1994) Control and responsibility: moral and religious issues in lay health accounts. *Sociological Review* 42, 414–437.

Mungabareena Aboriginal Corporation and Women's Health Goulburn North East (2008) Using a Health Promotion Framework with an 'Aboriginal Lens'. WHNGE. Available at: www.whealth.com.au (accessed 12 June 2020).

Murray, M., Pullman, D. and Heath Rodgers, T. (2003) Social representations of health and illness among 'baby-boomers' in Eastern Canada. *Journal of Health Psychology* 8, 485–499.

Nutbeam, D. (2019) Health education and health promotion revisited. *Health Education Journal* 78 (6), 705–709.

Nyamwaya, D. (2005) Trends and factors in the development of health promotion in Africa 1973–2003. In: Scriven, A. and Garman, S. (eds) *Promoting Health: Global Perspectives*. Palgrave Macmillan, Basingstoke, UK.

Omonzejele, P.F. (2008) African concepts of health, disease and treatment: an ethical inquiry. *Explore* 4, 120–126.

Onditi, F. and Odera, J. (2017) Gender equality as a means to women empowerment? Consensus, challenges and prospects for post-2015 development agenda in Africa. *African Geographical Review* 36(2), 146.

Orme, J., Powell, J., Taylor, P., Harrison, T. and Grey, M. (2003) *Public Health for the 21st century*. Open University Press, Buckingham, UK.

Orton, L. and Anderson de Cuevas, R.M. (2019) Roma populations and health inequalities: a systematic review of multiple intersecting determinants. *European Journal of Public Health* 29 (4), doi: 10.1093/eurpub/ckz186.662

Panter-Brick, C. and Eggerman, M. (2018) The field of medical anthropology in social science & medicine. *Social Science & Medicine* 196, 233–239.

Park, J.D. (2019) *Re-Inventing Africa's Development*. Springer, eBook. Available at: https://link.springer.com/book/10.1007/978-3-030-03946-2 (accessed 6 August 2020).

Pederson, A., Rootman, I. and O'Neill, M. (2005) Health promotion in Canada: back to the past or towards a promising future? In: Scriven, A. and Garman, S. (eds) *Promoting Health: Global Perspectives*. Palgrave Macmillan, Basingstoke, UK.

Petersen, P.E. and Kwan, S. (2010) The 7th WHO Global Conference on Health Promotion: towards integration of oral health (Nairobi, Kenya 2009). *Community Dental Health* 27 (Supplement 1), 129–136.

Pickett, K.E. and Wilkinson, R.G. (2015) Income inequality and health: a causal review. *Social Science & Medicine* 128, 316–326.

Pierret, J. (1993) Constructing discourses about health and their social determinants. In: Radley, A. (ed.) *Worlds of Illness: Biographical and Cultural Perspectives on Health and Disease*. Routledge, London, pp. 9–26.

Pihl, G.T., Johannessen, H., Ammentorp, J., Jensen, J.S. and Kofoed, P.E. (2017) 'Lay epidemiology': an important factor in Danish parents' decision of whether to allow their child to receive a BCG vaccination: a qualitative exploration of parental perspective. *BMC Pediatrics* 17, 194. https://doi.org/10.1186/s12887-017-0944-3

Pill, R. and Stott, N. (1982) Concepts of illness causation and responsibility: some preliminary data from a sample of working class mothers. *Social Science & Medicine* 16, 43–52.

Pill, R. and Stott, N. (1987) The stereotype of 'working class fatalism' and the challenge for primary care health promotion. *Health Education Research* 2, 105–114.

Popay, J. and Dhooge, Y. (1989) Unemployment, cod's head soup and radical social work. In: Langan, M. and Lee, P. (eds) *Radical Social Work Today*. Routledge, London, pp. 140–164.

Potter, I. (1997) Looking back, looking ahead – health promotion: a global challenge. *Health Promotion International* 12, 273–277.

Public Health England (2018) *Public Health Outcomes Framework*. Available at: https://fingertips.phe.org.uk/profile/public-health-outcomes-framework (accessed 6 August 2020).

Pugliese-Garcia, M., Heyerdahl, L.W., Mwamba, C., Nkwemu, S., Chilengi, R., Demolis, R., Guillermet, E.

and Sharma, A. (2018) Factors influencing vaccine acceptance and hesitancy in three informal settlements in Lusaka, Zambia. *Vaccine* 36, 5617–5624.

Raeburn, J.M. and Rootman, I. (1998) *People Centered Health Promotion*. John Wiley & Sons, Chichester, UK.

Randell, E., Jerdén, L., Öhman, A. and Flacking, R. (2016) What is health and what is important for its achievement?: A qualitative study on adolescent boys' perceptions and experiences of health. *Open Nursing Journal* 10, 26–35.

Rappaport, J. (1985) The power of empowerment language. *Social Policy* 15, 15–21.

Ratcliffe, T. (2020) *Fair Health in the Time of Covid-19*. Available at: www.fairhealth.org.uk (accessed 30 April 2020).

Raworth, K. (2017) *Doughnut Economics: Seven Ways to Think Like a 21st-Century Economist*. Chelsea Green Publishing, Vermont.

Riddell, R.C. (2008) *Does Foreign Aid Really Work?* Oxford University Press, Oxford, UK.

Rifkin, S (2003) A framework linking community empowerment and health equity: it is a matter of CHOICE. *Journal of Health, Population and Nutrition* 21(3), 168.

Riger, S. (2002) What's wrong with empowerment? In: Revenson, T.A., D'Augelli, A.R., French, S.E., Hughes, D., Livert, D.E., Seidman, E., Shinn, M. and Yoshikawa, H. (eds) *Quarter Century of Community Psychology: Readings from the American Journal of Community Psychology*. Kluwer Academic/Plenum, New York.

Rissel, C. (1994) Empowerment: the holy grail of health promotion? *Health Promotion International* 9, 39–47.

Robertson, S. (2006) Not living life in too much of an excess: lay men understanding health and well-being. *Health* 10, 175–189.

Rootman, I., Goodstadt, M., Hyndman, B., McQueen, D.V., Potvin, L., Springett, J. and Ziglio, E. (eds) (2001) *Evaluation in Health Promotion. Principles and Perspectives*. WHO, Geneva.

Sanders, D. with Carver, R. (1985) *The Struggle for Health: Medicine and the Politics of Underdevelopment*. Macmillan Educational, Basingstoke, UK.

Schrecker, T. (2019) The Commission on Social Determinants of Health: Ten years on, a tale of a sinking stone, or a promise yet unrealised? *Critical Public Health* 29 (5), 610–615.

Seedhouse, D. (1997) *Health Promotion: Philosophy, Prejudice and Practice*. John Wiley & Sons, Chichester, UK.

Seedhouse, D. (2001) *Health: The Foundations for Achievement*, 2nd edn. John Wiley & Sons, Chichester, UK.

Seedhouse, D. (2004) *Health Promotion: Philosophy, Prejudice and Practice*, 2nd edn. London, John Wiley & Sons, Ltd.

Sen, A. (1993) Capability and well-being. In: Nussbaum, M. and Sen, A. (eds) *The Quality of Life*. Oxford University Press, Oxford.

Serrata, J., Hernandez-Martinez, M. and Macias, R. (2016) Self-empowerment of immigrant Latina survivors of domestic violence: a promotora model of community leadership. *Hispanic Health Care International (Women's Health for Women's History Month)* 14(1), 37–46.

Sidell, M. (2010) Older people's health: applying Antonovsky's salutogenic paradigm. In: Douglas, J., Earle, S., Handsley, S., Jones, L., Lloyd, C. and Spurr, S. (eds) *A Reader Promoting Public Health, Challenge and Controversy*, 2nd edn. Sage, London, pp. 27–32.

Small, N., Gardiner C., Barnes, S., Gott, M., Halpin, D., Payne, S. and Seamark, D. (2012) 'You get old, you get breathless, and you die': chronic obstructive pulmonary disease in Barnsley, UK. *Health & Place* 18, 1396–1403.

Smith, C. (2000) Healthy prisons: a contradiction in terms? *The Howard Journal of Criminal Justice* 39, 339–353.

Smith, J., Griffiths, K., Judd, J., Crawford, G., D'Antoine, H., Fisher, M., Bainbridge, R. and Harris, P. (2018) Ten years on from the World Health Organization Commission of Social Determinants of Health: Progress or procrastination? *Health Promotion Journal of Australia*, 29, 3–7.

Solomon, B.B. (1976) *Black Empowerment: Social Work in Oppressed Communities*. Columbia University Press, New York.

Spencer, G. (2015) Troubling moments in health promotion: unpacking the ethics of empowerment. *Health Promotion Journal of Australia: Official Journal of Australian Association of Health Promotion Professionals* 26(3), pp. 205–209.

Stainton-Rogers, W. (1991) *Explaining Health and Illness: An Exploration of Diversity*. Harvester/Wheatsheaf, London.

Staples, L.H. (1990) Powerful ideas about empowerment. *Administration in Social Work* 14, 29–42.

Svalastog, A.L., Donev, D., Kristoffersen, N.J. and Gajović, S. (2017) Concepts and definitions of health and health-related values in the knowledge landscapes of the digital society. *Croatian Medical Journal* 58 (6), 431-435.

Swami, V., Arteche, A., Chamorro-Premuzic, T., Maakip, I., Stanistreet, D. and Furnham, A. (2009) Lay perceptions of current and future health, the causes of illness, and the nature of recovery: explaining health and illness in Malaysia. *British Journal of Health Psychology* 14, 519–540.

Swanson, A. (2015) Does foreign aid always help the poor? Available at: www.weforum.org (accessed 30 April 2020).

The Aldridge Foundation and Johnson, M. (2008) *The User Voice of the Criminal Justice System*. The Aldridge Foundation, London.

Thompson, S., Watson, M.C. and Tilford, S. (2018) The Ottawa Charter 30 years on: still an important standard for health promotion. *International Journal of Health Promotion and Education* 56 (2), 73–84.

Tones, K. (1997) Health promotion as empowerment. In: Sidell, M., Jones, L., Katz, J. and Peberdy, A. (eds) *Debates and Dilemmas in Promoting Health: A Reader*. The Open University, Milton Keynes, UK, pp. 33–42.

Tones, K. and Tilford, S. (2001) *Health Promotion: Effectiveness, Efficiency and Equity*. 3rd edition. Nelson Thornes, Cheltenham, UK.

UBI Lab Leeds (2020) *What is UBI?* Available at: www.ubilableeds.co.uk (accessed 30 April 2020).

UN (1948) Universal Declaration of Human Rights. Available at: http://www.un.org/events/human rights/2007/hrphotos/declaration%20_eng.pdf (accessed 24 January 2012).

Wallerstein, N. (1992) Powerlessness, empowerment, and health: implications for health promotion programs. *American Journal of Health Promotion* 6, 197–205.

Wallerstein, N. (2002) Empowerment to reduce health disparities. *Scandinavian Journal of Public Health* 30, 72–77.

Wallerstein, N. (2006) What is the evidence on effectiveness of empowerment to improve health? *Report for the Health Evidence Network (HEN)*. Available at: http://www.ama.lu/docs/E88086.pdf (accessed 6 August 2020).

Wang, W., Chen, J., Sheng, H., Wang, H., Yang, P., Zhou, X. and Bergquist, R. (2017) Infectious diseases of poverty, the first five years. *Infect Dis Poverty* 6 (96), doi: 10.1186/s40249-017-0310-6

Ward, D. and Mullender, A. (1991) Empowerment and oppression: an indissoluble pairing for contemporary social work. *Critical Social Policy* 11, 21–29.

Warwick-Booth, L., Cross, R. and Lowcock, D. (2021) *Contemporary Health Studies: An Introduction*. 2nd edn. Polity Press, Cambridge, UK.

Whitehead, M. (1992) The concepts and principles of equity and health. *International Journal of Health Services* 22, 429–445.

Whitehead, M. and Dahlgren, G. (2007) *Concepts and Principles for Tackling Social Aocial Inequities in Health. Levelling Up Part 1*. Studies on Social and Economic Determinants of Health, No. 2. WHO Collaborating Centre for Social Determinants of Health, University of Liverpool, UK.

WHO (World Health Organization (1986a) Healthy cities: promoting health in the urban context. WHO, Copenhagen. Available at: http://www.who.dk/healthy-cities/ (accessed 18 July 2011).

WHO (1986b) Ottawa Charter for health promotion. *Health Promotion* 1, iii–v.

WHO (1995) *Health in Prisons. Health Promotion in the Prison Setting. Summary Report on a WHO meeting, London, 15–17 October* 1995. WHO, Copenhagen.

WHO (2005) *The Bangkok Charter for Health Promotion in a Globalised World*. WHO, Geneva. Available at: www.who.int/healthpromotion/conferences/6gchp/bangkok_charter/en/index.html (accessed 25 August 2020).

WHO (2008) *Closing the Gap in a Generation: Health Equity Through Action on Social Determinants of Health*. WHO, Geneva.

WHO (2009) *Milestones in Health Promotion: Statements from Global Conferences*. WHO, Geneva.

WHO (2013) *The Helsinki Statement on Health in All Policies*. WHO, Geneva.

WHO (2016) *The Shanghai Declaration*. WHO, Geneva.

WHO (2017) Human rights and health. Factsheet. Available at: www.who.int (accessed 30 April 2020).

WHO (2018) Noncommunicable disease: key facts. Available at: www.who.int (accessed 30 April 2020).

WHO (2019) Immunization coverage: key facts. Available at: www.who.int (accessed 24 April 2020).

Wilkinson, R. and Pickett, K. (2009) *The Spirit Level. Why More Equal Societies Almost Always Do Better*. Allen Lane, London.

Wills, J. and Woodhead, D. (2004) The glue that binds: articulating values in multidisciplinary public health. *Critical Public Health* 14, 7–15.

Williams, E., Buck, D. and Babalola, G. (2020) What are health inequalities? The King's Fund, London, UK. Available at: https://www.kingsfund.org/publications/what-are-health-inequalities (accessed 7 April 2020).

Wise, S. (1995) Feminist ethics in practice. In: Hugman, R. and Smith, D. (eds) *Ethical Issues in Social Work*. Routledge, London.

Woodall, J., Raine, G., South, J. and Warwick-Booth, L. (2010) *Empowerment & Health and Well-being: Evidence Review*. Centre for Health Promotion Research, Leeds Metropolitan University, Leeds, UK.

Woodall, J., Warwick-Booth, L. and Cross, R. (2012) Has empowerment lost its power? *Health Education Research* 27(4), 742–745.

World Bank (2019a) Life Expectancy at Birth. Available at: https://data.worldbank.org (accessed 24 April 2020).

World Bank (2019b) Mortality rate, infant (per 1,000 live births). Available at: www.data.worldbank.org (accessed 7 April 2020).

World Economic Forum (2015) How should we measure wellbeing? Available at: https://www.weforum.org (accessed 3 February 2020).

Wills, J. and Woodhead, D. (2004) The glue that binds: articulating values in multidisciplinary public health. *Critical Public Health* 14, 7–15.

Yang, Y., Bekemeier, B. and Choi, J. (2018) A cultural and contextual analysis of health concepts and needs of women in a rural district of Nepal. *Global Health Promotion* 25 (1), 15–22.

2 People, Power and Communities

LOUISE WARWICK-BOOTH AND SALLY FOSTER[1]

This chapter aims to:
- explore 'the community' as a vital context for health promotion;
- explore different meanings of community participation, engagement, community involvement and community development;
- discuss the importance of social capital;
- explore the role of lay involvement in health promotion; and
- suggest that working *with* communities and not merely *in* communities is essential for resilience and wellbeing.

Introduction

In the previous chapter, a view of health promotion was developed that emphasized a focus on the social determinants of health, social justice, empowering and participatory approaches. This chapter addresses the central importance of community and healthy communities in such a view of health promotion, and of people as active producers of health and agents of change. In it, we argue that there is a need to see the world through the community's eyes, to appreciate the contribution that people and communities can make to improve their health without placing full responsibility for health upon community members. We start by exploring both the term 'community' and the centrality of community involvement to health promotion; we then discuss the health-enabling community, through networks and social capital, before moving on to explore the growing recognition of the importance of lay people's health knowledge and the contribution they can make in terms of health care and health promotion. There are many ways of involving and working with communities and we explore various models, especially the community development approach, before concluding with a consideration of other ways in which people may address health issues, wellbeing and resilience through social action.

Communities as a Context for Health Promotion Practice

Although the community is the central focus for health promotion practice, the term community itself, is debated and used to mean different things (Laverack and Wallerstein, 2001). The notion of community is frequently linked to place – thus a community can be understood to be a setting; however, it is too simplistic to say that community is just neighbourhood (Green *et al.*, 2019). Communities are also formed upon the basis of collective identity, sense of belonging, shared values and network membership (Piper, 2009). Advances in technology mean that virtual communities exist and are perceived as real communities to those who are members (De Leeuw, 2000). 'Community' is a term used to describe the relationships, bonds, identities and interests that join people together and/or give them a shared interest in a place, service, culture or activity (Yerbury, 2011). The notion of community and other related terms (participation, empowerment, involvement, social action and coproduction) remain fuzzy concepts, hard to define (Sarrami-Foroushani *et al.*, 2014). Mayo (1994, p. 48) says of the term community, 'it is not just that the term has been used ambiguously. It has been contested, fought over and appropriated for different uses and interests to justify different politics, policies and practices.' The term can be used at both descriptive and evaluative levels and is defined as much by community members as by academics (Shaw, 2004); therefore, the notion of community continues to be contested. Despite these issues with understanding communities, health promoters continue to work in communities as part of their work in addressing the broader social determinants of health (Kinder *et al.*, 2000) because communities are fundamentally linked to both health and health inequalities (Warwick-Booth *et al.*, 2021) and in building healthy, resilient, connected and empowered communities, the health of the population can be improved (PHE and NHS England, 2015; NICE, 2016).

Debates about the nature of work in communities are central to health promotion practice. Many professionals have the word community in their title: community suggesting the location of their work, for instance community nurses, community care workers and police community support officers. But to say one works in the community is not necessarily to say one works with the community. McKnight (2003), for instance, talks about the relationship many professionals have with their clients, and points out that the word client is derived from the Greek, and means 'one who is controlled', whereas he argues strongly for a model of practice that frees people from medical clienthood to act as 'citizens', meaning those who hold power. Indeed, McKnight argues that health is a political communal issue and that to 'convert a medical problem into a political issue is central to health improvement' (1978, p. 39). More recently, Silva and Sena (2013) argue that health promotion within communities can be seen critically as a form of social control to manage vulnerable populations.

Criticisms aside, this focus on community health action is reflected in various global initiatives and statements from the WHO, such as the Alma-Ata Declaration: '… people have a right and a duty to participate individually and collectively in the planning and implementation of their health care' (WHO, 1978, p. 1). The Ottawa Charter states:

> Health promotion works through effective community action in setting priorities, making decisions, planning strategies and implementing them to achieve better health. At the heart of this process is the empowerment of communities, and the ownership and control of their endeavours and destiny.
>
> (WHO, 1986a, b)

The eighth global health promotion in Shanghai (WHO, 2016) noted the political nature of health, as well as the importance of wellbeing (WHO, 2017). The conference built upon the already established healthy cities approach (WHO, 1986a, b) in which a network of places had already been created in an attempt to get health on the social, economic and political agenda of local government, as well as demonstrating the influence of all policy sectors upon health and wellbeing. This programme is focused upon community as a geographical location requiring attention to improve health and tackle injustices (Box 2.1).

Developing healthy communities and healthy cities is seen as an important tool to tackle inequalities, develop resilience and improve wellbeing with community participation used as a starting point for action within health promotion practice. Health policies across Europe and more globally attempt to encourage this agenda, recognizing the important role of civil society in achieving health equity (WHO, 2011, 2012). The reason why community is so central is because this is the level of social experience where the possibilities of action and the constraints of structures meet (Popple and Shaw, 1997). In

---

Box 2.1. The concept of a healthy city.

- A healthy city is defined by a process, not an outcome.
- A healthy city is conscious of health and is trying to improve it, so any city can be a healthy city.
- The requirements of being a healthy city are simply a commitment to health and a process and structure to achieve it.
- A healthy city is one that continually creates and improves its physical and social environments and expands the community resources that enable people mutually to support each other in performing all the functions of life and developing to their maximum potential.
- The most successful healthy cities have the commitment of local community members, have a clear vision, demonstrate the ownership of policies, involve a wide array of stakeholders and have processes for institutionalizing their approach.

(Adapted from WHO 2011, 2020)

communities, we see the interface between the social, economic and environmental determinants of health and individuals' lives. South *et al.* (2012) argue that there is a need to reframe community-based health promotion to reflect a shift from 'intervention driven' approaches to 'people-centred' delivery. Indeed, in relation to health inequalities, Baum (2007) talks about the 'nutcracker effect' and makes a case for an approach to tackling such inequalities, which has not only top-down actions involving policies, but also bottom-up involvement from civil society. Health can be promoted though the efforts of communities within civil society, but advocacy is also needed to ensure that the necessary infrastructure is in place to enable rather than control the growth of community assets (South, 2014a).

The rest of this chapter explores key issues in such control, and debates about participation, community development and empowerment. In addressing issues of control and participation, we stress throughout the vital importance of the lay perspective, of seeing the world through people's eyes, and acknowledging and valuing people's contribution.

However, our starting point is communities themselves, and evidence about what makes a health-enabling community (Campbell, 2001), as well as a healthy community. In regard to health promotion within community contexts, social capital emerges as an important concept (Eriksson, 2011). Despite a lack of consensus about both the definition and measurement of it, ecological studies suggest that social capital is a collective resource and an important determinant of health at the community level (Poortinga, 2006).

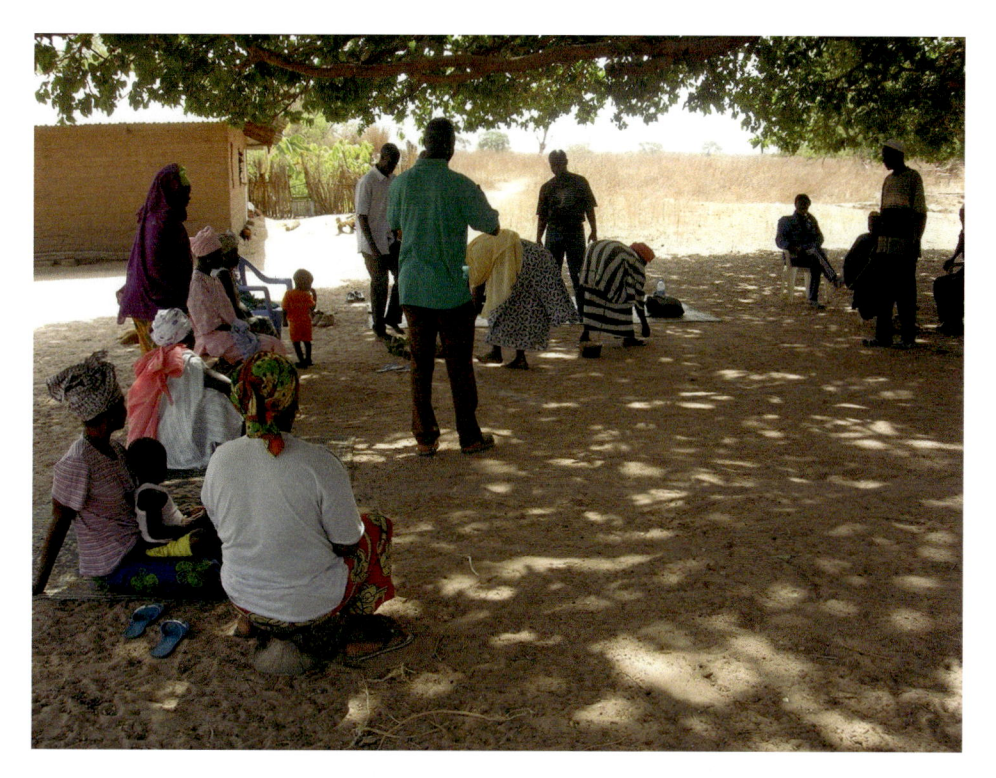

Students in The Gambia undertaking a community mapping exercise.

Communities are People Working Together: Social Capital and Health

Social capital has been given much attention within academic literature, policy circles and health promotion research in recent years. Particular attention has been afforded to the concept in relation to how it affects health and communities via social support mechanisms (Eriksson, 2011); Maass *et al.* (2016) explore how social capital experienced on a neighbourhood level influences life satisfaction and self-rated health. Bagnall *et al.* (2018) argue that social relations are now widely recognized as an important determinant of individual and community wellbeing. Several definitions of the concept suggest

> **Box 2.2. Social capital, social support and health.**
>
> There is a large amount of evidence showing social capital as an important determinant of health (Szreter and Woolcock, 2002; Eriksson, 2011). Social capital has been empirically linked to:
>
> - increased mental health (Kawachi and Berkman, 2001; Wind and Komproe, 2012);
> - reduced mortality (Kawachi *et al.*, 1997);
> - improved health behaviours (Weitzman and Kawachi, 2000; Lindstrom *et al.*, 2000);
> - self-reported health improvements and increased life satisfaction (Maass *et al.,* 2016); and
> - less inequality – income inequality leads to poorer health outcomes via disinvestment in social capital (Kawachi *et al.*, 1997; Marmot, 2015).
>
> Overall, social capital is an individually positive health determinant if trusting people live in areas with high community social capital (Rocco and Suhrcke, 2012).

that it has positive consequences for members of communities (Box 2.2), achieved through shared norms, networks and trust. As different theorists highlight a variety of interpretations of the concept, these will be considered now, with particular attention being paid to how health relates to each.

Communities Are Connections and Social Obligations

Bourdieu describes social capital as a potential resource linked to networks and relationships of mutual acquaintance and recognition, giving members collectively owned capital (Schuller *et al.*, 2000). Bourdieu (1999) identified the superimposition of social and physical space, and the associated disadvantages that are bestowed upon less powerful social groups by their residence in poorer communities. Research suggests that levels of social capital and associated health benefits are context dependent (Oshio, 2016), therefore the structural constraints on individuals and the unequal access that people have to resources based on class, gender and race (Everingham, 2003) require recognition. For Bourdieu (1999), access to resources and issues of power within society are the key to social capital (Harper, 2001). Social capital effectively viewed as connections and social obligations in Bourdieu's (1986) understanding can be converted under certain conditions into economic capital. Evidence about area effects upon health have grown in recent years especially literature on the beneficial nature of social capital for communities and community health (Wind *et al.*, 2011; Wind and Komproe, 2012). Atkinson and Kintrea (2004) argue that individuals living within deprived communities are held back because of where they live rather than by their individual characteristics. Hence, what is important from this perspective is the way in which individual networks operate to enhance or constrain health outcomes within specific communities. Furthermore, where communities are unequal, health outcomes are poorer (Marmot and Wilkinson, 2001; Marmot, 2015; Pickett and Wilkinson, 2015). The importance of social capital levels within communities in relation to health is illustrated through the example of Roseto (Box 2.3).

The Roseto example highlights the importance of the function of social capital in relation to health within a community context. A later study conducted in the M-region of Japan illustrates how people sharing the same workplace had stronger solidarity and improved health (Hanibuchi *et al.*, 2012), highlighting the function of work and historical context in creating social capital. Coleman (1998) defines social capital by its function, describing it as a resource to be drawn upon with social relations constituting useful capital resources for actors through processes such as obligations, expectations, trust, information channels and setting norms. Coleman (1998) sees these resources as less exclusionary than Bourdieu (1999). According to Coleman (1990), social capital takes three forms:

- first, the obligations and expectations, which depend upon the trustworthiness of the social environment;
- secondly, the capacity of information to flow through the social structure in order to provide a basis for action; and
- finally, it is the presence of norms accompanied by effective sanctions.

> **Box 2.3. The Roseto effect.**
>
> - From 1955 to 1965, Roseto, an Italian American community in Eastern Pennsylvania, displayed a high level of social capital through ethnic and social similarities, close family networks and good community cohesion (Stout *et al.*, 1964).
> - Roseto community members had a very low rate of myocardial infarction (heart attacks) in comparison with nearby communities (Bruhn and Wolf, 1979).
> - It was suggested that the stable and supportive structure of the community and strong family cohesion may have led to a protective effect against heart attacks (Bruhn and Wolf, 1979).
> - As the community evolved and changed during the 1960s and 1970s, family and community ties became less important. Greater rates of heart attacks were seen as well as higher mortality rates. This shows the importance of social networks and community ties in relation to health because there were no significantly different risk factors for Roseto and its neighbouring communities (Egolf *et al.*, 1992).

Social capital differs from other forms of capital in that it does not necessarily bring benefits just to the individual; rather, it brings benefits to all of those who are part of the social structure including community members.

Despite this recognition of the wider benefits of the concept, Coleman's theorizing primarily focuses upon individuals and the family. Coleman also argues that social capital creation is a largely unintentional process (Schuller *et al.*, 2000), and later research has not been able to evidence the specific mechanisms through which positive or indeed negative social capital is created (Villalonga-Olives and Kawachi, 2017). Hence, if social capital production is unintentional, how can it be encouraged or developed within the context of communities for health promotion (Eriksson, 2011)? Furthermore, Coleman's concept, if applied in practice, would lead researchers to focus upon social capital as inherently good (Everingham, 2003), but critics say that social capital can also be health damaging (Villalonga-Olives and Kawachi, 2017). Clearly, the uncritical stance taken by Coleman requires caution. Even if human capital can be increased, this does not necessarily ensure better community-level prospects because structural factors also need to be considered. For example, social capital levels within communities relate to economic and political contexts as well as material resources (Campbell, 2019), yet if social capital benefits the community as a whole and can be developed through effective social policy, it can consequently serve as a useful tool in health promotion practice.

Communities Are Networks of People

According to Putnam (2000), social capital refers to the connections among individuals, social networks and other forms of reciprocity and trust, which arise from them. Networks, norms and trust dominate his definition of the concept whilst activity is situated at the heart of civic life and therefore is a crucial aspect of his conceptualization (Schuller *et al.*, 2000). Putnam (1993a, b) suggests that the more people work together, the more that social capital is produced. This relates to the notion that communities that work together are indeed healthier, and this has been evidenced in Japan (Hanibuchi *et al.*, 2012). Putnam's work imbues community with highly positive connotations portraying an image of helpful, friendly interactions between individuals based upon personal knowledge and face-to-face contact. This ignores the downside of community life in which negative relationships may be detrimental to both physical and mental health. Villalonga-Olives and Kawachi (2017) point out that social capital does have a 'dark side', therefore researchers need to be careful to avoid the trap of presenting community solidarity, social control and collective sanctions as the catch-all in solving health-related problems.

Central to Putman's (2000) conceptualization of social capital is his description of different types of networks, all of which operate within communities to produce differential health effects.

1. Bonding networks – bonding social capital is essentially related to a common identity with group members having some factors in common (Jochum,

2003). The literature highlights the potential negative impact of excessive bonding social capital because it can serve to create exclusivity (Taylor, 2000a, b), and social contagion of negative health behaviours such as smoking and drinking (Takakura, 2015).

2. Bridging networks – these are the weak connections between people such as business associates and acquaintances. Bridging social capital is likely to be greater in communities and organizations that have a collaborative approach (Jochum, 2003). Narayan (1999) pays particular attention to the potential for less powerful and more socially excluded groups to benefit from bridging ties and links to wider resources. Kamphuis *et al.* (2019) found that bridging social capital had differential relations with health behaviour among low and high educational groups, and therefore suggest that less community segregation is important for improving health.

3. Linking networks – these are the connections

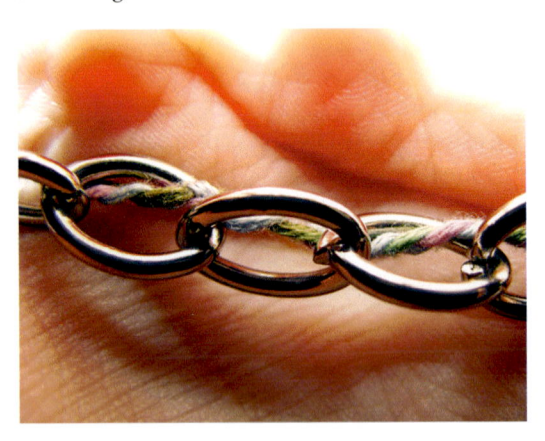

Hand-held friendship representing bonding social capital (by imma-ty-grr; this image was marked with a CC BY-ND 2.0 license. Creative Commons.)

made to those in positions of power by those less powerful (Putnam, 2000). Linking social capital is useful in terms of enlisting and engaging support from key agencies and key players within community contexts and for designing targeted health promotion interventions (Villalonga-Olives and Kawachi, 2017).

These different types of social capital are also said to interact with each other. However, there is some debate about whether this interaction occurs automatically and recent empirical findings suggest that moving from bonding to bridging social capital is beset with contradictions. Thus, the interaction between the different types of social capital requires further exploration and is not as simple as some suggest, especially when designing health promotion programmes (Villalonga-Olives and Kawachi, 2017). Despite complexities, evidence does show that network membership and related social support are important in relation to health, as Box 2.4 demonstrates.

There is some contradictory evidence here in the sense that network membership can detrimentally affect health. For example, network phenomena are relevant to obesity because obesity appears to spread through social ties (Christakis and Fowler, 2007), and membership of some networks may increase risk-taking behaviour that is damaging to health (Villalonga-Olives and Kawachi, 2017). Furthermore, the mechanism of action between social support activities, membership of networks and health outcomes remains unclear.

Communities Are People That Trust Each Other

Fukuyama primarily presents social capital as trust by defining the concept as 'a set of informal values or norms shared amongst members of a group that permits co-operation between them' (1999, p. 16). Most social capital definitions pay attention to trust and give equal weight to trust and networks, but some prioritize one over the other (Berman and Phillips, 2003). For Fukuyama (1999), trust leads to cooperation, which makes both groups and networks operate smoothly. Central to this conceptualization is the radius of trust, where it is argued that the further trust expands outside of the family then the more likely it is to be based upon moral resources and ethical behaviours (Fukuyama, 2001). Zarychta (2015) argues that people who trust more feel safer in their communities, and therefore have better emotional wellbeing, enabling them to be more open to accessing networks around them – all of which is likely to lead to better health outcomes. Where groups have a narrow radius of trust, their in-group solidarity reduces their ability to cooperate with both insiders and outsiders. It is arguably difficult for people to trust those outside of narrow circles, especially in the absence of weak ties. This argument

> **Box 2.4. Are community networks positive for health?**
>
> - Being socially connected to other people is good for health and wellbeing (Mittlemark, 1999; Cacioppo and Patrick, 2008; Bagnall et al., 2018).
> - One large-scale international study demonstrated that, during a 7-year period, those with adequate social relationships had a 50% greater survival rate compared with people who reported having poor social relationships (Holt-Lunstad et al., 2010).
> - Smoking behaviour spreads through networks with interconnected people often stopping smoking in unison (Christakis and Fowler, 2008). Elements of social capital such as 'trust' and 'social participation' are independently and positively associated with smoking cessation (Giordano and Lindstrom, 2010).
> - Networks can provide opportunities for peer identities to be re-negotiated, which in turn influence health-related behavioural norms (Campbell, 2001); networks of solidarity can be useful in working as a launch pad for protests and the creation of social movements; marginalized groups can confront those with power and work to gain health-related resources (Campbell, 2019).

about in-group trust reflects parallels to Putnam's emphasis on close, tight-knit networks not always being beneficial. Communities with broader networks of trust are more likely to care about individual members and to support them in ways that are beneficial for their health. Households that trust their neighbours and are surrounded by trusting community members report better health statuses (Zarychta, 2015). Furthermore, in communities with higher levels of trust, wider interactions between people are likely to be more cooperative and less stressful. Family, neighbours and friends are likely to provide more social support as a result of higher levels of trust (Halpern, 2005), and social support has already been shown to be beneficial for health. In comparison, social isolation is now understood to be detrimental to health; social isolation and loneliness combined with low socio-economic status, leads to increased health-risk behaviours in such communities (Holst Algren et al., 2020).

Social Capital and Health Promotion within a Community Context

These definitions of social capital all highlight elements such as trust and associational linkages, although they give different weight to their importance. The different definitions also emerge from a variety of theoretical traditions. Bourdieu draws upon Marxism, Coleman is concerned with function, Putnam politically locates his interpretation and Fukuyama's discussion is inherently conservative. Yet all of these interpretations suggest that the concept is useful for understanding communities and in achieving positive health outcomes. The benefits of social capital in relation to health can seemingly be conferred upon individuals and communities via several different pathways (Kawachi and Berkman, 2001), which are still not fully understood despite on-going research in this area. If social capital can provide community-level benefits then it is important for health promotion practice (Box 2.5).

However, a cautious approach is required when examining the links between health promotion and social capital. There are complex and subtle ways in which inequality manifests itself within community relationships, which on the surface seem to be based upon trust and reciprocity (Leonard, 2004). For example, inclusion and exclusion occurs based upon gender, ethnicity, age and religious affiliation, as well as the broader community context, because the social environment of trust within any community context affects individuals' levels of trust (Zarychta, 2015). The key lesson to be drawn from the empirical evidence for health promoters is that, although social capital can have positive health outcomes, it is not a 'thing' that can be promoted via public health interventions and simply 'given' to people. Health promoters need to get to grips with the concept because 'understanding social capital is part of understanding the operations of power in daily life and how social structure as practiced in daily life creates and perpetuates inequalities' (Stevens, 2008, p. 1182). Maass et al. (2016) argue that more locally and contextually rooted knowledge on the concept is needed in order to deliver effective health promotion across different contexts. Understanding the concept involves examining its complexities, including the problems and criticisms highlighted within the literature.

Box 2.5. Social capital and health promotion practice.

- Social capital is important for community development, which is central for health promotion practice (Wakefield and Poland, 2005). Using assets-based approaches to map health needs has been successfully piloted in some communities (Greetham, 2011). Community development and community commissioning approaches focus upon helping communities to improve their health themselves (Buck and Wensell, 2018).
- Involvement and empowerment are central to health promotion practice; similarly, associating together and engaging in community affairs are crucial to social capital development for Coleman (1998), all of which can be promoted via volunteering as a mechanism of inclusion and network expansion (South et al., 2012).
- Social capital is a resource that may have positive use in relation to health promotion initiatives, because it is an important protective factor for some physical health outcomes (Rodgers et al., 2019). For example, trust plays an important role in people's health-seeking behaviours, so those with higher levels of trust are likely to engage in health-promoting activities (Shahbari et al., 2020). Musavengane and Kloppers (2020) highlight the importance of strong social capital in promoting the realization of community resilience when communally managing natural resources.
- Putnam (2000) marshals evidence to demonstrate that in high social capital areas, public spaces are cleaner, people are friendlier and the streets are safer. In some communities, more positive levels of health are achieved when social capital is developed to a higher level (Zarychta, 2015). Kingsley et al. (2020) note the importance of community spaces to encourage social interaction, following their research into community gardens in Australia.
- Kim et al. (2017) argue that bridging social capital is essential to rebuild post-disaster communities, because it is a 'catalyst' of co-production. Bonding social capital is crucial for short-term disaster recovery in the form of support from close community members and bridging social capital supports the creation of co-production, leading to increased opportunities for community-oriented development.
- The concept may be useful in explaining collective action in terms of mutual involvement and the creation of alliances to achieve group and community goals, including those related to health improvement (Campbell, 2019).

Problems with the Concept of Social Capital

There are a number of criticisms of the concept of social capital, with many commentators recognizing that inadequate attention has been paid to the power inequalities that drive poor health and the macro-forces that structurally determine community health (Campbell, 2019). Others have noted issues with its definitional diversity (Portes and Landolt, 1996; Schuller et al., 2000; Everingham, 2003), lack of precision (Flora, 1998; Wall et al., 1998; Everingham, 2003) and measurement (Portes and Landolt, 1996; Green et al., 2000; Walker and Wigfield, 2003). Fukuyama's (1999) approach has again been criticized because of his monoculturalist standpoint in which he asserts that societies need to share the same language, norms and moral values in order to avoid disintegration. Other commentators such as Kymlicka (1995a, b) offer a more multiculturalist perspective. Davies (2002) also suggested that the concept is gender blind and ethnocentric. With specific reference to health contexts, the way in which policy makers view social capital can involve victim blaming, because poor people may be viewed as unhealthy as a result of not participating enough in community activities (Muntaner and Lynch, 1999), and responsibility is then placed back onto communities without attention being paid to inequalities (Campbell, 2019). Box 2.6 outlines some of the complexity of building social capital in the community.

Thus, social capital creation in the context of healthy communities needs both a considered and critical approach. Social capital development is certainly not a magic bullet for health promoters nor is it a cheap option, because the quality of relationships is important within networks. Indeed, 'taking social capital seriously in the context of health promotion in rich or poor countries is therefore not in any sense a cheap option; it is an additional dimension – and one necessarily requiring additional costs – which has been too neglected

> **Box 2.6. Issues with attempts to build social capital at a community level.**
>
> 1. Trust within any neighbourhood is not guaranteed. The impact of historical divisions within areas, contemporary housing policies, intense deprivation and the sudden presence of streams of money can all act to undermine levels of trust between individuals and groups within neighbourhoods (Hibbitt *et al.*, 2001). The key point here is that the nature of relationships matters for health outcomes (Zarychta, 2015).
> 2. Secondly, building social capital may not be a suitable goal for all community contexts or purposes. Social capital is highly context dependent (Jochum, 2003), different factors in different places create success (Groves *et al.*, 2003) and as a result, consideration must be paid to the socio-economic situation and the institutional environment within any community (Jochum, 2003). Evidence about how various aspects of social capital affect different health outcomes for community members remains unclear (Eshan *et al.*, 2019).
> 3. Some individuals are better placed within a community to lead others forward in developing social capital. Despite this suggestion, the literature on social capital has largely ignored the importance of leadership (Purdue, 2001).
> 4. Social capital is only valuable to the extent that community members and policy makers recognize and sustain its value. There is growing evidence that social networks and social capital increase people's resilience to and recovery from illness. Increasingly, the impact of health promotion interventions is measured in economic terms, yet the evidence of the monetary benefits associated with social capital related investments remains lacking (Buck and Wensall, 2018).

in the past' (Szreter and Woolcock, 2002, p. 26). All of this ultimately begs the question of how social capital relates to the concept of a healthy community.

Healthy Communities and Social Capital

There is no simple answer to what a healthy community will look like when measured against the concept of social capital because of the many complexities already discussed. The key lessons for health promoters in relation to social capital as part of healthy communities are now outlined.

- Healthy communities are not necessarily those with more social capital.
    - Cohesive communities can also be characterized by distrust, fear and racism as well as exclusion of outsiders (Baum, 1999). Health promoters should therefore carefully examine the types of social capital present when engaged with community work (Zarychta, 2015).
    - Enhancing social capital in neighbourhoods is assumed to be a beneficial strategy in terms of promoting life satisfaction, as well as strengthening sense of coherence even in communities that are already understood to be healthy (Maass *et al.*, 2016).
- Healthy communities are more likely to have the right kind of social capital in which network access serves to link to resources that help improve situations (Gibson, 2010), the community environment is trusting (Zarychta, 2015) and community members can support wellbeing (Atkinson *et al.*, 2020).
    - Building bridging social capital will not necessarily lead to healthier communities because only particular individuals are likely to participate and so this becomes exclusionary (Wakefield and Poland, 2005). In segregated communities divided along many lines such as race, class and gender, developing shared norms and networks is difficult (Gibson, 2006; Kamphuis *et al.*, 2019).
    - Healthy communities have health-promoting social relations and understanding of assets-based approaches to supporting improved health (Greetham, 2011). Bagnall *et al.* (2018) outline that there is a range of intervention approaches to community infrastructure that can be used to boost social relations and wellbeing in community contexts: for example, involving community members in the organization and planning of community infrastructure changes and the provision of a focal point or reason to interact.
- Healthy communities are happy communities.
    - There are links between happiness and health with subjective wellbeing strongly influencing health and all-cause mortality (Deiner and Chan, 2011). Holistic definitions of health examine the interaction and

relationship between the self, the community and the environment. Thus, being part of happy communities is important for individual mental health.
- There are many determinants of happiness but whether a person is happy depends upon if others in that person's individual networks are also happy, suggesting that happiness is related to groups and levels of social capital (Fowler and Christakis, 2008). Interventions to enhance subjective wellbeing are therefore useful tools for public health practitioners (Deiner and Chan, 2011). The people, the place and power relations are important components of community wellbeing (Atkinson et al., 2017).
- Whilst deprivation, median income and unemployment are associated with higher wellbeing inequality in some communities, higher levels of engagement in heritage activities and the use of green space (for example for exercise) are associated with less wellbeing inequality (What Works Wellbeing, 2017).

- Healthy communities are salutogenic.
  - Antonovsky (1996) raised questions about the origin of health, asking health promoters to explore this rather than focusing upon the causes of disease. He argues that an individual sense of coherence, the way in which people view their lives, has a positive influence upon health. This definition of health is at the individual, group or societal level; therefore, communities that enable people to build a sense of coherence are salutogenic and healthier. An assets-based model of health fits well with salutogenesis since it emphasizes the positive capacity of communities to promote the health of its members (Kawachi, 2010).

- Healthy communities are resilient.
  - Cinderby et al. (2014) conducted an action research project exploring the effect of different interventions to facilitate civic engagement and a more resilient and environmentally sustainable community in a low-income neighbourhood in the UK. They found that linking sustainability to community interests was important in engaging people, and that sustained engagement is essential in embedding change. They noted that improvements in social capital are a significant aspect of increasing community resilience but that supportive governance is still required.
  - Tobin et al. (2014) argue that bonding social capital works at the community level to enable long-term recovery from shock events (such as global pandemics). O'Sullivan et al. (2013) also demonstrate that social networks and infrastructure can be mutually reinforced during a crisis.

- Healthy communities have assets (assets model).
  - Communities have numerous assets – individual and community resources that they can draw upon – that are useful in protecting against negative health outcomes. Community-level resources include social capital such as networks, solidarity and community cohesion. These are health promoting irrespective of the level of inequality and disadvantage within the community (Morgan and Ziglio, 2007). Health promoters therefore should work in ways to develop assets in community-centred approaches (South et al., 2012), which involves focusing upon health promotion, drawing on assets, promoting equity in health by working with those experiencing barriers to health and by using participatory methods to involve community members (South, 2014b).

Given increasing environmental challenges to communities, the concept of social capital remains an important element of health promotion practice, as well as political discourse (Box 2.7; see Chapter 3). We now turn to the issue of working with communities as a central component of health promotion practice, by exploring lay knowledge and the lay contribution, and various models of community participation.

Communities Are People Working Together: The Lay Contribution

Much of the preceding discussion has indicated that a focus on healthy communities requires an approach that goes beyond seeing people as 'passive recipients of paternalistic professional efforts to improve their health' (Taylor, 2007, p. 98) and instead regards them as an essential resource in enhancing their own health and that of their community. As a way of highlighting this, Box 2.8 offers two examples of projects that focus on grandmothers. In these projects, the health knowledge and experience that grandmothers have is valued and integrated into the programmes, allowing the grandmothers to take a vital role in helping others.

> **Box 2.7. Social capital and community responses to emerging public health issues.**
>
> Social capital is an important resource that can used to support health in times of crisis, for example, in enabling health outcomes and supporting resilience. Covid-19 was declared as a global pandemic by the WHO on 11 March 2020, with several community responses emerging at the same time across the UK:
>
> - networks of community volunteers working together to provide aid and support to those in need in the form of food parcels, befriending at a social distance and online resources;
> - educational networks (universities) providing training, expert advice, research evidence and equipment to support learning about the new disease;
> - voluntary sector organizations launching co-ordinated approaches to provide support, with a specific focus upon vulnerable and disadvantaged community members; and
> - statutory sector responses, local authority services such as the health, social care and housing sector working to meet community need.
>
> These responses all occurred in a national environment in which the government was also adapting policy to support citizens. Whilst social capital is evident here in network responses, and possibly increased trust in some areas, communities and broader infrastructure systems have varying resources and capacity to draw upon in their responses. Furthermore, evidence from Rao and Greve (2018) suggests that in instances where disaster causation is attributed to other community members, this can weaken ties and increase suspicion and distrust. Blame and anger were reported in national news bulletins detailing increased racism towards Chinese health-care workers because of the virus first being identified in Wuhan, China, as well as in negative responses to people perceived not to be adhering to new social-distancing guidelines.

One place where there has been increasing recognition of lay expertise is in encounters with health professionals. In 1985, Tuckett *et al.* talked about the medical encounter as the meeting of two experts: not only the health professional but also the patient, who had considerable experiential knowledge of their own body, health and illness. Debates about this professional–patient relationship have centred on the frequently used terms 'compliance' and 'adherence', both of which connote a relationship of inequality and obedience; proponents of a more patient-centred approach have suggested terms like 'concordance', as well as 'shared decision-making' and 'collaboration' to signify this different kind of relationship (Britten and Maguire, 2016). In addition, the term 'lay expert' has entered the vocabulary of health care, particularly with the initiatives associated with 'expert patients' in chronic disease management (DOH, 2001). This is further developed in the more recent focus on 'co-production', which 'describes the participation of service users (patients) in the healthcare system. Patients are recognised as shaping its processes and outcomes, thereby challenging typical depictions of them as either passive service receivers or active only to "self-manage" their own health issues' (Baim-Lance *et al.*, 2019, p. 129). Such initiatives are partially rooted in the growing focus on lay health knowledge and behaviour, outlined in Chapter 1; but they are also linked to the rising consumerism in welfare services, critiques of medical power (e.g. Illich, 1976; Kelleher *et al.*, 2006) and pragmatic efforts to respond to the increasing pressure felt in health services worldwide.

We also have considerable evidence of the role of people in self-care and unpaid care of family, friends and neighbours. The Parliamentary Office of Science and Technology (POST) (2018) reported that there were 6.5 million unpaid carers in the UK, with around 25% of them providing more than 50 hours of such care a week. Recognition of the enormous contribution of such unpaid care for health and social care policy is clearly important, but the lay contribution is wider even than this and covers lay roles in the services themselves, as volunteers and lay health workers, and it is to these roles we now turn.

As noted above, people engage in health-care work all the time, in looking after their own health, or that of family and neighbours. In the past, and even today in deprived communities, people often had no access to other forms of care; women, for example, have assisted in childbirth, often combining what Kleinman (1980) calls the 'popular' and 'folk' sectors. However, the development of programmes for lay or community health workers

> **Box 2.8. Grandmothers as a resource: two examples.**
>
> **1.** Grandmother Project (GMP) is a non-profit organization that works with communities in developing countries to improve the lives of women and children, especially girls. Its central focus is the recognition of the authority and influence that grandmothers have in many cultures. Adopting a 'Change through Culture' approach, two of its key pillars are:
>
> - Building on cultural roles, values and traditions
> - Recognizing the wisdom and authority of elders and involving them in all programmes, especially the grandmothers (https://grandmotherproject.org/)
>
> The Executive Director of GMP is Judi Aubel, who founded the organization as a result of her experiences of projects involving grandmothers. In a co-authored paper in 2004 she describes a community intervention in Senegal that involved grandmothers and older women and inspired her subsequent work (Aubel *et al.*, 2004). The authors are critical of what they call the dominant transmission–persuasion paradigm in health education and communication. As a result of a study, which highlighted the significant role played by grandmothers and older women in the community in relation to maternal and child health, a 'grandmother strategy' was developed. Working in communities that were very traditional in their ideas and practices in relation to health, the strategy:
>
> - aimed to develop existing human resources in the community and enhance social networks;
> - focused on encouraging 'learners' to actively and critically analyse both their own experience and alternative solutions and construct their own strategies to deal with everyday problems (p. 950).
>
> This approach was participatory and empowering, with activities such as songs and problem-posing 'stories-without-an-ending', which encouraged 'discussion of problematic nutrition-related situations and possible solutions' (p. 951). After initial scepticism, the grandmothers were won round by the respect shown for their roles, ideas and experiences, and they participated enthusiastically. Both quantitative and qualitative findings suggested the strategy had been successful, with not only improved nutritional practices but strengthened family and community ties. Whilst there are various factors in this success, a key one was the acknowledgement of the lay perspective, and the integration of this.
>
> The grandmothers themselves said:
>
> - 'We feel much stronger now because not only do we have our traditional knowledge'; but, in addition,
> - 'We have acquired the knowledge of the doctors' (p. 954).
>
> (Aubel *et al.*, 2004)
>
> **2. The Friendship Bench**
>
> Dr Dixon Chibanda, a Zimbabwean psychiatrist, started the project as an inexpensive way of helping people with mental health problems in a resource-poor setting; those with mental health problems, especially anxiety and depression, literally sit on a bench outdoors and talk to a grandmother, who uses her training in problem-solving therapy to help them. But Chibanda (2017, p. 344) points out the grandmothers 'contributed to the team's understanding of local concepts of common mental disorder, including indigenous idioms of distress used to navigate through the therapy sessions' and this 'contributed towards the development of a local mental health lexicon and cultivated community ownership of the intervention'.

(CHWs) has its origins in the shift to primary health care (PHC) from the late 1970s onwards, and the community health movements of the 1970s. The PHC movement that arose post Alma-Ata grew out of critiques of the nature of urban hospital-focused health care systems (e.g. Sanders with Carver, 1985), and the alternatives being developed in post-colonial and socialist countries such as Tanzania and China, with a focus on poor communities and the use, for example, of barefoot doctors. Thus, PHC was seen to address two agendas: one was that of creating an alternative to the high-cost urban health systems with highly trained health professionals; the other was the 'transformative agenda, which saw ill-health as rooted in the poverty and inequality in people's lives' (Standing *et al.*, 2008, p. 2097). Community mobilization and the training of local people to provide basic services was seen as central to PHC, and as a result, CHW programmes proliferated, although Standing *et al.* (2008) point to their decline from the late 1980s onwards. Perry *et al.* (2014) attribute this decline to problems with the implementation of CHW programmes and a changing political and economic climate that did not support comprehensive PHC; however, they do point to the emerging evidence of the success of programmes in countries such as Brazil, Bangladesh and Nepal in achieving rapid reductions in the under-5 child mortality rate. In fact, from the late 1990s there has been a renewed interest in CHWs and 'compelling evidence that CHWs are critical for helping health systems achieve their potential, regardless of a country's level of development (Perry *et al.*, 2014, p. 399).

So what are CHWs? They go by many names (Taylor *et al.*, 2018, list 131 terms to describe CHWs in the global literature) and, as we shall see, they are surrounded by many issues, but the WHO defines them thus:

> Community health workers should be members of the communities where they work, should be selected by the communities, should be answerable to the communities for their activities, should be supported by the health system but not necessarily a part of its organization, and have shorter training than professional workers.
>
> (WHO, 1989, as cited by Lehman and Sanders 2007, p. 3)

This definition suggests that CHWs are seen as embedded in communities, as well as performing an important linking role between health-care systems and their communities (Lehman and Sanders, 2007). However, the issues that surround them are many and a summary of these can be seen in Box 2.9. Much of the research on CHWs has been carried out in countries of the global South. However, in the global North, the use of lay health workers is also advocated and has been well researched, for instance in the UK and the USA, although often in relation to very different agendas. There are two key questions – is the main motivation for the use of lay health workers that they are able to stand in for health professionals and thus offer 'an extension of a resource-constrained health service' (Rifkin, 2014, p. 775), or is there a positive value to the use of their knowledge and skills 'that allows lay health workers to serve as change agents to others within their community' (Canadian Health Services Research Foundation, 2007, p. 2)?

The first of these questions is primarily functional in terms of service delivery and seems to be stressed in the 2019 resolution passed by the World Health Assembly that 'recognized that community health workers play an important role in delivering quality primary health care services as part of inter-disciplinary teams' (https://www.who.int/hrh/news/2019/health-worker-momentum-wha72/en/).

However, the second question is more relevant to health promotion and recognizes the particular advantages of the use of CHWs in reaching communities; this has meant that the use of CHWs in the global North is very much associated with accessing 'hard-to-reach' groups. For instance, in North America, where there are estimated to be nearly 200,000 CHWs (Perry *et al.*, 2014), CHWs have been used to encourage underserved groups to access preventative services; for example, encouraging Vietnamese-American women to attend for cancer screening (Mock *et al.*, 2007) or delivering mental health interventions to recent immigrants to the USA (Weaver and Lapidos, 2018). A more radical approach is that of Poder es Salud/Power for Health in Oregon, USA, where a project worked with CHWs from local African American and Latino communities to address the root causes of health disparities (Farquhar *et al.*, 2008). In their paper, Farquhar *et al.* (2008) explore the experiences of the CHWs themselves, rather than the communities, and they describe the multiple roles of the CHWs, their work as community organizers and their experiences as members of the Steering Committee for the project. What comes through vividly in their account is the activist roles of the CHWs and the importance of an increasing sense of power; not only do the participating families and neighbours 'have a greater sense of community … and now because of that they know they have the power to change things' (Farquhar *et al.*, 2008, p. 4), but the CHWs themselves felt empowered by the project.

In 2004, a role similar to a CHW, the health trainer, was introduced in England (DOH, 2004) and health trainer programmes now exist in most parts of the country, albeit on a small scale. Health trainers are recruited to work with communities with the poorest health, and the majority are drawn from those communities. They do outreach work in order to engage with communities that professionals have found 'hard to reach', offer one-to-one support for people who want to make a change to improve their health, and connect them to activities in their local area. A study in England entitled People in Public Health (South *et al.*, 2010a) explored the many public health roles lay people are taking and the myriad ways they are contributing to improving the health of their communities, and it concluded that a particular strength of lay people in health roles is their ability to act as such a bridge to communities, to deliver health

> **Box 2.9. CHWs.**
>
> **1.** Who volunteers and who selects? The issues here relate to power in the community, as well as the possible use of patronage to select particular members for training.
>
> **2.** What are the 'person characteristics' of CHWs? What knowledge and skills do they have (are they literate, or educated to some degree?) Are there particular personal qualities they should have, and how similar are they to their client groups? There seems to be a degree of consistency across programmes in relation to some of these issues, but still CHWs are a diverse group.
>
> **3.** Should they be paid and, if so, by whom? The general evidence is that volunteering does not sustain most CHW schemes, as by definition they are often in poor communities. Thus, most CHWs are remunerated, and more usually by the state rather than the local community. However, does this change the nature of the relationship of CHWs with their local community?
>
> **4.** What are their roles – and who are their recipients? Questions here relate to how specialized or generic their work is, and whether they are preventing disease or promoting access to services. CHWs might be offering clinical or social support for a particular client group, or be acting as mediators or be engaged in more activist roles for a community.
>
> **5.** What training do they receive? Again, by definition, training is short, but without ongoing training and support, CHWs may be put in situations where they cannot meet the expectations of the communities in which they work. This may be particularly true where the CHWs have specialist roles in relation to, for example, TB, or maternal and child care. There is also the issue of how much CHWs are trained as community mediators, rather than as health-care practitioners.
>
> **6.** To whom are they accountable? On the one hand, CHWs may become embedded in the government services of which they are a part and struggle then to obtain status and recognition within this service (this may lead them, for example, to seek further training and remuneration to enhance their professional status). On the other hand, if CHWs see themselves as embedded in the community, their roles and actions may bring them into conflict with the very government services that pay them.
>
> **7.** How sustainable and durable are CHW programmes? The evidence suggests that, without the support of both established services and the communities themselves, the failure rate of CHW programmes is high. Also, what affects the attrition rate of CHWs?
>
> (Lehman and Sanders, 2007; Standing *et al.*, 2008; South *et al.*, 2013; Rifkin, 2014; Perry *et al.*, 2014; Kane *et al.*, 2016; Olaniran *et al.*, 2017; Gale *et al.*, 2018)

messages and offer support in appropriate ways to people who might otherwise be disengaged or who face barriers to participation.

There are a number of issues with CHWs, however, as was noted earlier. Evaluations of local services have consistently shown that the peer-led, person-centred approach adopted by, for example, health trainers is hugely popular and is helping people make changes that they want to make to improve their health (Kinsella *et al.*, 2011; White *et al.*, 2010). However, there can be challenges in combining community engagement with achieving public health targets for behaviour change (Cook and Wills, 2011). Indeed, a report on health trainers in England stated that, with health services under pressure and a target focused commissioning environment, the health trainer services have become polarized, with some adopting a more clinical approach (e.g. conducting health checks or supporting clients with specific medical conditions), whilst at the other end of the spectrum there has been resistance to this and a continuing focus on sustainable community development (Royal Society for Public Health, 2015).

Similarly, Attree *et al.* (2012) point out that whilst health trainers address inequity of access to services and engage with many diverse, disadvantaged communities, they do not address structural inequalities in health. This point is also stressed by Gale *et al.* (2018) in their study of pregnancy outreach workers in the UK, where they comment that for pregnant women deemed at 'risk', such workers 'do not have any significant impact on the "upstream" inequalities and structures that are causing the problem in the first place' (p.103). Finally, Weaver and Lapidos (2018) raise similar issues in their review of CHWs in mental health interventions in the USA. They conclude that involvement of CHWs may 'favour medically oriented roles over socially oriented roles promoting justice and equity within communities' (Weaver and Lapidos, 2018, p. 175).

South *et al.* (2012) also explore the challenges for health professionals working with lay health workers; for a number of years, there have been suggestions that a process of de-professionalization might be occurring in relation to the medical profession in particular (Cooper *et al.*, 2011). De-professionalization has been linked to, among other trends, the changing nature of health professionals' relationships with their patients, and a more knowledgeable and demanding public. Clearly, having lay people acting in public health or health care roles, together with the shift we saw earlier to recognizing lay ideas about health as a form of knowledge, suggests a possible challenge to the idea of the all-knowing and all-powerful professional. For example, Glenton *et al.* (2013) found, in their systematic review of lay health worker programmes globally, that health professionals working with lay health workers feared a 'loss of authority'. There are also issues about how professionals and lay health workers work together and how much they value each other. In a study of five community partnerships in South Africa, El Ansari *et al.* (2002) outline five key domains of partnership working, which include educational competencies, partnership fostering skills, community involvement expertise, proficiency as change agents, and strategic and management skills. They conclude from their study that whilst community members valued the skills of professionals especially in relation to proficiency as change agents and strategic and management skills, professionals had limited appreciation of community skills in all domains. Whilst this study was not specifically about CHWs, it does suggest potential problems in valuing those without professional training.

South *et al.* (2010a) also found that there were concerns about acceptance by health professionals:

> I think some of the professionals boo hoo us. (L25)
>
> I think they [lay workers] need credibility, I think they need that, I think a lot of … a lot of health care professionals see themselves as the professionals and they know best. (P23)
>
> (South *et al.*, 2010a, p. 193)

Another dimension of this is the fact that most CHWs are women and Kane *et al.* (2016) suggest the gendered nature of such lay health work needs to be examined, especially in terms of the value attached to it by health professionals. The other issue for lay health workers is their own potential professionalization, the possibility of pursuing further training and gaining greater remuneration and the challenges of working within bureaucratic institutions. An example of the ways in which a lay health project goes 'mainstream' is shown by the Fag Ends project (Box 2.10). Kane *et al.* (2016) also point out that failure to address some of these

---

Box 2.10. Fag Ends Smoking Cessation Service.

The Fag Ends Service had its origins in a community development self-help project, started in Everton in 1994 in a deprived area of Liverpool, in which ex-smokers volunteered to help others give up smoking. Over time, there were changes in the project and by 1999 it had become the main smoking cessation service for Liverpool, with the lay advisers working as employees. Springett *et al.* (2007) provide an account of the way in which the service used local knowledge to provide a successful service, appropriate and responsive to users' needs, whilst also meeting the requirements from national guidance. The critical role of the lay health workers is clear; as the workers themselves said, their clients:

> … want real people, don't they. People they meet every day, on the same level, talking in everyday terms. Sometimes they get frightened of too much medical jargon. Most of our clients don't understand that. (p. 251)

(Springett *et al.*, 2007)

At the heart of the account is the recognition of the tensions between the lay world and the professional world, and the conflicting ideologies of bottom-up and top-down provision:

> What lay beneath the Fag Ends experience … is an issue of conflicting ideologies that still reverberate at the centre of health promotion and public health, situated as it is in the dominant discourse of medical science … many established power relationships including the devaluing of local knowledge by the professional remain undisturbed. (p. 254)

Yet the Fag Ends Service offers a glimpse into how a service can manage to be responsive to its users, recognizing their own knowledge, culture and complex lives, and retaining the ethos of a self-help group.

issues may account for high attrition rates among CHWs in some programmes.

Clearly, there are challenges in engaging lay people in public health roles, and there are also many variations in the types of lay worker programmes, which need to be borne in mind in assessing them. However, CHW programmes themselves have also been challenged as a diversion from addressing structural inequalities in health and as part of a right wing agenda to 'shrink the state' and replace paid workers with volunteers. South *et al.* (2013) address these challenges and put forward a strong argument in support of engaging lay people as part of a more people-centred public health, and this is reinforced in the book entitled *People Centred Public Health*, which sets out a radical vision for a different public health system with citizen engagement at its core (South *et al.*, 2012). Lay engagement is not about saying there can be individual solutions to structural problems, and it need not undermine professionals or replace paid jobs. Rather, it is a way of people gaining more control over their health and is supported by a growing evidence base, which demonstrates that lay engagement can make a real difference to health at a community level.

Community Participation

The claim earlier that the public are now no longer seen as 'passive recipients of paternalistic efforts to improve their health (Taylor, 2007, p. 98) is nowhere more evident than in the emphasis on community participation in promoting health. The previous discussion of lay health work is a reflection of this focus, but community participation can also be seen to go further than this by involving communities in processes relating to the identification of health problems and action on these. Central to debates about community participation and health are issues of power and empowerment, and the concepts of community participation and empowerment have become central tenets of health promotion in the years since the 1978 Alma-Ata Declaration. They have also been reaffirmed in the recent Declaration of Astana, which links the Alma-Ata Declaration and the 2030 Agenda for Sustainable Development, by emphasizing: 'enabling and health-conducive environments in which individuals and communities are empowered and engaged in maintaining and enhancing their health and well-being' (WHO and UNICEF, 2018).

So what is meant by community participation in health? If people have a 'right and a duty to participate individually and collectively in the planning and implementation of their health care' (WHO, 1978) and if at the heart of health promotion is 'the empowerment of communities, and the ownership and control of their endeavours and destiny' (WHO, 1986a, b), what does this mean in practice? Public Health England and NHS England (2015) talk about community-centred approaches and South *et al.* (2019, p. 357) comment that 'community participation is a multi-dimensional and somewhat nebulous concept'. One way of addressing this has been to develop models of participation that reflect the degree of actual involvement and power of lay people. Perhaps the most used are those of Brager and Specht (1973, as cited by Tones and Tilford, 2001) and Arnstein (1969), who uses a ladder to demonstrate how participation may move from the lower rungs of manipulation, therapy and informing, to middle rungs of consulting and placating; only the top three rungs of partnership, delegated power and citizen control demonstrate citizen power. Hart (1992) later adapted this to develop a ladder applicable to assessing children's participation and all of this has been built on by the International Association of Public Participation in their spectrum of participation (IAP2, 2018) (Fig. 2.1). Similarly, Green *et al.* (2019) link degrees of participation to degrees of empowerment, suggesting that often what is called participation is really about involving communities in health promotion initiatives that come from professional agendas and are professionally led. In a similar vein, Rifkin *et al.* (2000) identified three different approaches to community participation and health; the medical approach, the health planning approach and the community development approach. In the medical approach, community participation is envisaged as communities responding to professional directives and taking action to improve their health. In the health planning approach, community participation is again professionally led, with the community participating in planning and delivering appropriate health care. In the final approach, that of community development, the focus goes beyond health services to the wider determinants of health and it is the community that identifies and acts on the conditions affecting their health. McKnight (1978) offers a classic account of such an approach in Chicago (Box 2.11).

Spectrum of Public Participation

Inform · Consult · Involve · Collaborate · Empower

Source: International Association for Public Participation

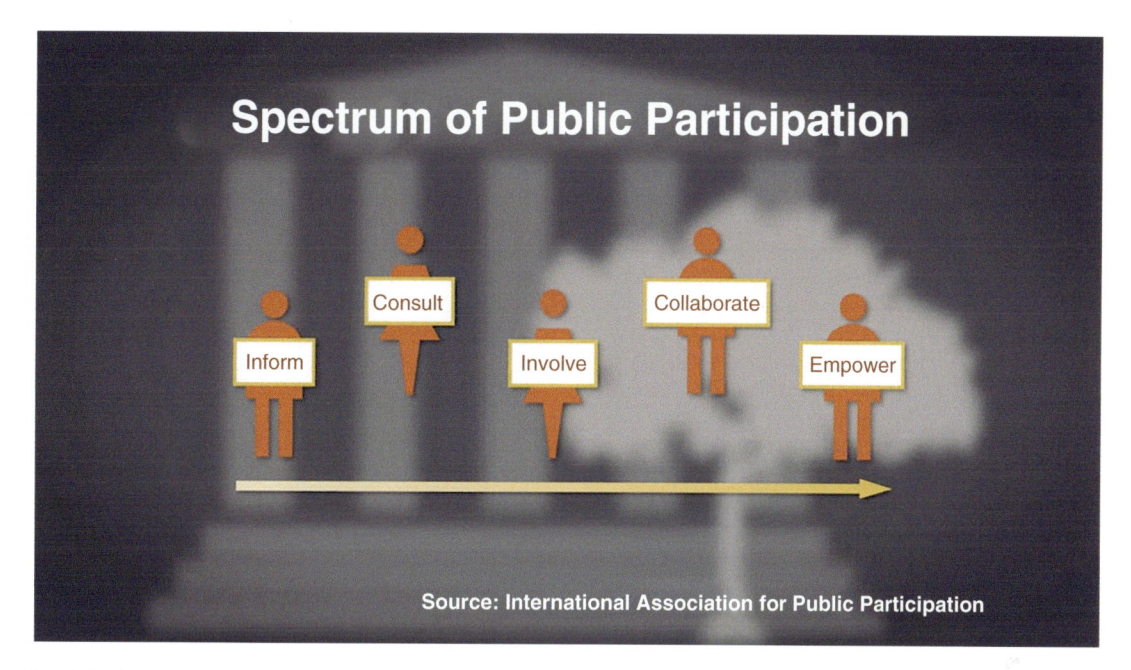

Fig. 2.1. Spectrum of Participation (CC BY-NC-SA 2.0).

The example, later in this chapter, of the community development approach to participation and health illustrates the centrality of empowerment to such participation, and the move from a model of clients to one of citizens who, rather than being controlled, are actually wielding power themselves. It also stresses the importance of associations rather than institutions in promoting health in communities, and this issue has been explored earlier in this chapter in relation to social capital. Finally, this approach is firmly rooted in a recognition of the social determinants of health that require action beyond the provision of health services, and again, as an approach to community participation, it is explored more in a later section.

However, it is clear that this more radical understanding of what is involved in community participation and health is not always reflected in programmes or policies. Whilst participatory approaches in health found favour in the 1970s, when the progressive agenda reflected the greater power of Third World countries and the socialist world (De Vos *et al.*, 2009), the 1980s ushered in a 'lost decade' of debt and structural adjustment programmes, and the health planning and medical approaches to community participation gained popularity, with an emphasis on the 'cultural sensitivity' and appropriateness of health services and initiatives, which could be achieved by involving the community in issues of design and delivery. Such programmes were also often about cost sharing or cost cutting, as illustrated by the Bamako initiative and community control and financing of health centres, making them essentially about 'rural development on the cheap' (Jewkes and Murcott, 1998). The World Bank's enthusiastic support of community participation is seen as further evidence of this association with cost reduction, and Rifkin (1996) describes such community participation programmes as being products of a 'target oriented framework', rather than an 'empowerment framework', i.e. community participation is seen as a means to improve service delivery, in what is a utilitarian model of community participation (Morgan, 2001), rather than as a form of mobilization that will lead to the 'increased ability of marginalized communities to control key processes that influence their lives' (De Vos *et al.*, 2009, p. 123). In the latter framework, community participation is both a means and an end, and it is inescapably political, involving a paradigm shift to a bottom-up rather than top-down approach to health promotion and placing power relations at the centre. Such an understanding of community participation and empowerment recognizes the potential for conflict with both professionals and their health agenda, as

Box 2.11. Community action in Chicago.

McKnight's example centres on a community of about 60,000 mainly poor and black people in Chicago. Their initial efforts were focused on 'recapturing' the two hospitals, which had originally serviced the community when it was a predominantly white community, and which were not accessible to the current residents of this poor, black community. Yet after gaining access to these hospitals and changing their policies, there was little evidence of improvements in health, so the community set about getting information about the nature of the problems for which people were being hospitalized. The seven most common (in order of frequency) were:

- automobile accidents;
- interpersonal attacks;
- accidents (non-auto);
- bronchial ailments;
- alcoholism;
- drug-related problems; and
- dog bites.

The community organization was struck by the fact that the problems were mainly social rather than medical ones, and they set about tackling the one they felt they could most successfully addressed, that of dog bites. Drawing on community resources, they set up a scheme to pay 'dog bounties' and over a short period of time, a number of stray dogs were caught, and the cases of dog bites decreased. The sense of achievement here led to the next action: dealing with car accidents. By mapping where the accidents had taken place, the community organization identified places where they could take action (e.g. the entrance to the parking area for a local store) and places where the community had less power (e.g. major highways for suburban commuters dissected their community). In the case of the latter, it became clear that communities affected by such through traffic would need to coordinate efforts to convince the city authorities to change policies.

The third issue to be addressed was that of 'bronchial problems' and one factor in these: good nutrition. To address the problem of affordable fruit and vegetables, a greenhouse was erected on the roof of an apartment building where fruit and vegetables could be grown. Not only did this provide a source of income, but an unexpected advantage of this greenhouse was that it conserved heat in the building; it also became a popular place with older people from a local retirement home, who came to help, and began to feel more useful in the community.

McKnight concludes that:

> Health action must lead away from dependence on professional tools and techniques, towards community building and citizen action. Effective health action must convert a professional-technical problem into a political, communal issue.

(McKnight, 1978, p. 39)

---

well as with those who have economic and other resources, and whose power may be challenged. Indeed South *et al.* (2018, p. 14) point out that 'community-centred approaches for health and wellbeing involve shifts in power, as the practice of public health becomes joint action routinely designed and delivered with, not done to, people'.

These conflicts are illustrated well in the account of participatory budgeting (PB) in the city of Porto Alegre in Brazil, by Guareschi and Jovchelovitch (2004). Improvements in indicators such as sanitation, housing, health and education in Porto Alegre have been linked to the implementation in the city of such PB, which allows democratically elected representatives of communities to carry forward their communities' views about allocation of public resources; in addition, most city departments have participatory councils where any citizen could discuss issues to do with city services. These processes were not imposed from above, but were the outcome of community participation, and have created a 'new public sphere' and 'a real redistribution of power in the city' (Guareschi and Jovchelovitch, 2004), which has mobilized primarily poor people in the struggle against health inequalities. Yet in the process of participation, difficulties have been encountered in terms of the political culture, the power structures of the city's budget definition, and the resistance of professionals, especially health professionals, to accepting community involvement in what were deemed to be specialist areas. In addition, differences within and between communities also became clear, and those who became very involved in the participatory processes were themselves criticized for becoming too close to those in power (issues about the degree to which community representatives can, or do, actually represent their communities have long been a theme in the literature about community participation, e.g. Jewkes and Murcott,

1998; Saguin, 2018). Overall, Guareschi and Jovechelovitch (2004) conclude that:

> Through participation individuals develop competencies for both themselves and their communities to achieve real gains in all areas deemed essential for health. As individuals become vocal and active, they emerge as conscious actors of their own culture.
>
> The capacity of communities for effective participation generates gains at the personal, community and political levels. It not only empowers individuals and the community, but also poses to the institutional structures of the state the need to incorporate and take into account the insights and demands coming from grassroots movement.
> (Guareschi and Jovechelovitch, 2004, p. 319).

Since the publication of their research, however, others have been more questioning of the success of PB. Rocha Franco and Teixeira Assis (2019) concluded that, whilst there was evidence of positive impacts of PB in terms of measures of wellbeing and infant and child mortality in the city they focused on, Belo Horizonte (also in Brazil), PB had not been as radically transformative as hoped; whilst it has had redistributive effects on public spending, there 'seems to be little transformation in the unequal sociospatial order on which PB was supposed to have a levelling effect' (p. 89).

This account of PB focuses attention on the outcomes of participation and, in the case of health, the shared assumptions that the 'involvement of communities enhances the delivery and uptake of health interventions to address inequalities' (Draper et al., 2010, pp. 1102–1103). There are many problems in evaluating community participation; as it is both a process and an outcome, involving different degrees of power in different contexts, capturing the complexity of community participation can be difficult in evaluation studies, and the same issues arise when looking at replicating and scaling up strategies. One attempt to capture this complexity can be seen in Rifkin, Muller and Bichmann (1988, as cited in Rifkin et al., 2000), where five factors that characterize community participation are identified: needs assessment, leadership, organization, resource mobilization and management. For each of these factors, there is an assessment of the degree of community participation, from narrow (almost exclusively professionally or externally controlled) to wide (community 'ownership'), and a diagram is constructed to represent this. In a more recent development of this approach, Draper et al. (2010) disaggregate five different components or indicators of community participation, with much more importance attached to community participation in evaluation, and to women's involvement generally (they link the latter to their focus on maternal and child health, but this might be seen as significant for many community health programmes). The five components are:

1. Who leads (community or professionals?).
2. Planning and management (to what extent is there a partnership between professionals and the community?).
3. Women's involvement (seen as critical for maternal and child health, the issue here being the degree of active participation by women).
4. Support for programme development in terms of finance and programme design (to what extent does the community mobilize and control resources?).
5. Monitoring and evaluation (to what extent is involved the community in this?).

Using the participation continuum to create process indicators for these five factors, they are then able to create a spidergram (Fig. 2.2), which maps participation for all five factors in a simple, yet powerful way and then links these to outcome measures such as health indicators, uptake of services and sustainability. However, Draper et al. (2010) note that whereas, from the case studies offered, there is significant evidence for the critical role of community participation, it is not possible to offer firm prescriptions about the nature of such participation, given the heterogeneity of communities and the impact of local contexts. Indeed, Rifkin (2009) suggests that trying to define terms such as 'community' and 'participation', and creating a standard model for community participation in health, is unrealistic; all will depend on the context, and especially the political context. In her 2014 update of this work, she explores this further, noting that too many evaluations focus on Randomized Controlled Trials (RCTs) and outcomes, which are situational and not generalizable. In looking at the kind of research that might be useful, she draws on the work of Pawson et al. (2005, p. 21) on realist reviews 'aimed at discerning what works for whom, in what circumstances, in what respects and how'. Rifkin thus proposes that more attention needs to be paid to 'examining community participation as a process and dealing with critical issues around empowerment, ownership, cost-effectiveness and sustainability of health improvements' (Rifkin, 2014, p. 103). Chuah et al. (2018) reach a similar

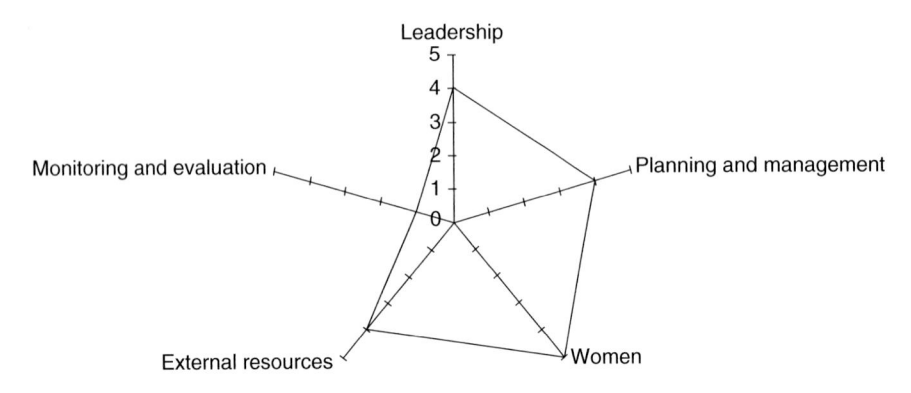

Fig. 2.2. Spidergram of participation (adapted from Rifkin *et al.*, 1988).

conclusion in their systematic review of community participation in general health initiatives in high and upper-middle income countries. Bagnall *et al.* (2018) review a range of community interventions to promote health and wellbeing and note that the better-quality evidence in the studies they looked at tended to be qualitative. Finally, South *et al.* (2019) and Orton *et al.* (2019) also address the issue of evaluation, and propose the application of complex systems thinking so that, as South *et al.* (2019, p. 11) put it: 'community context should not be seen as a static backdrop to an intervention, but as a dynamic feature of a wider system'.

Given that the success of community participation may be situational, attempts to replicate particular programmes on a massive scale may be futile. However, there is one oft-cited example of the replication and scaling up of a successful initiative – that of the Tostan approach in Senegal (Easton *et al.*, 2003) in Box 2.12.

The spread of the Tostan approach allows us to see the central role of participation in the bottom-up approach adopted, and to contrast this with the top-down legislative approach. Monkman *et al.* (2007) also suggest that there is a potential in the process of such programmes to move from *mediated empowerment*, which in this case relates to the key role of the non-governmental organizations (NGOs) involved, to a form of *socio-political empowerment*, with 'the transformation of the community from an object that is acted upon by outside forces, to a subject capable of acting upon and transforming its world' (Rocha, 1997, as cited by Monkman *et al.*, 2007, p. 461). Not only does such action no longer require the aid of intermediaries, but also its very nature suggests a degree of

empowerment, which Laverack (2004) places at the far end of the community empowerment continuum, and we will return to social action and social movements at the end of the chapter. Participation and empowerment are central concepts for health promoters working with communities and fundamental components, too, of community development approaches.

Strengthening Communities: Community Development and Assets-based Approaches

The previous section focused on issues in community participation, but this term is often interchangeable with terms such as 'community engagement' and 'community development'. Community development has a long history, which raises important issues that we will now explore as an approach to building healthy communities. The National Institute for Health and Clinical Excellence (NICE) in the UK defines it thus:

> Community development is about building active and sustainable communities based on social justice, mutual respect, participation, equality, learning and co-operation. It involves changing power structures to remove the barriers that prevent people from participating in the issues that affect their lives.
> (NICE, 2008, p. 38)

Just as in community participation, the principles and values underlying community development distinguish it from other community-based work. Key principles revolve around a belief in and respect for people and of what they are capable, asserting that people have skills as well as needs and have the right to participate in things that affect their lives.

> **Box 2.12. The Tostan approach.**
>
> Tostan is a rural village empowerment programme (VEP) that originated in Senegal. The word *tostan* means 'breakthrough' or 'coming out of the egg' in Wolof, and the programme, which started in the late 1980s, focused on non-formal education and literacy for rural women, although men were not excluded, and some did enrol. The orientation of the education programme was participatory, and the curriculum, which was problem focused, responded to women's expressed interests and needs.
>
> The initial education modules led to follow-up activities and there was demand for more continuing education, so that further modules were added. The most popular were those on human rights and women's health and soon men began to join the modules too, and men's health was included as an issue. It was after these two modules that one community resolved to address the issue of female genital cutting (FGC), a centuries-old practice that had both short- and long-term effects on the health of girls and women, but which was a requisite for marriage. In a very short time, the community publicly renounced the practice, and others showed interest, including a 'cutter', who had seen herself the consequences of FGC. However, the critical turning point came when a locally respected imam became involved. Whilst initially concerned about the threat to tradition, tales from his own female relatives changed his mind, and he supported the women. However, he pointed out that efforts to eradicate such an embedded practice might only divide communities where actually it needed to unite them as, unless all the intermarrying communities renounced the practice, those who had not experienced FGC would not be marriageable. The decision was made to speak to other communities avoiding explicit and condemnatory language – indeed to invite the communities themselves to go through some of the processes experienced by the initial community. The outcome of this process was that more villages joined the opposition to FGC, and the movement started to spread through Senegal.
>
> At this point, the President of Senegal became involved, and a law was introduced abolishing FGC and punishing violators, but this was counterproductive, leading to resistance and greater difficulties for those attempting to follow Tostan's approach and initiate changes from below. Indeed, key elements of the success of the approach were that it was collectively owned, grounded in the local context and empowering. However, requests for Tostan to develop initiatives in other areas and countries has tended to go along with a more goal-orientated approach to participation, which has led to selecting only elements of the original approach to achieve social change. For instance, where the original focus was on literacy and non-formal education, this was replaced with a more limited focus on health and human rights, reflecting the particular focus of the donors behind these new programmes, which was FGC. However, the authors report success in other countries, especially Sudan and Mali, and in the case of the latter, Monkman *et al.* (2007) write of the way in which the revised VEP retained key elements that have empowered the communities involved and its 'transformatory potential' for gender relations.
>
> In a recent update, Tostan (now the name of an international NGO with its headquarters in Dakar, Senegal) says that its programme since 1991 has sparked nearly 9000 communities across Africa to publicly abandon FGC, affecting an estimated >5.5 million people (https://medium.com/tostan-stories/naima-dido-human-rights-activist-fgc-d090dc4279a9).

Community development is founded on values of equity and social justice and the need to address inequalities in order to build a fairer world.

As we have seen throughout this chapter, the *process* of community development is very important, with empowerment at both individual and community levels being central. According to Green *et al.* (2019, p. 52) the three key features of an empowered community are: 'a sense of community – that is, a therapeutic feel of identification with fellow community members; an active commitment to achieve community goals; and what is increasingly termed 'social capital'. Laverack (2009) describes community empowerment as developing along a continuum from personal action, development of small mutual groups, community organization around key issues, partnership work with other organizations through to social and political action. Community development is a way in which community activists, health promoters, community development workers and others can work with people, either in a geographical/neighbourhood setting, or with a community of interest, to help them progress along this continuum.

The major theorist and activist whose work underpins community development was Paulo

Freire. His influence was mentioned in Chapter 1, and his educational ideas will be referred to in Chapter 4, but it is important to mention his work here, too, as it relates to working with communities. Central to Freire's approach is the concept of 'conscientization', which Ledwith (2005, p. 95) describes as 'the process of becoming critically aware of structural forces of power which shape people's lives as a precondition for critical action for change'. Freire developed his ideas through years of practice as an educator and an activist. He believed in 'praxis', which is the constant interaction of theory and practice. He was a passionate advocate for poor communities and believed that through a process of critical dialogue people become empowered and that this would in turn lead to them taking collective action to improve their lives. Freire's ideas have been criticized by Marxists for insufficient analysis by class, by feminists for his lack of attention to patriarchy and by those who considered him a dangerous revolutionary, but his ideas have prevailed and are still central to community development thinking and practice.

The case study in Box 2.13 illustrates how a primary school teacher who became a 'community organizer' took a Freirian approach to engaging with people in the community where he was based. This involved moving over a number of months from getting to know the community by doing a lot of listening and networking, through to helping them identify the things that most concerned them and work out what they wanted to do about them. Then, when the community felt sufficiently empowered, moving on to supporting collective action by community members to address the things they had prioritized. Box 2.14 outlines a community development and health improvement programme in the UK.

Whilst community development work may not be recognized as requiring great skills, in the view of Twelvetrees (2017) this form of practice is, in fact, highly skilled. Part of the skill set community development workers employ is in using many and varied methods to engage communities, as the example on the use of storytelling as a way of engaging very marginalized communities in Box 2.15 illustrates.

Community development is often linked to an assets-based approach to work in communities; this approach has gained currency in recent years and Assets Based Community Development (ABCD)

> is considered as one method among many which aims to mobilise and harness the skills, resources and talents of individuals and communities. The central thrust is that communities should drive the development process themselves though identifying and mobilising existing – often unrecognised – assets and, in the process, respond to and create local economic opportunities.
>
> (Roy, 2017, p. 456) (see Fig. 2.3).

Overall, we can see that community development can be an effective way of engaging communities and ultimately of improving health and reducing inequalities; in England, for example, government policy increasingly supports community engagement to promote health (Brunton *et al.*, 2017; South *et al.*, 2018) and this support seems to be growing worldwide. However, the concern is that such initiatives, in stressing what people and

---

Box 2.13. Using a community development approach in practice.

This case study centres on the story of a primary school teacher who became a community organizer. His training taught him how to listen and really hear what people are saying and feeling. He worked on a farm but spent as much time as possible getting closely involved in the life of the community. He listened for 'generative themes', topics that people have strong feelings about. He gained the confidence of a number of village people and was soon invited to a number of meetings of women's groups, church meetings, etc. He prepared 'codes' on the generative themes and presented these in picture form or through story and drama. He engaged the people in dialogue about the possibilities of change. One theme considered particularly important was the lack of money to buy vegetables from wealthy landowners. As a result, the group pooled their savings and rented land on which they grew their own vegetables. The best product of the garden, however, was the discovery that they could work together to solve a problem.

(Tones and Tilford, 2001, p. 402)

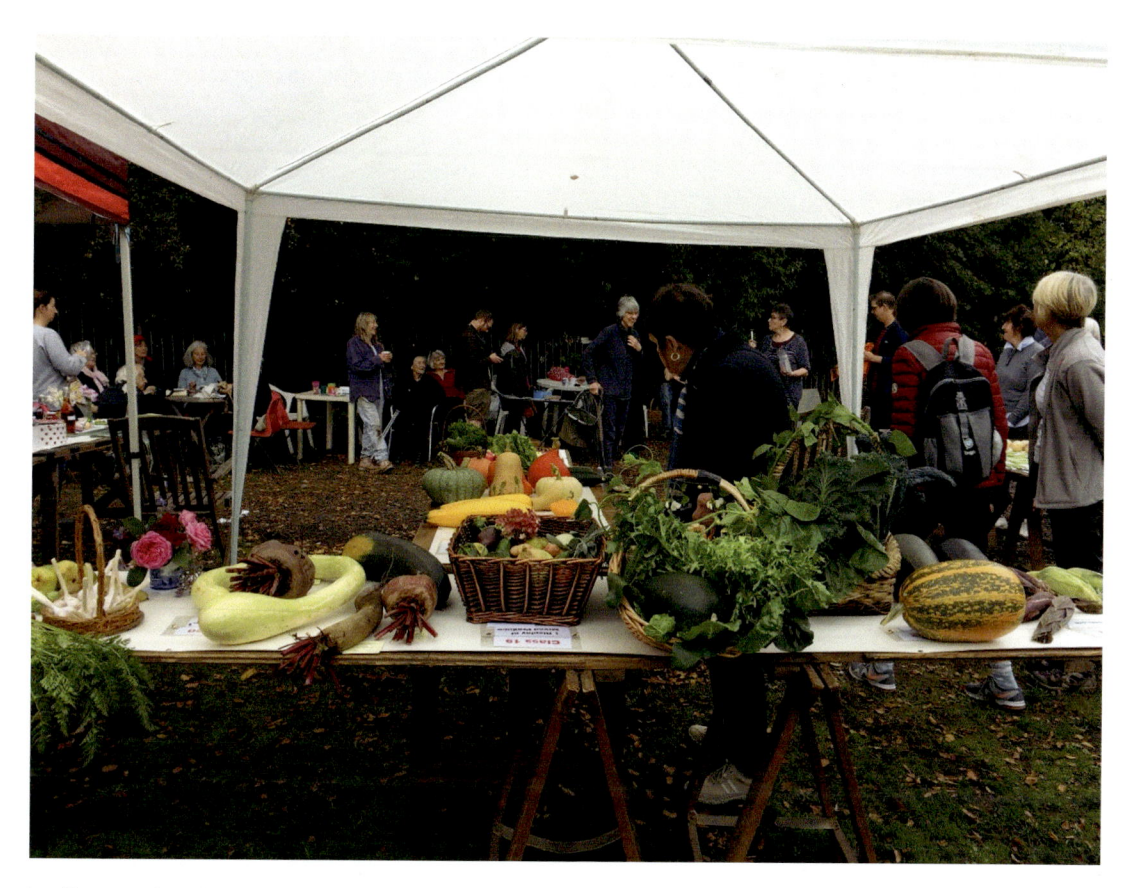

An allotment show in Leeds, England.

> **Box 2.14. Community development route to health improvement in Aylesbury, UK.**
>
> The aims of this Community Development and Health Improvement programme include:
>
> - to co-produce a range of health improvement projects based upon preventative and early health interventions that aim to enable individuals and communities to take responsibility for their own health;
> - to work in collaboration with the local statutory and voluntary sectors to enable and enhance community ownership, capacity, resilience and cohesion by building the confidence and skills of local people.
>
> The programme operates from a Healthy Living Centre and offers a range of different community and health improvement programmes, a nursery, community café and the hire of a community centre, managed on behalf of the local housing trust. The delivery methodology of all these programmes is community engagement, recognition of community resources and joint problem solving.
>
> (PHE, 2018)

Box 2.15. Storytelling, an example of an effective tool for community development.

Katrice Horsley uses storytelling to work with many and varied groups of people from Bangladeshi women to young male offenders in the UK. She has also worked in Ghana. Through recounting both traditional and current stories, people can explore a range of feelings within a safe space through drawing parallels between the situation within the story and their experience. Sometimes telling stories can be part of another activity such as sewing and collage making and the narratives can be woven into the textile being made. This helps to build confidence and connections between people. Storytelling can also be a non-threatening way to challenge discrimination and prejudice, and to develop self and political awareness.

> Every culture has a story to tell but few people have the confidence or platform to share them. Storytelling projects can promote the telling and sharing of both personal and traditional stories challenging negative stereotypes and assumptions in a positive and non-threatening way. Every culture has a history of storytelling and this shared link makes storytelling powerful as a tool in exploring conflict and diversity.

(Horsley, 2007, p. 4)

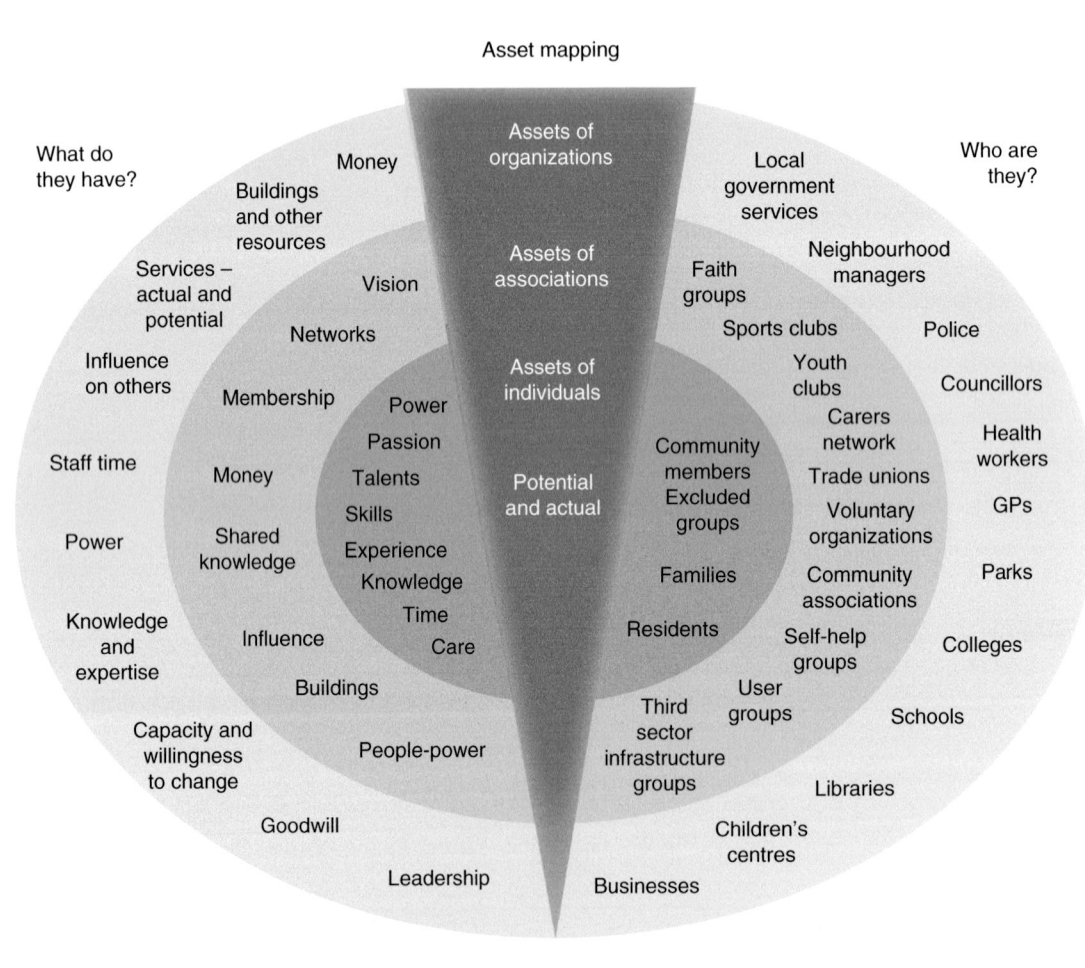

Fig. 2.3. Partnership with individuals and communities – an asset-based approach (from A glass half-full: how an asset approach can improve community health and well-being. ©IDeA 2010).

communities can do for themselves at a micro-level, may neglect the wider macro-level social determinants of their health (Roy, 2017; Blickem *et al.*, 2018). They may encourage individualization and marketization, so essentially becoming a tool of neoliberalism (Roy, 2017), and reflecting the interests of big business and the financial sector, i.e. the rich and powerful, rather than the interests of the poor and marginalized. Community development, which leads to those with least power trying to assert some control over their lives, is unsurprisingly not favoured by those with a vested interest in the system as it is. Hence, community development has had a somewhat chequered history across the world, with practice often falling out of favour with funders and those in power, when people become empowered and question the status quo. It does not fit comfortably as an approach with a focus on achieving narrow targets around disease reduction and behaviour change, which originate with managers, funders and politicians, not with communities, and so may remain a marginal activity in many countries. If it *is* adopted as an approach, we have seen that this may be partly for utilitarian reasons; for instance, in the UK, this is suggested when South *et al.* (2015, p. 9) point out that the NHS Five Year Forward View makes clear that 'harnessing the renewable energy of patients and communities is no longer a 'discretionary extra' but instead is key to the sustainability of health and care services'. The challenge facing activists who believe in equity and social justice is to reclaim ideas like 'community engagement', 'community development' and 'community empowerment', and emphasize a social justice perspective (Wilson and Mavhandu-Mudzusi, 2019) to challenge hollow rhetoric and the imposition of 'top-down' approaches that have to grow 'bottom-up' if they are to be true to their real meaning and serve the interests of disadvantaged people.

Health Activism

The focus of health promotion is on building healthy, resilient and connected communities (Mapplethorpe, 2020). The concept of 'resilience' is increasingly seen in the literature about public health (Ziglio *et al.*, 2017) but, in their work, DeVerteuil and Golubchikov (2016, p. 148) stress that 'resilience' relates to processes that 'can stimulate social activism, social movements and networks that are essential seeds of transformations'. Indeed, Laverack (2004) sees social and political action as the end of the continuum of community empowerment, and much of this chapter has touched on ways in which community participation may involve such action; Zoller (2005) coins the term *health activism* to imply 'at some level, a challenge to the existing order and power relationships that are perceived to influence some aspects of health negatively, or to impede health promotion' (Zoller, 2005, p. 344). Defined thus, health activism not only encompasses community development models of community participation, but it might also be seen as an example of a social movement, an attempt to build a new social order. An example of this widened focus is seen in the work of Campbell (2019) in writing about social capital and health promotion in marginalized settings. She argues that a focus on community level mobilization to build bonding and bridging social capital needs integrating with attention to 'social movements fighting to create macro-social contexts that enable and support individual-level behaviour change' (Campbell, 2019). In a similar vein, Wallerstein *et al.* (2011, p. 234) caution against a focus on social capital and social mobilization that 'might by default manipulate participation toward joining the status quo, versus social movements that embrace important moments of conflict to challenge socioeconomic systems that replicate inequities'.

Social movements that focus on health offer 'collective challenges to medical policy and politics, belief systems, research and practice that include an array of formal and informal organizations, supporters, networks of co-operation and media' (Brown *et al.*, 2004, p. 52), although we might wish to expand that definition to include health policy more broadly. Various typologies of health social movements (HSMs) have been offered, distinguishing them in terms of their focus; in health promotion, there has been interest in constituency-based HSMs such as the women's health movement, or grass-roots-based organizations and community development projects addressing local health problems. However, formal alliances such as IBFAN (International Baby Food Action Network), which lobbies and advocates to promote breastfeeding, is an example of another type of HSM, as are groups demanding access to, for example, antiretroviral therapy (ART). Indeed, Zoller (2005) points out that, with a broader conceptualization of health, health activism may go beyond HSMs; examples might be the protests of the Occupy Movement

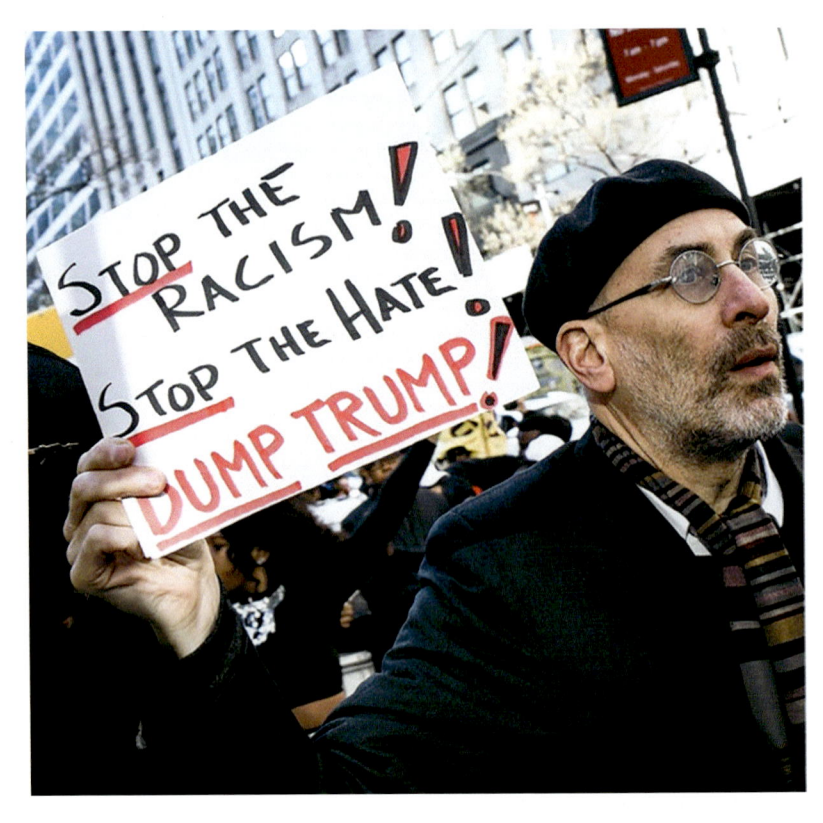

Community activism and protest against racism ('New York Protest' © KarlaAnnCoté).

against social and economic inequality, or the growing climate movement. What is key here, however, is that all such movements, and health activism, are evidence of the contribution that people make and their participation in forms of action that address health issues.

Summary

The central focus of this chapter has been on the engagement and empowerment of people and communities in promoting health. A useful way of illustrating community-centred approaches can be seen in Fig. 2.4. It offers UK examples of approaches to strengthening communities, from community development to building social capital, and it illustrates various ways of involving people as volunteers and lay health workers. Finally, there are examples of how libraries and social prescribing can be used as ways of accessing community resources, and also of how the Healthy Cities initiative and participatory budgeting can build collaborations and partnerships.

The role of communities in global health promotion has been stressed from Alma-Ata in 1978 to Astana in 2018. This is being written in 2020, in the midst of the Covid-19 pandemic, and writing about another epidemic, that of HIV, Valdiserri and Holtgrave (2019, p. 2902) contend that 'without the active involvement of communities affected by HIV, it will not be possible to end the virus' epidemic spread in the US'. Surely the same must be true of the coronavirus pandemic, with both Marston *et al.* (2020) and Yardley *et al.* (2020) talking of the need to involve communities in managing the Covid-19 pandemic, and Mackworth-Young *et al.* (2020) also stressing the importance of engaging with community perspectives in designing locally effective interventions for Covid-19 in Zimbabwe.

Throughout this chapter we have agreed with Taylor (2007), who pointed out that health promotion that is imposed on people is rarely effective, and needs to be done not *to* people, but *with* and *by* them. However, such participatory approaches raise important issues for the practice of health promotion. Some of these issues relate to professional practice, models of working

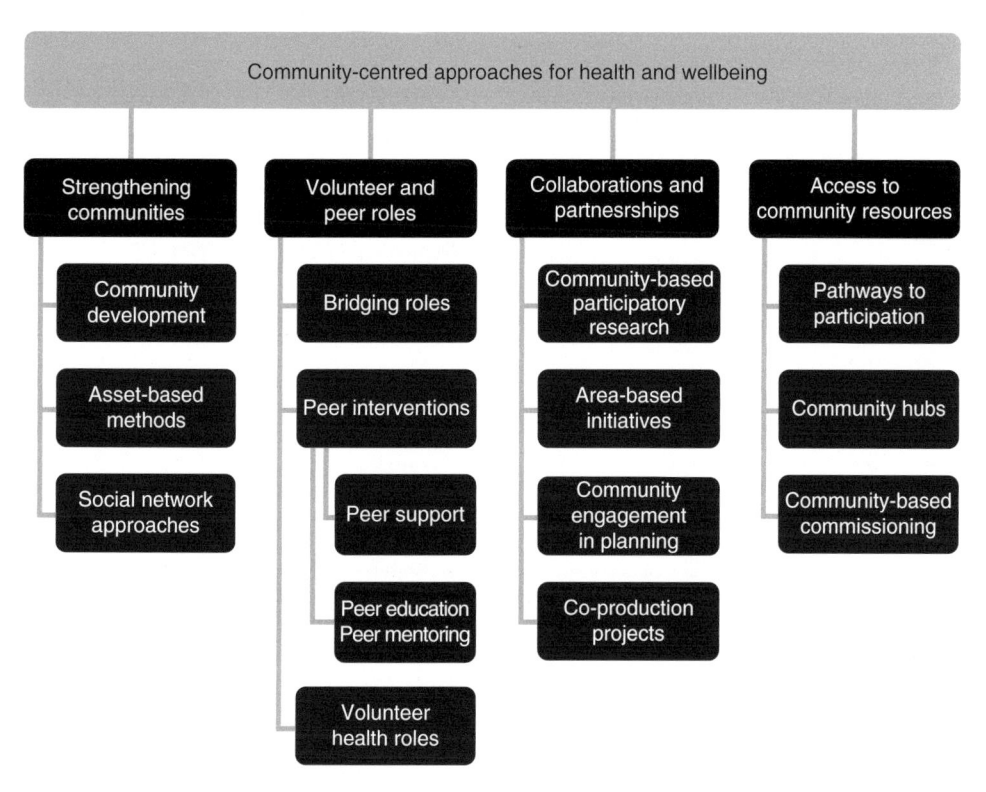

Fig 2.4. The family of community-centred approaches with examples of common UK models (PHE and NHS England, 2015).

and the skills required, and these are explored further in Chapter 5. However, perhaps more importantly, such approaches raise issues of power and control. As we have seen in this chapter, both agency and structure need to be taken into account in health promotion (Roy, 2017). So if the causes of health problems are to also to be found at the level of macro-social and economic policies, then we need to move beyond the community to look at such wider policies, the question of power, and their relevance for health (De Vos *et al.*, 2009). The next chapter will therefore explore Health in All Policies (HiAP) and the policy process, with a focus on the importance of these for health promotion; however, in recognizing the role of people as health activists and stakeholders in relation to the policies that affect health, the question of participation and empowerment will remain a key issue.

Note

[1] The previous version of this chapter entitled 'Healthy Communities' was written by Louise Warwick-Booth, Sally Foster and Judy White.

Further Reading

Cook, I.G., Halsall, J.P. and Wankhade, P. (2016) *Sociability, Social Capital, and Community Development. A Public Health Perspective.* Springer, New York.

Laverack, G. (2019) *Public Health: Power, Empowerment and Professional Practice.* 4th edn. Red Globe Press, London.

Ledwith, M. (2016) *Community Development in Action: Putting Freire into Practice.* The Policy Press, Bristol, UK.

Ledwith, M. and Springett, J. (2009) *Participatory Practice: Community Based Action for Transformative Change.* The Policy Press, Bristol, UK.

South, J., White, J. and Gamsu, M. (2012) *People Centred Public Health.* The Policy Press, Bristol, UK.

References

Antonovksy, A. (1996) The salutogenic model as a theory to guide health promotion. *Health Promotion International* 11, 11–18.

Arnstein, S. (1969) A ladder of citizen participation. *Journal of the American Institute of Planners* 35, 216–224.

Atkinson, R. and Kintrea, K. (2004) Opportunities and despair, it's all there: practitioner experiences and explanations of area effects and life chances. *Sociology* 38, 437–455.

Atkinson, S., Bagnall, A.M.B., Corocan, R., South, J. and Curtis, S. (2020) Being well together: individual subjective and community wellbeing. *Journal of Happiness Studies* 21, 1903–1921.

Attree, P., Clayton, S., Karunanithi, S., Nayak, S., Popay, J. and Read, D. (2012) NHS health trainers: a review of emerging evaluation evidence. *Critical Public Health* 22 (1), 25–38.

Aubel, J., Touré, I. and Diagne, M. (2004) Senegalese grandmothers promote improved maternal and child nutrition practices: the guardians of tradition are not averse to change. *Social Science and Medicine* 59, 945–959.

Bagnall, A.M., South, J., Di Martino, S., Southby, K., Pilkington, Mitchell, B., Pennington, A. and Corcoran, R. (2018) Places, spaces, people and wellbeing: full review. A systematic review of interventions to boost social relations through improvements in community infrastructure (places and spaces). What Works Wellbeing. Available at: https://whatworkswellbeing.org/wp-content/uploads/2020/01/Places-spaces-people-wellbeing-full-report-MAY2018-1_0119755600.pdf (accessed 11 August 2020).

Baim-Lance, A., Tietz, D., Lever, H., Swart, M. and Agins, B. (2019) Everyday and unavoidable coproduction: exploring patient participation in the delivery of healthcare services. *Sociology of Health & Illness* 41 (1), 128–142.

Baum, F. (1999) The role of social capital in health promotion: Australian perspectives. *Health Promotion Journal of Australia* 9, 171–178.

Baum, F. (2007) Cracking the nut of health equity: top down and bottom up pressure for action on the social determinants of health. *Promotion & Education* 14, 90–95.

Berman, Y. and Phillips, D. (2003) Indicators for social cohesion. Paper submitted to the European Network on Indicators of Social Quality of the European Foundation on Social Quality, Amsterdam.

Blickem, C., Dawson, S., Kirk, S., Vassilev, I., Mathieson, A., Harrison, R., Bower, P. and Lamb, J. (2018) What is asset-based community development and how might it improve the health of people with long-term conditions? A realist synthesis. *SAGE Open* 8 (3), 1–13.

Bourdieu, P. (1986) The forms of capital. In: Richardson, J. (ed.) *Handbook of Theory and Research for the Sociology of Education*. Greenwood Press, New York, pp. 241–258.

Bourdieu, P. (1999) *The Weight of the World: Social Suffering in Contemporary Society*. Cambridge University Press, Cambridge, UK.

Britten, N. and Maguire, K. (2016) Lay knowledge, social movements and the use of medicines: personal reflections. *Health* 20(2), 77–93.

Brown, P., Zavestoski, S., McCormick, S., Mayer, B., Morello-Frosch, R. and Altman, R.G. (2004) Embodied health movements: new approaches to social movements in health. *Sociology of Health and Illness* 26, 50–80.

Bruhn, J.G. and Wolf, S. (1979) *The Roseto Story: An Anatomy of Health*. University of Oklahoma Press, Norman, Oklahoma.

Brunton, G., Thomas, J., O'Mara-Eves, A., Jamal, F., Oliver, S. and Kavanagh, J. (2017) Narratives of community engagement: a systematic review-derived conceptual framework for public health interventions *BMC Public Health* 17, 944. https://doi.org/10.1186/s12889-017-4958-4

Buck, D. and Wensell, L. (2018) Communities and health. The Kings Fund. Available at: https://www.kingsfund.org.uk/publications/communities-and-health (accessed 28 April 2020).

Cacioppo, J. and Patrick, W. (2008) *Loneliness: Human Nature and the Need for Social Connection*. WW Norton and Co., London.

Campbell, C. (2001) Social capital and health: contextualizing health promotion withi local community networks. In Baron, S., Field, J. and Schuller, T. (eds) *Social Capital: Critical Perspectives*. Oxford University Press, Oxford, UK, pp. 182–196.

Campbell, C. (2011) Embracing complexity: towards more nuanced understandings of social capital and health. *Global Health Action* 4, 1–3.

Campbell, C. (2019) Social capital, social movements and global public health: fighting for health-enabling contexts in marginalised settings. *Social Science and Medicine* 112–153.

Canadian Health Services Research Foundation (2007) Incorporate lay health workers to promote health and prevent disease. Evidence boost for quality. September 2007, Ontario, Canadian Health Services Research Foundation. Available at: http://www.chsrf.ca/publicationsandresources/pastseries/evidenceboost/07-09-01/b672cd4e564a-4f10-8f96-679c1109eb41.aspx.

Chibanda, D. (2017) Reducing the treatment gap for mental, neurological and substance use disorders in Africa: lessons from the Friendship Bench in Zimbabwe. *Epidemiology and Psychiatric Sciences* 26, 342–347.

Christakis, N.A. and Fowler, J.H. (2007) The spread of obesity in a large social network over 32 years. *New England Journal of Medicine* 357, 370–379.

Christakis, N.A. and Fowler, J.H. (2008) The collective dynamics of smoking in a large social network. *New England Journal of Medicine* 358, 2249–2258.

Chuah, F.L.H., Srivastava, A., Singh, S.R., Haldane, V., Koh, G.C.H., Seng, C.K.. McCoy, D. and Legido-Quigley, H. (2018) Community participation in general health initiatives in high and upper middle income countries: a systematic review exploring the nature of participation, use of theories, contextual drivers and power relations in community participation. *Social Science & Medicine* 213, 106–122.

Cinderby, S., Haq, G., Cambridge, H. and Lock, K. (2014) *Practical Action to Build Community Resilience. The Good Life Initiative in New Earswick.* Joseph Rowntree Foundation, York, UK.

Coleman, J.S. (1990) *Foundations of Social Theory*. The Belknap Press of Harvard University Press, Cambridge, Massachusetts.

Coleman, J.S. (1998) Social capital in the creation of human capital. *American Journal of Sociology* 94, 95–120.

Cook, T. and Wills, J. (2011) Engaging with marginalised communities: the experience of London health trainers. *Perspectives in Public Health* 132, 221–227.

Cooper, R.J., Bissell, P., Warde, P., Murphy, E., Anderson, C., Avery, T., James, V., Lymn, J., Guillaume, L., Hutchinson, A. and Ratcliffe, J. (2011) Further challenges to medical dominance? The case of nurse and pharmacist supplementary prescribing. *Health* 20, 1–19.

Davies, R. (2002) Monitoring and evaluation NGO achievements. In: Desai, V. and Potter, R.B. (eds) *The Companion to Development Studies*. Arnold, London.

Deiner, E. and Chan, M.Y. (2011) Happy people live longer: subjective wellbeing contributes to health and longevity. *Applied Psychology: Health and Well-Being* 3, pp. 1–43, doi:10.1111/j.1758 0854.2010.01045.x.

De Leeuw, E. (2000) Commentary – beyond community action: communication arrangements and policy networks. In: Poland, B., Green, L.W. and Rootman, I. (eds) *Settings for Health Promotion*. Sage, Thousand Oaks, California.

DeVerteuil, G. and Golubchikov, O. (2016) Can resilience be redeemed? *City* 20 (1), 143–151.

De Vos, P., Malaise, G., De Ceukelaire, W., Perez, D., Lefevre, P. and Van der Stuyft, P. (2009) Participation and empowerment in primary health care: from Alma Ata to the era of globalization. *Social Medicine* 4, 121–127.

DOH (2001) *The Expert Patient: A New Approach to Chronic Disease Management for the 21st Century*. DOH, London.

DOH (2004) *Choosing Health: Making Healthier Choices Easier*. The Stationery Office, London.

Draper, A., Hewitt, G. and Rifkin, S. (2010) Chasing the dragon: developing indicators for the assessment of community participation in health programmes. *Social Science and Medicine* 71, 1102–1109.

Easton, P., Monkman, K. and Miles, R. (2003) Social policy from the bottom up: abandoning FGC in sub-Saharan Africa. *Development in Practice* 13, 445–458.

Egolf, B., Lasker, J., Wolf, S. and Potvin, L. (1992) The Roseto effect: a 50-year comparison of mortality rates. *American Journal of Public Health* 82, 1089–1092.

El Ansari, W., Phillips, C.J. and Zwi, A.B. (2002) Narrowing the gap between academic professional wisdom and community lay knowledge: partnerships in South Africa. *Public Health* 116, 151–159.

Eshan, A., Klaasa, H.S., Bastianena, A. and Spinia, D. (2019) *Social capital and health: a systematic review of systematic reviews SSM – Population Health* 8, 100425.

Everingham, C. (2003) *Social Justice and the Politics of the Community*. Ashgate, Aldershot, UK.

Farquhar, S.A., Wiggins, N., Michael, Y.L., Luhr, G., Jordan, J. and Lopez, A. (2008) 'Sitting in different chairs': roles of the community health workers in the Poder es Salud/Power for Health Project. *Education for Health* 21, 39.

Flora, J.L. (1998) Social capital and communities of place. *Rural Sociology* 63, 481–506.

Fowler, J.H. and Christakis, N.A. (2008) Dynamic spread of happiness in a large social network: longitudinal analysis over 20 years in the Framingham heart study. *British Medical Journal* 337, 1–9.

Fukuyama, F. (1999) *Social Capital and Civil Society*. Conference paper prepared for the IMF Conference on Second Generation Reforms.

Fukuyama, F. (2001) Social capital, civil society and development. *Third World Quarterly* 22, 7–20.

Gale, N.K., Kenyon, S., MacArthur, C., Jolly, K. and Hope, L. (2018) Synthetic social support: theorizing lay health worker interventions. *Social Science & Medicine* 196, 96–105.

Gibson, A. (2006) *Health and community: is the concept of social capital helpful?* PhD thesis, Faculty of Health and Social Care, Open University, Milton Keynes, UK.

Gibson, A. (2010) Does social capital have a role to play in the health of communities? In: Douglas, J., Earle, S., Handsley, S., Jones, L., Lloyd, C.E. and Spurr, S. (eds) *A Reader in Promoting Public Health. Challenge and Controversy*, 2nd edn. Sage, London.

Giordano, G.M. and Lindstrom, N. (2010) The impact of social capital on changes in smoking behaviour: a longitudinal cohort study. *European Journal of Public Health* 21, 347–354.

Glenton, C., Colvin, C.J., Carlsen, B., Swartz, A., Lewin, S., Noyes, J. and Rashidian, A. (2013) Barriers and facilitators to the implementation of lay health worker programmes to improve access to maternal and child health: qualitative evidence synthesis (Review). *Cochrane Database Syst Rev.*10: CD010414.

Green, G., Grimsley, M., Syolcas, A., Prescott, M., Jowitt, T. and Linacre, R. (2000) *Social Capital, Health and Economy in South Yorkshire Coalfield Communities*. Centre for Regional Economic and Social Research, Sheffield Hallam University, Sheffield, UK.

Green, J. and Tones, K. (2010) *Health Promotion: Planning and Strategies*, 2nd edn. Sage, London.

Green, J., Cross, R., Woodall, J. and Tones, K., (2019) *Health Promotion: Planning and Strategies*. 4th edn. Sage, London, UK.

Greetham J (2011) Growing Communities from the Inside Out: Piloting an asset based approach to JSNAs within the Wakefield district: Methods and findings [online]. Available at: http://www.asset-basedconsulting.net/uploads/publications/Growing%20Communities%20from%20the%20Inside%20Out.pdf (accessed 28 April 2020).

Groves, R., Middleton, A., Murie, A. and Broughton, K. (2003) *Neighbourhoods that Work. A Study of the Bournville Estate, Birmingham*. The Policy Press, Bristol, UK.

Guareschi, P. and Jovchelovitch, S. (2004) Participation, health and the development of community resources in southern Brazil. *Journal of Health Psychology* 9, 311–322.

Halpern, D. (2005) *Social Capital*. Polity Press, Cambridge, UK.

Hanibuchi, T., Murata, Y., Ichida, Y., Hirai, H., and Kondo, K. (2012) Place-specific constructs of social capital and their possible associations to health: a Japanese case study. *Social Science and Medicine* 75, 1, 225–232.

Harper, R. (2001) *The Measurement of Social Capital in the United Kingdom*. Office for National Statistics, London.

Hart, R. (1992) *Children's Participation from Tokenism to Citizenship*. UNICEF.

Hibbitt, K., Jones, P. and Meegan, R. (2001) Tackling social exclusion: the role of social capital in urban regeneration on Merseyside – from mistrust to trust. *European Planning Studies* 9, 141–161.

Holst Algren, M., Ekholma, O., Nielsena, L., Kjær Ersbølla, A., Kronborg Bak, C., Tanggaard Andersen, P. (2020) Social isolation, loneliness, socioeconomic status, and health-risk behaviour in deprived neighbourhoods in Denmark: a cross-sectional study *SSM. Population Health* 10, 100546.

Holt-Lunstad. J., Smith, T.B, and Layton, J.B (2010) Social relationships and mortality risk: a meta-analytic review. *PLoS Medicine*, 7, 7, e1000316, doi:10.1371/journal. pmed.1000316.

Horsley, K. (2007) Storytelling, conflict and diversity. *Community Development Journal* 10, 109.

IAP2 (2018) *Spectrum of Public Participation*. International Association for Public Participation. Available at: https://cdn.ymaws.com/www.iap2.org/resource/resmgr/pillars/Spectrum_8.5x1_Print.pdf

Illich, I. (1976) *Limits to Medicine*. Marion Boyars, London.

Jewkes, R. and Murcott, A. (1998) Community representatives: representing the 'community'? *Social Science and Medicine* 46, 843–858.

Jochum, V. (2003) *Social Capital: Beyond the Theory*. NCVO Publications, London.

Kamphuis, C. M., Groeniger, J.O., Poelman, M.P., Beenackers, M.A and van Lenthe, F.J. (2019) How does bridging social capital relate to health-behavior, overweight and obesity among low and high educated groups? A cross-sectional analysis of GLOBE-2014. *BMC Public Health* 19, 1635.

Kane, S., Kok, M., Ormel, H., Otiso, L., Sidat, M., Namakhoma, I., Nasir, S., Gemechu, D., Rashid, S., Taegtmeyer, M., Theobald, S. and de Koning, K. (2016) Limits and opportunities to community health worker empowerment: a multi-country comparative study. *Social Science & Medicine* 164, 27–34.

Kawachi, I. (2010) The relationship between health assets, social capital and cohesive communities. In: Morgan, A.,. Davies, M. and Ziglio, E. (eds) *Health Assets in a Global Context*. Springer, New York, pp. 167–179.

Kawachi, I. and Berkman, L. (2001) Social ties and mental health. *Journal of Urban Health Bulletin of the New York Academy of Medicine* 78, 458–467.

Kawachi, I., Kennedy, B.P., Lochener, K. and Prothrow-Stith, D. (1997) Social capital, income inequality and mortality. *American Journal of Public Health* 87, 1491–1498.

Keleher, H. (2004) Why build a health promotion evidence base about gender? *Health Promotion International* 19, 3. doi: 10.1093/heapro/dah313.

Kelleher, D., Gabe, J. and Williams, G. (2006) *Challenging Medicine*. 2nd edn. Routledge, London.

Kim, C., Nakanishi, H., Blackman, D., Freyens, B. and Benson, A.M. (2017) The effect of social capital on community co-production: towards community-oriented development in post-disaster recovery. *Procedia Engineering* 180, 901–911.

Kinder, G., Cashman, S.B., Siefer, S.D., Inouye, A. and Hagopian, A. (2000) Integrating healthy communities concepts into health professions training. *Public Health Reports* 115, 266–270.

Kingsley, J., Foenandera, E. and Bailey, A. (2020) "It's about community": exploring social capital in community gardens across Melbourne, Australia *Urban Forestry and Urban Greening* 49, 126640.

Kinsella, K., White, J. and South, J. (2011) *East Riding Health Trainer Service: An Evaluation Report*. Bridlington, UK.

Kleinman, A. (1980) *Patients and Healers in the Context of Culture*. University of California Press, London.

Kymlicka, W. (1995a) *Multicultural Citizenship*. Clarendon Press, Oxford, UK.

Kymlicka, W. (ed.) (1995b) *The Rights of Minority Cultures*. Open University Press, Oxford, UK.

Laverack, G. (2004) *Health Promotion Practice: Power and Empowerment*. Sage, London.

Laverack G. (2009) *Public Health, Power, Empowerment and Professional Practice*, 2nd edn. Palgrave Macmillan, Basingstoke, UK.

Laverack, G. and Wallerstein, N. (2001) Measuring community empowerment: a fresh look at organizational domains. *Health Promotion International* 16, 179–185.

Ledwith, M. (2005) *Community Development: A Critical Approach*. The Policy Press, Bristol, UK.

Lehman, U. and Sanders, D. (2007) *Community Health Workers: What do we know about them? The State of the Evidence on Programmes Activities, Costs and Impact on Health Outcomes of using Community Health Workers*. Department of Human Resources for Health, Evidence and Information for Policy. WHO, Geneva.

Leonard, M. (2004) Bonding and bridging social capital: reflections from Belfast. *Sociology* 38, 927–944.

Lindstrom, M., Hanson, B.S., Ostergren, P.O. and Berglund, G. (2000) Socio-economic differences in smoking cessation: the role of social participation. *Scandinavian Journal of Public Health* 28, 200–208.

Maass R.B., Christian, K.A., Bengt Lindstrømd, M. and Lillefjella, B. (2016) The impact of neighborhood social capital on life satisfaction and self-rated health: a possible pathway for health promotion? *Health and Place* 42, 120–128.

Mackworth-Young C.R.S, Chingono R., Mavodza C., McHugh G., Tembo M., Dziva Chikwari. C. et al. (2020) 'Here, we cannot practice what is preached': early qualitative learning from community perspectives on Zimbabwe's response to COVID-19 [submitted]. *Bull World Health Organ*. E-pub: 20 April 2020, doi: http://dx.doi.org/10.2471/BLT.20.260224

Mapplethorpe, T. (2020) Can we build healthier, more resilient and connected communities? Available at: https://publichealthmatters.blog.gov.uk/2020/01/14/can-we-build-healthier-more-resilient-and-connected-communities/ (accessed 18 May 2020).

Marmot, M. (2015) *The Health Gap: The Challenge of an Unequal World*. Bloomsbury, London.

Marmot, M. and Wilkinson, R.G. (2001) Psychosocial and material pathways in the relation between income and health: a response to Lynch et al. *British Medical Journal* 322, 1233–1236.

Marston, C., Renedo, A. and Miles, S. (2020) Community participation is crucial in a pandemic. Comment. *The Lancet* 395 (10238), 1676–1678.

Mayo, M. (1994) *Communities and Caring: The Mixed Economy of Welfare*. Macmillan, Basingstoke, UK.

McKnight, J.L. (1978) Politicizing health care. *Social Policy* 9, 36–39.

McKnight, J.L. (2003) Regenerating community: the recovery of a space for citizens. The IPR Distinguished Public Policy Research Lecture Series, Institute for Policy Research, Northwestern University. Available at: www.abcdinstitute.org/docs/abcd/regenerating.pdf (accessed 3 November 2012).

Mittlemark, M.B. (1999) Social ties and health promotion: suggestions for population based research. *Health Education Research* 14, 447–451.

Mock, J., McPhee, S.J., Nguyen, T., Wong, C., Doan, H., Lai, K.Q., Nguyen, K.H., Nguyen, T.T. and Bui-Tong, N. (2007) Effective lay health worker outreach and media-based education for promoting cervical cancer screening among Vietnamese American women. *American Journal of Public Health* 97, 1693–1700.

Monkman, K., Miles, R. and Easton, P. (2007) The transformatory potential of a village empowerment program: the Tostan Replication in Mali. *Women's Studies International Forum* 30, 451–464.

Morgan, A. and Ziglio, E. (2007) Revitalising the evidence base for public health: an assets model. *IUHPE –Promotion and Education Supplement* 2, 16–22.

Morgan, L.M. (2001) Community participation in health: perpetual allure, persistent challenge. *Health Policy and Planning* 16, 221–230.

Muntaner, C. and Lynch, J. (1999) Income inequality, social cohesion and class relations: a critique of Wilkinson's neo-Durkheimian research programme. *International Journal of Health Services* 29, 59–81.

Musavengane, R. and Kloppers, R. (2020) Social capital: an investment towards community resilience in the collaborative natural resources management of community-based tourism schemes. *Tourism Management Perspectives* 34, 100654.

Narayan, D. (1999) *Bonds and Bridges: Social Capital and Poverty*. World Bank, Washington, DC.

NICE (National Institute for Health and Clinical Excellence) (2008) Community Engagement. NICE, London.

NICE (National Institute for Health and Care Excellence) (2016) Community Engagement: improving health and wellbeing and reducing health inequalities, in NICE guideline NG 44. NICE, London.

Olaniran, A., Smith, H., Unkels, R., Bar-Zeev, S. and van den Broek, N. (2017) Who is a community health worker? – a systematic review of definitions. *Global Health Action* 10, doi: 10.1080/16549716.2017.1272223

Orton, L., Ponsford, R., Egan, M., Halliday, E., Whitehead, M. and Popay, J. (2019) Capturing complexity in the evaluation of a major area-based initiative in community empowerment: what can a multi-site, multi team, ethnographic approach offer? *Anthropology & Medicine* 26 (1), 48–64.

Oshio, T. (2016) The association between individual-level social capital and health: crosssectional, prospective cohort and fixed-effects models. *Journal of Epidemiology and Community Health* 70, 25–30.

O'Sullivan, T., Kuziemsky, C. and Corneil, W. (2013) Unravelling the complexities of disaster management: a framework of critical social infrastructure to promote population health and resilience. *Social Science and Medicine* 93, 238–236.

Parliamentary Office of Science & Technology (POST) (2018) *Unpaid Care*. PN 582, July 2018.

Pawson, R. and Tilley, N. (1997) *Realistic Evaluation*. Sage, London.

Pawson, R., Greenhalgh, T., Harvey, G. and Walshe, K. (2005) Realist review: a new method of systematic review designed for complex policy interventions. *Journal of Health Services Research & Policy* 10(Suppl. 1), 21–34.

Perry, H.B., Zulliger, R. and Rogers, M.M. (2014) Community health workers in low-, middle-, and high-income countries: an overview of their history, recent evolution, and current effectiveness. *Annual Review of Public Health* 35, 399–421.

PHE (Public Health England) (2018) Community development route to health improvement in Aylesbury. Available at: https://www.gov.uk/government/case-studies/community-development-route-to-health-improvement-in-aylesbury (accessed 18 May 2020).

PHE and NHS England (2015) *A Guide to Community-Centred Approaches for Health and Wellbeing*. PHE, London.

Pickett, K. and Wilkinson, R.G. (2015) Income inequality and health outcomes: a causal review. *Social Science and Medicine* 128, 316–326.

Piper, S. (2009) *Health Promotion for Nurses. Theory and Practice*. Routledge, Oxford, UK.

Poortinga, W. (2006) Social relations or social capital? Individual and community health effects of bonding social capital. *Social Science and Medicine* 63, 255–270.

Popple, K. and Shaw, M. (1997) Editorial introduction. Social movements: re-asserting 'community'. *Community Development Journal* 32, 191–198.

Portes, A. and Landolt, P. (1996) Unsolved mysteries; the Tocqueville files II. The downside of social capital. *The American Prospect* 7, 18–21.

Purdue, D. (2001) Neighbourhood governance: leadership, trust and social capital. *Urban Studies* 38, 2211–2224.

Putnam, R.D. (1993a) *Making Democracy Work. Civic Traditions in Modern Italy*. Princeton University Press, Princeton, New Jersey.

Putnam, R.D. (1993b) The prosperous community. *The American Prospect* 4, 35–42.

Putnam, R.D. (2000) *Bowling Alone. The Collapse and Revival of American Community*. Simon and Schuster, New York.

Rao, H. and Greve, H. (2018) Disasters and community resilience: Spanish flu and the formation of retail cooperatives in Norway. *Academy of Management Journal* 61, 5–25.

Rifkin, S.B., Muller, R.F. and Bichmann, W. (1988) Primary health care: on measuring participation. *Social Science Medicine* 26 (9), 931–940.

Rifkin, S.B. (1996) Paradigms lost: toward a new understanding of community participation in health programmes. *Acta Tropica* 61, 79–92.

Rifkin, S.B. (2009) Lessons from community participation in health programmes: a review of post Alma-Ata experience. *International Health* 1, 31–36.

Rifkin, S.B. (2014) Examining the links between community participation and health outcomes: a review of the literature. *Health Policy Plan* 29, ii98–ii108.

Rifkin, S.B., Lewando-Hunt., G. and Draper, A.K. (2000) *Participatory Approaches in Health Promotion and Health Planning: a Literature Review*. Health Development Agency, London.

Rocco, L. and Suhrcke, M. (2012) Is social capital good for health? A European perspective. WHO, Copenhagen.

Rocha Franco, S.H. and Teixeira Assis, W.F. (2019) Participatory budgeting and transformative development in Brazil. *Geoforum* 103, 85–94.

Rodgers, J., Valuev, A.V., Hswena, Y. and Subramanianc, S.V. (2019) Social capital and physical health: an updated review of the literature for 2007–2018. *Social Science and Medicine* 236, 112360.

Roy, M.J. (2017) The assets-based approach: furthering a neoliberal agenda or rediscovering the old public health? A critical examination of practitioner discourses. *Critical Public Health* 27 (4), 455–464 https://doi.org/10.1080/09581596.2016.1249826.

Royal Society for Public Health (2015) Indicators of change: the adaptation of the health trainer service in England. Available at: https://www.rsph.org.uk/uploads/assets/uploaded/128c70d4-2a0c-4289-be00249b10c520f0.pdf (accessed May 18 2020).

Saguin, K. (2018) Why the poor do not benefit from community-driven development: lessons from participatory budgeting. *World Development* 112, 220–232.

Sanders, D. with Carver, R. (1985) *The Struggle for Health: Medicine and the Politics of Underdevelopment*. Macmillan Educational, Basingstoke, UK.

Sarrami-Foroushani, P., Travaglia, J., Debono, D. and Braithwaite, G. (2014) Key concepts in consumer and community engagement: a scoping meta-review. *BMC Health Services Research*, 14, 250.

Schuller, T., Baron, S. and Field, J. (2000) Social capital: a review and a critique. In: Baron, S., Field, J. and Schuller, T. (eds) *Social Capital. Critical Perspectives*. Oxford University Press, Oxford, UK, pp. 1–38.

Shahbari, N.A.E., Gesser-Edelsburg, A. and. Mesch, G.S. (2020) Perceived trust in the health system among mothers and nurses and its relationship to the issue of vaccinations among the Arab population of Israel: A qualitative research study *Vaccine* 38, 29–38.

Shaw, M. (2004) *Community Work: Policy, Politics and Practice*. Working Papers in Social Science and Policy, The University of Hull, Hull, UK.

Silva, K. and Sena, R. (2013) Health promotion: criticism of everyday life medicalization practices. *Journal of Nursing Education and Practice* 3, 9, 83–92.

South, J. (2014a) Health promotion by communities and in communities: current issues for research and practice. *Scandinavian Journal of Public Health* 42 (Suppl 15), 82–87.

South, J. (2014b) The family of community-centred approaches for health and wellbeing. Presentation at NICE PHAC on community engagement, 11 December 2014.

South, J., Meah, A., Bagnall, A.-M., Kinsella, K., Branney, P., White, J. and Gamsu, M. (2010a) People in public health – a study of approaches to develop and support people in public health roles. Final report. NIHR Service Delivery and Organisation programme. Available at: https://fundingawards.nihr.ac.uk/award/08/1716/206 (accessed 25 August 2020).

South, J., Raine, G. and White, J. (2010b) *Community Health Champions: Evidence Review. Centre for Health Promotion Research*, Leeds Metropolitan University, Leeds, UK.

South, J., Meah, A. and Branney, P. (2011) 'Think differently and be prepared to demonstrate trust': findings from public hearings, England on supporting lay people in public health roles. *Health Promotion International* 27(2), 284–294.

South., J, White, J. and Gamsu, M. (2012) *People-centred Public Health*. The Policy Press, Bristol, UK.

South, J., Meah, A., Bagnall, A-M. and Jones, R. (2013) Dimensions of lay health worker programmes: results of a scoping study and production of a descriptive framework. *Global Health Promotion* 20(1), 5–15.

South, J., Connolly, A.M, Stansfield, J.A., Johnstone, P., Henderson, G. and Fenton, K.A. (2018) Putting the public (back) into public health: leadership, evidence and action. *Journal of Public Health* 41 (1), 10–17.

South, J., Bagnall, A.M., Stansfield, J.A., Southby, K.J. and Mehta, P. (2019) An evidence-based framework on community centred approaches for health. *Health Promotion International* 34, 356–366.

Springett, J., Owens, C. and Callaghan, J. (2007) The challenge of combining 'lay' knowledge with 'evidence-based' practice in health promotion: Fag Ends Smoking Cessation Service. *Critical Public Health* 17, 243–256.

Standing, H., Mushtaque, A. and Chowdhury, R. (2008) Producing effective knowledge agents in a pluralistic environment: what future for community health workers? *Social Science and Medicine* 66, 2096–2107.

Stevens, C. (2008) Social capital in its place: using social theory to understand social capital and inequalities in health. *Social Science and Medicine* 66, 1174–1184.

Stout, C., Morrow, J., Brandt, E.N. and Wolf, S. (1964) Study of an Italian–American community in PA; unusually low incidence of death from myocardial infarction. *Journal of the American Medical Association* 188, 845.

Szreter, S. and Woolcock, M. (2002) *Health by Association? Social Capital, Social Theory and the Political Economy of Public Health*. Von Hugel Institute Working Paper, Cambridge, UK.

Takakura, M. (2015) Relations of participation in organized activities to smoking and drinking among Japanese youth: contextual effects of structural social capital in high school. *International Journal of Public Health* 60, 679–689.

Taylor, B., Mathers, J. and Parry, J. (2018) Who are community health workers and what do they do? Development of an empirically derived reporting taxonomy. *Journal of Public Health (Oxf)* 40(1),199–209.

Taylor, M. (2000a) Communities in the lead: power, organisational capacity and social capital. *Urban Studies* 37, 1019–1035.

Taylor, M. (2000b) Maintaining community involvement in regeneration: what are the issues? *Local Economy* 15, 251–267.

Taylor, P. (2007) The lay contribution to public health. In: Orme, J., Powell, J., Taylor, P., Harrison, T. and Grey, M. (eds) *Public Health for the 21st Century. New Perspectives on Policy, Participation and Practice*, 2nd edn. Open University Press, Maidenhead, UK, pp. 98–117.

Tobin, G. Whiteford, L. Murphy, A. Jones, E. and McCarty, C. (2014) Modeling social networks and community resilience in chronic disasters: case studies from volcanic areas in Ecuador and Mexico. In: Gasparini, P. *et al.* (eds), *Resilience and Sustainability in Relation to Natural 13 Disasters: A Challenge for Future Cities*. Springer Briefs in Earth Sciences.

Tones, K. and Green, J. (2004) *Health Promotion: Planning and Strategies*. Sage, London.

Tones, K. and Tilford, S. (2001) *Health Promotion, Effectiveness, Efficiency and Equity*, 3rd edn. Nelson Thornes, Cheltenham, UK.

Tuckett, D., Boulton, M., Olson, C. and Williams, A. (1985) *Meetings Between Experts*. Tavistock, London.

Twelvetrees, A. (2017) *Community Development, Social Action and Social Planning*. 5th edn. Macmillan Education, UK.

Valdiserri, R.O. and Holtgrave, D.R. (2019) Ending HIV in America: not without the power of community. *AIDS and Behavior* 23(11), 2899–2903.

Villalonga-Olives, E. and Kawachi, I. (2017) The dark side of social capital: a systematic review of the negative health effects of social capital *Social Science and Medicine* 194, 105–127.

Wakefield, S.E.L. and Poland, B. (2005) Family, friend or foe? Critical reflections on the relevance and role of social capital in health promotion and community development. *Social Science and Medicine* 60, 2819–2832.

Walker, A. and Wigfield, A. (2003) *Social Quality, Social Capital and Quality of Life.* Discussion Paper for ENIQ, February 2003.

Wall, E., Ferrazzi, G. and Schryer, F. (1998) Getting the goods on social capital. *Rural Sociology* 63, 300–322.

Wallerstein, N., Mendes, R., Minkler, M. and Akerman, M. (2011) Reclaiming the social in community movements. *Health Promotion International* 26 (S2), ii226-ii236.

Warwick-Booth, L., Cross, R. and Lowcock, D. (2021) *Contemporary Health Studies; An Introduction,* 2nd edn. Polity Press, Cambridge, UK.

Weaver, A. and Lapidos, A. (2018) Mental Health Interventions with Community health workers in the United States: a systematic review. *Journal of Health Care for the Poor and Underserved* 29 (1), 159–180.

Weitzman, E.R. and Kawachi, I. (2000) Giving means receiving: the protective effect of social capital on binge drinking on college campuses. *American Journal of Public Health* 90, 1936–1939.

What Works Wellbeing (2017) What drives wellbeing inequality at the local level across Great Britain? Community Wellbeing Evidence Programme What Works Centre for Wellbeing. Available at: www.whatworkswellbeing.org (accessed 11 August 2020).

White, J., South, J., Woodall, J. and Kinsella, K. (2010) *Altogether Better Thematic Evaluation – Community Health Champions and Empowerment. Centre for Health Promotion Research*, Leeds Metropolitan University, Leeds, UK.

WHO (World Health Organization) (1978) *Declaration of Alma-Ata, International Conference on Primary Health Care, Alma-Ata, USSR, 6–12 September 1978.* WHO, Geneva. Available at: http://www.who.int/publications/almaata_declaration_en.pdf (accessed 3 November 2012).

WHO (1986a) Ottawa Charter for health promotion. *Health Promotion* 1, iii–v.

WHO (1986b) *Ottawa Charter for Health Promotion. First International Conference on Health Promotion*, Ottawa, 17–21 November. WHO Regional Office for Europe, Copenhagen.

WHO (2011) *What is a Healthy City?* Available at: https://www.euro.who.int/en/health-topics/environment-and-health/urban-health/who-european-healthy-cities-network/what-is-a-healthy-city (accessed 25 August 2020).

WHO (2012a) *Rio Political Declaration on Social Determinants of Health. World Conference on Social Determinants of Health, Rio de Janeiro, Brazil* 2011.

WHO (2012b) Health 2020: a European policy framework supporting action across government and society for health and wellbeing. WHO, Copenhagen.

WHO (2016) 9th Global Conference on Health Promotion. Shanghai, China.

WHO (2017) Promoting health in the SDGs. Report on the 9th Global Conference for Health Promotion: All for Health, Health for All, 21–24 November 2016, WHO, Geneva.

WHO (2018) Astana declaration on primary health care: from Alma-Ata towards universal health coverage and sustainable development goals. WHO, Geneva.

WHO (2020) Types of healthy settings healthy cities. Available at: https://www.who.int/healthy_settings/types/cities/en/ (accessed 22 April 2020).

WHO (World Health Organization) and the United Nations Children's Fund (UNICEF) (2018) Declaration on Astana. Available at: https://www.who.int/docs/default-source/primary-health/declaration/gcphc-declaration.pdf (accessed 11 August 2020).

Wilson, P. and Mavhandu-Mudzusi, A.H. (2019) Working in partnership with communities to improve health and research outcomes. Comparisons and commonalities between the UK and South Africa. *Primary Health Care Research & Development* 20(e129),1–9.

Wind, T.R. and Komproe, I.H. (2012) The mechanisms that associate community social capital with post-disaster mental health: a multilevel model. *Social Science and Medicin.* 75, 1715–1720.

Wind, T.R., Fordham, M. and Komproe, I.H. (2011) Social capital and post-disaster mental health. *Global Health Action* 4. Available at: https://doi.org/10.3402/gha.v4i0.6351

Yardley, L., Amlôt, R., Rice, C., Robin, C. and Michie, S. (2020) How can we involve communities in managing the covid-19 pandemic? *Bmjopinion.* Available at: https://blogs.bmj.com/bmj/2020/03/17/how-can-we-involve-communities-in-managing-the-covid-19-pandemic/ (accessed 18 May 2020).

Yerbury, H. (2011) Vocabularies of community. *Community Development Journal* 47, 184–198.

Zarychta, A. (2015) Community trust and household health: a spatially based approach with evidence from rural Honduras. *Social Science and Medicine* 146, 85–94.

Ziglio, E., Azzopardi-Muscat, N. and Briguglio, L. (2017) Resilience and 21st century public health, *European Journal of Public Health* 27 (5), 789–790.

Zoller, H.M. (2005) Health activism: communication theory and action for social change. *Communication Theory* 15, 341–364.

3 Policies for Health in the 21st Century

LOUISE WARWICK-BOOTH AND SIMON ROWLANDS[1]

This chapter aims to:

- demonstrate the importance of including health in all policies;
- explain the differences between health policy, social policy and health in all policy;
- explore the policy process;
- introduce key ideas from the policy analysis literature;
- show how ideology affects policy making; and
- discuss the role of advocacy within health promotion.

Introduction

This chapter will discuss the importance of health in all policies (HiAP) in relation to health promotion. The need to consider health in all policies as a core component of health promotion has been reaffirmed and redeveloped over many years since the Ottawa conference. Health promoters have consistently put health on the agenda of policy makers across all policy sectors and levels of government (Mohindra, 2007). The Jakarta Declaration (WHO, 1997) listed a number of priorities for 21st-century health promotion, which were underpinned by multi-sectoral and partnership working, as well as a strong commitment to the idea of healthy public policy. The Mexico Conference (WHO, 2000) described health promotion as a key part of public policy within all countries. The Bangkok Charter (WHO, 2005) then re-emphasized the importance of health promotion and called for global governance to address the harmful health effects of trade, marketing and specific products. The Helsinki Conference (WHO, 2013) introduced a framework for Health in all Policies for national adaptation. This framework places emphasis on the consequences of all policy making in relation to health systems, the social determinants of health, and wellbeing.

It is crucial that health promoters can make sense of policy processes if they are to ensure that a HiAP approach is taken. Therefore, in this chapter, the policy-making process is discussed to illustrate its complexity, demonstrating how policy is made and shaped, debating what policy can achieve and discussing how policy can act as an instrument to effect change. The ideological basis of policy is also discussed, illustrating how different ideological positions are likely to result in a variety of outcomes for health. Policy sectors are identified and explained to show the ways in which many areas of policy relate to and influence health in both positive and negative ways. Agenda setting is touched upon, as part of the policy process, discussing stakeholders and how they influence policy. Advocacy as part of policy making is discussed, together with how health promoters can work as advocates. The role of policy outside the health sector is also discussed, along with the importance of inter-sectoral collaboration. In short, the chapter attempts to offer a critical discussion throughout of the entire policy process, from how policy is made, who influences policy, the key players in world health policy and the implications of all of this for health promotion practice.

What is Health in All Policies (HiAP)?

'Health in All Policies' (Box 3.1) is policy that has a clear and explicit concern for health and so has arguably far broader scope than 'public health policy'. The World Health Organization (WHO, 2013, p. 7) describes health in all policies as

> 'an approach to public policies across sectors that systematically takes into account the health implications of decisions, seeks synergies, and avoids harmful health impacts in order to improve population health and health equity'.

Within a HiAP approach, the conceptualization of health is broad, along the lines of the social model of health discussed in Chapter 1, with a central feature of the HiAP framework being about improving societal conditions and creating an environment that is more equitable and therefore results in more positive health outcomes.

Concerns with healthy public policy partially emerged as a response to a perceived over-emphasis on curative medicine and policy approaches adopting behavioural strategies (Kickbusch et al., 1990). There are many examples of already enacted healthy public policies. The Framework Convention on Tobacco Control (FCTC; Labonté and Laverack, 2010), which was the world's first global public health treaty, negotiated by the WHO in 2005, is a good example of a healthy public policy. This framework aimed to support an internationally coordinated response to combating the use of tobacco, and later led to some countries (including the UK) banning smoking in almost all enclosed spaces and workplaces. These healthy public policies aimed to reduce exposure to second-hand smoke for workers and the general public, with the secondary objective of reducing overall smoking rates. Gagliani (2019) notes that the smoking ban has improved public health in a range of ways, with fewer people smoking, and lower rates of respiratory illnesses. Another global example of a healthy public policy is that of the Kyoto Protocol on Greenhouse Gas Emissions (Labonté and Laverack, 2010), which aimed to reduce the levels of emissions at country level and so reduce climate change and its associated health impacts. This was later followed by the Paris Agreement in 2016, to strengthen the global response to climate change (United Nations, 2020).

The policy discourse was then developed into a HiAP focus during the 2011 Rio Political Declaration on Social Determinants of Health (WHO, 2011), and the United Nations (UN) General Assembly Resolution on the Prevention and Control of Non-Communicable Diseases (United Nations, 2011). Here policy makers are encouraged to consider the potentially positive and negative impacts of any policy change, in relation to health. In tackling a major concern in westernized countries, obesity, for example, not only has it been recognized that an 'obesogenic environment' has emerged, but also the solutions lie beyond individuals and lifestyle changes. Brown (2018) argues that policy alternatives to moralization about unhealthy behaviours include the regulation of unhealthy products (tobacco, alcohol and food containing trans-fats), but all approaches require ethical reflection. It is necessary in those countries with an 'obesity epidemic' to create supportive environments that consider

---

Box 3.1. Health in All Policies

The Health in All Policies Framework states that:

- Policy across all sectors and levels can and does have a significant impact on population health and health equity.
- Many of the determinants of positive health and indeed inequalities are related to broader conditions in which people live (social, environmental and economic), which are beyond the scope of the health sector and specific health policies.
- Multisectoral action is needed – this refers to actions between two or more sectors within governments, for example, health, transport and environment.
- This approach provides a way to identify and avoid unintended impacts of policy that can be damaging to population health.
- There are six key components that need to be addressed in order to put the framework into action:
    - Establishing both need and priorities
    - Framing and planning action
    - Identifying supportive structures and processes
    - Facilitating assessment and engagement
    - Conducting monitoring, evaluation and reporting
    - Building capacity.

(Adapted from WHO, 2013)

health in all policies. For example, developing transport policies that promote healthier ways of moving around, using policy to control food advertising, and to regulate the food industry (taxes on sugar sweetened beverages are one such example) and developing school policies that promote healthier eating and exercise are all likely to impact positively upon obesity. Changes to modes of transport encouraged by policy may also positively impact upon both health and the environment in numerous ways. Air pollution is responsible for more deaths than smoking, AIDS, diabetes and traffic collisions combined, and many more people suffer ill-health due to the effects of this pollution on their hearts, lungs and brains. This public health issue has historically been invisible on many policy agendas (Gardiner, 2019), yet the recent Covid-19 global pandemic has highlighted this issue. Covid-19 has helped to expose this health crisis, with associated lockdowns showing that improvements to air quality are possible when global emissions are reduced (Monks, 2020). Thus, governments and businesses are now being encouraged to consider how things can be done differently, to hold on to these improvements in air quality, and indeed other environmental gains.

Whilst all of this sounds highly desirable, it remains incredibly difficult to predict the consequences of policies in relation to health, largely because their influence on health is indirect and often occurs through several complex and conflicting pathways (Kemm, 2001), and outcomes can take many years to appear, following implementation (Gardiner, 2019). Estimating the harm and the benefits that arise from the implementation of policies is difficult and contested, with the harmful and beneficial impacts being likely to affect parts of populations and communities differently, despite any health impact assessment. Due to the inherent complexity of the policy process, health promoters need to remain concerned with the effects on health of policy perhaps designed for other purposes (Green *et al.*, 2018). A new main road through a rural area of, say, Nigeria might enable people to access health care more promptly, but might also increase child pedestrian accidents or increase flooding of

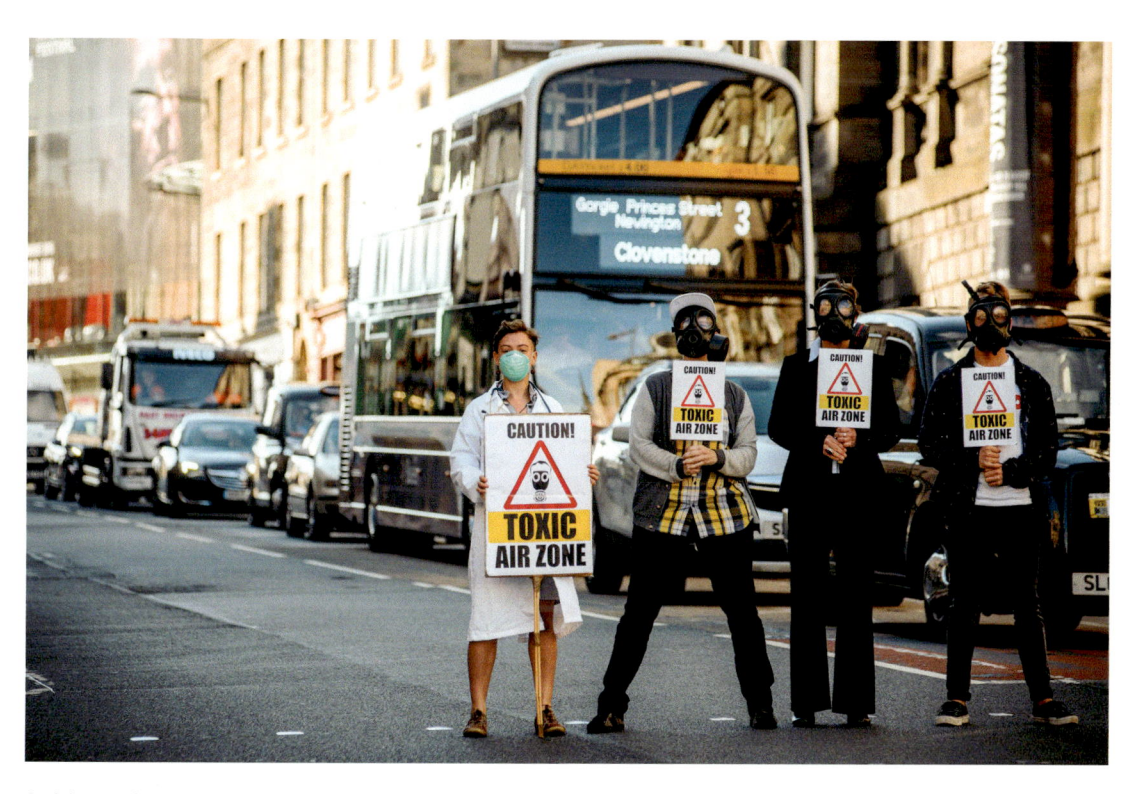

Activists gather to demand clean air in Edinburgh, Scotland (CC BY 2.0 license creative commons: https://search.creativecommons.org/photos/1d693a08-f18b-42ed-875b-11be9815e0c8).

homes, where the highway is built higher than dwellings (as is often the case). The World Bank's Structural Adjustment Policies received much criticism for their economic focus, which led to negative health outcomes (Easterly, 2003). Furthermore, governments may be reluctant to consider health in all policies on the grounds of costs and trade-offs; for example, there may be the loss of jobs associated with new trade policies and many governments remain concerned with being perceived as a 'nanny state' that interferes in people's lives through the policy process (Joffe and Mindell, 2004). There are many areas of life that citizens regard as 'private' and not suitable for policy interventions. This might include the number of children a family decides to have – though in China the opposite was the case, where the government, with its one-child policy, felt it could rightfully intervene!

Despite the complexity of using policy to promote health, there is evidence to show that health in all policies are helping to reduce inequities, especially as we know that policies that increase wealth inequality are more likely to damage health (Wilkinson, 1996; Wilkinson and Pickett, 2009; Marmot, 2015). Whilst Mantoura and Morrison (2016) acknowledge that policy in the global North tends to focus upon promoting healthier lifestyles and behaviour (sometimes called life-style drift), they argue that effective policy tools with a HiAP focus are available. These are summarized in Table 3.1.

All of these policy approaches, whether used individually or in combination, can address inequalities should there be political support to implement them. Influencing policy and achieving the implementation of more equitable societies is a central tenet of health promotion practice, although evaluating HiAP poses practical, theoretical and methodological challenges (Baum et al., 2016).

Social inequalities and health inequalities are widely documented and very well evidenced. Furthermore, despite improvements in overall health in many countries, inequalities persist. The 2008 Commission for the Social Determinants of Health emphasized the need to tackle the unequal distribution of power, money and resources. Marmot et al. (2020) highlight how the English national government has not prioritized health inequalities in its social policy approaches in the period 2010–2020, with a lack of health inequalities strategy evident, despite this being essential in their view because the amount of time people spend in poor health has been increasing in England since

Table 3.1. HiAP policy approaches.

Approach	Description
Political economy	Policy makers can use macro or structural level interventions to regulate markets and introduce labour market policies, and fiscal approaches to try to change the location of economic power, so that it is not held by dominant/rich groups at the expense of all others.
Macrosocial	This type of approaches focuses upon tackling unequal wealth distribution and increasing welfare support to those in need. Examples of this include establishing the provision of universal day care, universal health care or providing tax credits for those on lower incomes. These approaches attempt to mitigate against existing inequalities, so improve health outcomes as a consequence.
Intersectional	This approach advocates supporting specific groups of people deemed to be the most disadvantaged: for example, providing homeless-specific support for LGQBTI+ young people, to limit their exposure to health-damaging circumstances.
Life course	Policy approaches here focus upon key transition points during the life course. Examples include investment in early childhood development and education.
Living conditions	Policy approaches under this label acknowledge that people have differential access to material and psychological resources resulting in unequal health outcomes. Policy aims to reduce challenging conditions and to tackle environmental issues. Two examples include interventions to improve working conditions for those in low-paid occupations, and the provision of social housing for those in need.
Communities	Policy can seek to support disadvantaged and socially isolated communities who are likely to have worse health outcomes because of their circumstances. Participatory budgeting encourages community members to be involved in choosing the services that their communities require.

2010, and those living in more deprived areas spend more of their shorter lives in ill-health than those living in economically better-off regions. Previous English governments did try to use policy to tackle inequalities without success, primarily because such policies do not tackle the root cause of the problem (Wilkinson and Pickett, 2009). More recently, global recession and welfare state retrenchment have resulted in increased inequalities through those who can least afford it being affected the most (Cheetham et al., 2018). In the previous 2010 Marmot review, six areas were highlighted as important for policy makers in relation to tackling health inequalities:

1. Give every child the best start in life.
2. Enable all children, young people and adults to maximize their capabilities and have control over their lives.
3. Create fair employment and good work for all.
4. Ensure a healthy standard of living for all.
5. Create and develop healthy and sustainable places and communities.
6. Strengthen the role and impact of ill health prevention.

Bambra et al. (2005) previously argued that, because of the neo-liberal basis of Western economies, inequality needs to exist as part of the social structure, and therefore any specific policies to tackle 'inequalities' are tokenistic because no government will support a policy process that permits the full implementation of radical redistribution and the creation of a more equitable society. (A socialist regime would take a different view.) Thus, policy purporting to tackle health inequalities is simply minor reform, and so does not deal with the macroeconomic and structural causes of the problem. Bambra et al. (2005) argue that national-level policies to tackle inequalities also fail to consider the actions of global policy actors such as the WHO and the World Bank. Political ideology here clearly limits the formulation of effective policy for health and inequality reduction; ultimately 'the masking of the political nature of health, and the forms of the social structures and processes that create, maintain and undermine health, are determined by the individuals and groups that wield the greatest political power' (Bambra et al., 2005, p. 192). The World Bank operates according to a neoliberal model in which reduced government spending is a condition of lending money to developing economies (Easterly, 2003). Thus, the role of policy and its uses need to remain under critical scrutiny, as indeed do the strategies that are employed to build it.

Despite the challenges associated with using the policy process to tackle inequalities, health promoters remain engaged with tackling inequalities, with recent evidence suggesting the need for agencies such as the NHS, local government and other partners (including communities) to work together (Buck, 2018). Therefore, health promoters need to continue working on specific targeted initiatives to improve health, remain involved in research to build evidence around specific issues and ensure that they remain involved with strategies to build health in all policies.

What Is Social Policy?

A HiAP approach underpinning the formation and implementation of social policies leads us to consider more broadly what we mean by the term social policy. We are surrounded by social issues, some of which society feels there should be policies on, some of which are viewed as private issues (Mills, 1959). Issues such as gun control, the age of consent for marriage and human trafficking have all been subjected to *social* policy making. Other issues are more contentious as to whether they are suitable for policy making – reproductive rights and freedoms (e.g. the right to abortion) and parental discipline of children. (In the UK, parents and other caregivers are barred from smacking children in their care.) These two examples are more controversial, and some feel that they are 'private' matters and not conducive to 'social' policy making. Different views about individual choice and freedom result in variety of opinions here, leaving many areas of social policy mired in controversy and debate.

It may not always be clear what social policy is (Hudson et al., 2008). Social policy can be described as a field of activity decided upon and implemented by the government, a course of action and indeed a web of decisions rather than a single decision (Hill, 1997). The word 'policy' can be used very loosely in English, and Hogwood and Gunn (1984) characterize 'policy' in the following ways:

- as a label for a field of activity;
- as a statement of aspiration or purpose;
- as specific proposals;
- as (government) decisions;
- as formal authorization;
- as a programme;
- as an output(s);

- as an outcome(s);
- as a theory or model; and, finally,
- as a process.

'Social policy' is difficult to define and the scope of the field is extensive, typically covering social security, health, education, employment and housing. Platt (2019) describes social policy approaches as the mechanisms through which governments try to meet human needs for security, education, work, health and wellbeing, noting that policies focus upon areas defined as social problems, locally, nationally and globally. Furthermore, different nation-states adopt policies based upon various ideologies and principles so 'social' policies are by no means common to all nations (Esping-Anderson, 1990). Warwick-Booth et al. (2021) argue that policy can work in a variety of ways and hence affect health in both positive and negative ways. The policy-making process in which policy paths are determined is also complex and dynamic, itself subject to a range of influences from various groups and stakeholders who have an interest in directing policy.

What Is Health Policy?

All countries would recognize the need for 'health policy', usually housed in a Ministry of Health and actually concerned with disease, illness and threats to health. Health policy is described by Nutbeam (1998, p. 10) as 'a formal statement or procedure within institutions (notably government) which defines priorities and the parameters for action in response to health needs, available resources and other political pressures'. Warwick-Booth et al. (2021) state that health policy is often understood to involve the efforts of governments to improve health and provide medical care. Health policy covers many diverse areas such as the provision of health care services, approaches to tackle specific diseases such as confinement for TB sufferers and the lockdown of populations to prevent the spread of infection, and policy to deal with specific issues such as the right to die for the terminally ill and the reduction of incidences of teenage pregnancy. Many countries develop health policy to tackle particular challenges to health, especially where those areas are neglected or given low priority. Health policy is enacted through legislation but is distinguished from a health in all policies approach because *health policy* more narrowly focuses upon health (care) services and the provision of programmes such as immunization or screening (Nutbeam, 1998).

'Health policy' can therefore be distinguished from 'social policies that affect health' – the situation is complex, as health is obviously affected by many policy areas, not just health policy *per se*. Thus, numerous areas of *social* policy determine health outcomes even if they are not intended to. Policy regarding crime, employment, regulation of industry and many other examples all impact on health even if that is not their primary intention. More centrally in the health area, many government activities such as the taxation of products such as tobacco, sugar and alcohol, the regulation of air and water pollution, the safety of food and the working environment affect health and illness (Blakemore and Griggs, 2007). Joffe and Mindell (2004) argue that large health gains have emerged from a broad array of policies that often have not had health improvement as an objective at all. Thus, the provision of improved food supplies, sewerage and clean water resulted in the decline in infectious diseases (McKeown, 1979), historically, accounting to a large degree for the success of early public health in the UK.

There are many more government actions that have played a part in improving health and not all of these are encompassed under the remit of *health* policy specifically. For example, transport policy can have massive health benefits. Within the UK, the introduction of compulsory seatbelt wearing for those travelling in cars was enshrined in law during 1983. This transport policy had clear health benefits by reducing the number of deaths in car accidents significantly. Congestion charges in busy cities encouraging the use of public transport have inadvertently improved air quality and health (Green et al., 2018). Crammond and Carey (2017) note that policy interventions that improve overall educational attainment and break the association with disadvantaged childhood social position are likely to have beneficial effects on health equity. Conversely, the broader policy environment can be detrimental for health. For example, the use of pesticides for agricultural purposes affects health badly and has been well documented in The Gambia (Kuye et al., 2007). Road building potentially leads to more pollution (Gardiner, 2019) and higher levels of sedentariness (Roberts with Edwards, 2010). Thus, both our health and planetary sustainability are threatened as a result of some social policies. Austerity as policy approach

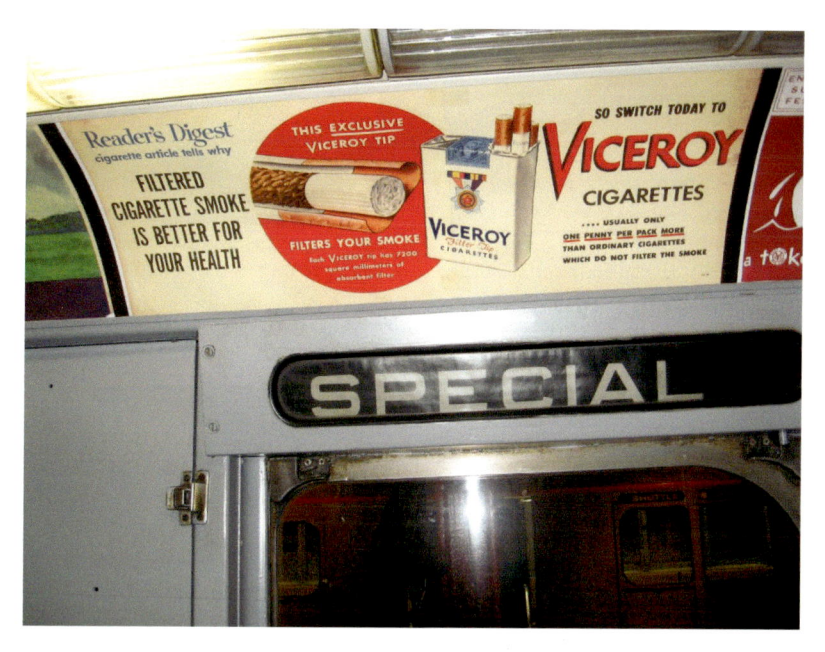

Tobacco marketing on the NY subway is now a museum exhibit, but not all countries have such restrictive advertising policies (copyright attribution 'Vintage NYC Subway Ad from NYC Transit Museum' by OliverN5 (https://www.flickr.com/photos/42907325@N00/96573666) CC BY-ND 2.0).

has been used across Europe following the 2007 recession and involved reduced social spending in combination with increased taxation. Roderick and Pollock (2018) argue that austerity has led to stalling life expectancy, increased infant and neonatal mortality and childhood poverty in the UK. Stenning and Hall (2018) highlight the impact of austerity policies on loneliness, especially for those already experiencing disadvantage, worsening their experiences of poverty, hardship and social isolation. Stuckler *et al.* (2017) report the impact of austerity on health system resilience, because of funding cuts. Any policies that increase inequality are likely to result in negative health impacts (Wilkinson and Pickett, 2009). Furthermore, any policies that are blind to inequalities also risk exacerbating them (Chastin *et al.*, 2018). Alston (2018, p. 22), in his analysis of UK austerity, states that 'poverty is a political choice…Resources were available to the Treasury at the last budget that could have transformed the situation of millions of people living in poverty, but the political choice was made to fund tax cuts for the wealthy instead.' Certainly, evidence about the social determinants of health and associated policy direction have not been acted upon in the UK (Marmot *et al.*, 2020).

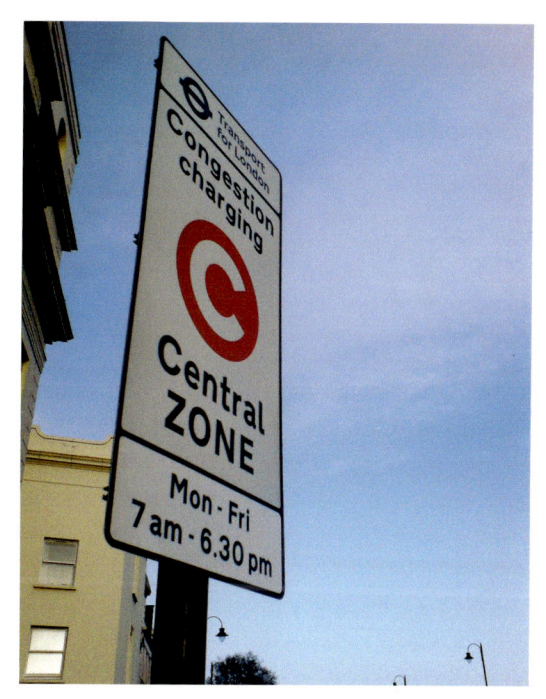

Transport policy has a major impact on health (copyright attribute 'The edge of the world.' by Andrew* (https://www.flickr.com/photos/26572975@N00/316457217) CC BY-SA 2.0).

We can therefore see that the field of social policy is a crucial determinant of health and this is now widely recognized. For example, Dahlgren and Whitehead's (1991) rainbow model frames policy as a determinant of health encompassed under general socio-economic, cultural and environmental conditions. It is also clear that the policy process is *political* and requires an understanding of who holds the ultimate power (Bambra *et al.*, 2005; Alston, 2018).

So far, we have discussed the necessity of health in all policies as a potential tool to tackle health inequalities and the complex health problems facing all societies; we have also tried to disentangle health policy, social policy and HiAP. We now turn to the process of policy making.

How Is Policy Formed and Shaped?

The policy process

Policy making is often conceived of in terms of a process or a cycle. This is a useful way of starting to look at policy as it breaks down the different stages of policy making. In addition, it signals that policy making is dynamic and about ongoing activity and change rather than focusing on set pieces such as legislation or formal documents. The policy process model can be used as both a descriptive approach (how policy *is* made) and a normative model (how policy *should be* made). Sometimes the policy-making process is presented as a simple cycle very similar to programme planning stages, which includes goals, methods, implementation and outcomes (Spicker, 2014).

Rationalist models of policy making are predicated on the idea of policy makers having good knowledge of problems and being able to choose different options, enabling rational decisions to be made. Policies can be made, implemented and evaluated in a linear way as suggested in the eight policy steps in Box 3.2.

In the literature, there are a number of theories of policy making and thus different theoretical perspectives regard the nature of the processes at work in diverse ways and present the extent of conflict and consensus in policy development again in disparate ways. In 'real life', policies rarely proceed smoothly through the stages and some theorists point out the incremental, piecemeal and 'messy' way that policies are actually developed. Some of these alternative ways of seeing policy making are presented in Table 3.2. Even when attempts to improve policy making are made, these have all suffered from a gap between theory and practice (Hallsworth *et al.*, 2011). For practitioners, the policy-making context and choices remain too complicated to enable them to inform recommendations. For researchers, too, there are gaps in their attempts to bridge the divisions between theory and practice (Cairney and Weible, 2017).

Debates therefore continue in relation to policy making and the contribution that theories of the process can make. Increasingly, the literature discusses policy making as a complex and chaotic process, influenced by certain groups and interests of policy actors, who are all invested and involved in the process (Cairney and Weible, 2017). Lindbolm described policy making in his seminal 1959 paper as the 'science of muddling through' and argued that there was a process of 'mutual partisan adjustment' (Parsons, 1995) in which policy making often occurs in a crowded arena where no single group is powerful enough to dominate the others. Consequently, policy emerges as a compromise between various interest groups who simply adjust their position to promote stability. Others, however, argue that contemporary Western political systems fail to operate in the interests of the people and instead operate as a deceptive branding force to promote underlying agendas (Reilly and McKee, 2012).

The role of evidence has also been described as increasingly important within policy-making circles

---

Box 3.2. The policy process.

1. Problem/state of society.
2. Agenda setting.
3. Issue processing/definition.
4. Selection of options.
5. Legitimation of options.
6. Allocation of resources.
7. Implementation.
8. Impact and evaluation.

(Adapted from Hogwood, 1987)

Table 3.2. Theories of policy making.

Theory about policy development	Explanation
Rationalist theories	• Policy making is a linear, sequence-based process in which a problem is identified and then solved, working through the stages of the process • This theory assumes that policy makers approach the problem rationally and go through the stages of the process logically
Incrementalist theories	• Policy makers never start with a blank sheet or perfect knowledge • Policy makers always react and respond to past policy change • Budget and resource decisions often result in incremental policy changes due to the constraints of shifting resources to and from different programmes and sectors • Policy change is always in small steps (incremental)
Marxist theories	• Policy is made by those in power to maintain the status quo • Power in policy making is held by those with money and business interests therefore policy is driven by them to meet their own goals
Network theories	• Policy is made by networks of actors who cluster together and focus upon specific interests • Networks can be formed when specific problems arise or they may already exist as part of dealing with ongoing policy problems
Pluralist theories	• Policy can be seen to emerge from the interaction of different parties at all stages of development and implementation • Colebatch (2002) refers to the horizontal and vertical dimensions of policy making to capture the pluralist aspects of policy making • Different groups hold brokerage positions and bargain for change according to their interests

with the emergence of evidence-based policy making discussed by both academics and governments. It would seem self-evident that policy making should be informed by research and the 'best evidence', in the same way that 'evidence-based practice' has emerged to inform practice more generally (a theme which is taken up in Chapter 5). However, there can be so much disagreement about what constitutes 'evidence' that policy making becomes impossible or is fraught with disagreements. The state of evidence about climate change is an example where there is such a divergent range of views from 'experts' and varying levels of acceptance of this amongst members of the public. Johnston and Deeming (2016) report that younger people and the better educated are more likely to accept policies designed to mitigate against climate change. Attitudes vary, however, and are influenced by media reports, which are often unwilling or indeed unable to communicate complex evidence about issues such as climate change. Therefore the rejection of 'evidence' can and does occur (Potts *et al*., 2007, 2008), but some policy theories do remain useful. Gavens *et al*. (2019) argue that using a policy transfer 'lens' offers insight into questions about 'robust' research evidence in relation to alcohol-related policy. However, in some instances (such as infectious disease outbreaks) policy makers are required to make speedy decisions under time pressure in situations of scientific uncertainty. The relationship between science and public health decision making remains in need of further study to support policy makers in delivering timely and effective crisis management (Salajan *et al*., 2020). Solving social and health problems is thus very complicated. Policy analysts (Chapman *et al*., 2009) have described 'wicked problems', which have the following characteristics:

1. Previously they have remained unsolved, thus policy has repeatedly failed to tackle the issues.
2. There are disagreements about the causes of the problem and therefore debate about how best to address it.
3. The issue has a large scope and is connected with several other issues that are also 'wicked'.
4. The issue is difficult in the sense that it can never be claimed to be solved.
5. There is much complexity involved and so the issue or problem may be unpredictable.

The characteristics of a 'wicked problem' can be seen in many areas related to health including inequalities, poverty and social exclusion.

Identifying influencing factors

Debates remain about how best to analyse the policy-making process (Walt *et al.*, 2002), and there are many factors that serve to influence the process, so understanding these is important for health promoters who wish to advocate for policy change. Much policy analysis is concerned with developing an understanding of the relative influence of different actors in a process characterized by conflict, consensus and power imbalances. Most policies are shaped by a variety of factors, although not all these influences will be visible or public.

Walt (1994) very usefully identifies a number of factors that influence policy:

- situational factors (such as politics and issues in the media);
- structural factors (relating to the organization of society and the political system of any given country);
- cultural factors (how society and individuals act and their value and belief systems); and
- environmental factors (events, structures and values that exist outside the boundaries of a political system but can influence decisions within it).

Crow and Jones (2018) argue that narratives are a central part of the policy process because they persuade both decision makers and the public, and therefore shape all stages of the policy process. Policy making involves a system of various actors who are all trying to achieve their preferred policy goals. Therefore, narratives are used by these actors to help them to achieve their goals and to communicate issues as well as solutions. Professionals and the wider public can also use narratives to communicate their preferences to those in power. Reilly and McKee (2012, p. 305) provide many examples of policy narratives used by those in power to 'profess their outward intentions in a manner that beguiles the electorate into thinking that they are aligned with "the common man", yet once elected, their true inclinations emerge'. For example, the English Conservative government offered a pre-election commitment to the NHS of no major re-organization, and then following their 2010 election victory unleashed a significant programme of change. In addition, they have offered various justifications to reduce the size of the state drastically. Narratives around the importance of community and responsibility are part of their branding to use the state in an increasingly neoliberal manner,

which has a significant challenge upon public health. The marketization of public health has led to a focus upon individual behaviour, whilst underplaying the significance of structural factors and social processes (Marmot, 2010; Williams and Fullagar, 2019). Ideology as an influencing factor in policy making is therefore in need of critical analysis.

Values and Ideology

The role of ideology

It is important when analysing policy to consider the ideological perspectives, political ideas and values that inform their development and shape how policy is structured. Ideologies are belief systems or ideas that frame the way policy makers respond to problems.

> Analysis of causes of disease distribution requires attention to the political and economic structures, processes and power relationships that produce societal patterns of health, disease, and wellbeing via shaping the conditions in which people live and work.
> (Krieger, 2011, p. 168)

Policy will always reflect societal, political and organizational values. These values may be expressed explicitly or, more often, be implied within policy. Political ideology includes assumptions, for example, about where the responsibility lies for health. Is health primarily the responsibility of the individual or of the government? Ideas about regulating behaviour and encouraging behaviour change are ideologically driven. Ideology is therefore an important aspect of policy making because belief structures make certain policies possible. Consequently, political will has to be examined and viewed in terms of its ideological underpinnings.

Table 3.3 gives a summary of key ideological positions and outlines how they influence policy. The description is simplified to illustrate how ideology can inform policy development, which in turn impacts upon health outcomes. Policy is driven by a variety of actors and stakeholders holding different ideological viewpoints. Which ideology dominates is usually bound up with who holds the balance of power in the national or local government.

An example of this can be seen in austerity policy responses to the global economic downturn of 2007. What was essentially a failure of the banking and housing sectors led ultimately to national governments underwriting commercial debts.

Table 3.3. Ideology and the direction of health policy.

Ideology	Key facets of the approach	Example policy
Conservatism	• Traditional order of society maintained • Recognizes inequalities but sees them as natural • Assumes that the role of the state should be minimal to avoid the creation of paternalism and welfare dependency • Values the private sector in service provision	• No policy focus upon dealing with health inequalities • Privatization of services including the provision of health care • Less public sector spending overall, with negative implications for such services • Increased inequalities
Liberalism	• Focuses upon freedom of choice and the importance of the individual • Individuals are seen as needing to behave responsibly • Neo-liberalism is a global economic approach scaling back the state and public spending and encouraging privatization	• Increased state intervention to control the market • Increased state intervention in relation to the provision of health care services • Individuals are responsible for their health • But neo-liberalism advocates reduced public spending, increased privatization and therefore increases inequalities
Socialism	• Broad ideology, with differing meanings • Originally associated with Marxism, and advocating revolution against the state • Contemporary socialism involves governments attempting to reform the state, and increasing state intervention in service provision	• Expansion of state involvement in public services including health care provision • Concerned with equality in both treatment and provision (the UK NHS was established upon the basis of socialist ideology)
Nationalism	• Rather than an ideology, this is a belief system • Nations should be self-governing, e.g. Scotland • Shared national identity is perceived as important in promoting social cohesion	• Difficult to say as the overall political context in which nationalism is employed will affect health • Scottish health policy has included more equalitarian policy within their NHS such as no prescription charges for everyone • Some nationalist approaches have been damaging for health due to cuts in public spending
Feminism	• There are a variety of different feminist approaches, e.g. liberals attempt to overcome discrimination via the legal system, whereas radicals focus upon the oppression within domestic relationships between men and women • Generally feminists are concerned with gender relationships	• Feminists draw attention to inequalities in health care provision in both diagnoses and treatment, arguing for changes in service provision
Environmentalism, 'Green ideology'	• Again this applies to a broad range of ideas • This school of thought focuses upon the global environmental crisis as well as the importance of the environment • Advocates sustainability and argues that policies should not damage the environment	• The environment and public health are seen as closely interconnected • The ecosystem should support public health rather than damage it • Policy should encourage sustainable development to reduce inequalities • Policy should encourage reduction in carbon usage and ecological footprints

Put differently, the privatization of profit and nationalization of risk (Kerasidou and Cribb, 2019). This served to exacerbate inequalities by protecting the occupations and income of the wealthy (financiers) at the expense those in most need (welfare recipients) (Castano et al., 2016; Ruckert and Labonté, 2017). The adverse impact on health and social outcomes are well documented

(Brand *et al.*, 2013), and disadvantaged health for the most marginalized though two key mechanisms:

1. Social risk effect – Impact on the social determinants of health through increased unemployment, homelessness and poverty whilst simultaneously reducing spending on social protection and welfare.
2. Healthcare effect – Cuts and more restricted access to healthcare services access.

(Stuckler *et al.*, 2017)

While Marmot (2020) lamented on Britain's '*lost decade*' and widening inequalities due to these unnecessary ideological choices, the previous year's Report of the UN Special Rapporteur on Extreme Poverty and Human Rights made the following claim of the UK:

> The social safety net has been badly damaged by drastic cuts to local authorities' budgets, which have eliminated many social services, reduced policing services, closed libraries in record numbers, shrunk community and youth centres and sold off public spaces and buildings. The bottom line is that much of the glue that has held British society together since the Second World War has been deliberately removed and replaced with a harsh and uncaring ethos. A booming economy, high employment and a budget surplus have not reversed austerity, a policy pursued more as an ideological than an economic agenda.
>
> Alston (2018, p. 1)

Austerity policies were at the time routinely framed by, largely conservative, politicians and media as 'the only choice in reducing national debt', insisting on a public responsibility to redress the deficit, despite the situation arising from a failure of commercial markets (Basu, 2019; Kerasidou and Cribb, 2019). In truth, the evidence for the effectiveness of austerity economics is limited and contested, whilst alternative stimulus approaches based on Keynesian economic models that encourage government spending have shown some success in specific countries and contexts (Karanikolos *et al.*, 2013; Karger *et al.*, 2014). These differing economic policy approaches reflect ideological positioning rather than best evidence. Some political analysts claim that austerity provided an ideal smokescreen for the furtherment of a long planned ideological journey toward reduced state intervention, increased competition and private sector provision, where the financial crisis is reduced to an opportunistic mechanism to 'achieve a neoliberal goal by the back door' (Wren-Lewis, 2016).

A more recent example of the ideological tension between economic and health policy can be seen in the Covid-19 debate over when and how 'lockdown' should end, and 'normal business' resume. It is rare that the health impact of economic policy on vulnerable groups, and the ideological interests behind them, has been so overtly discussed in the public sphere (Horton, 2020; Nunes, 2020). Competitive market ideology inevitably creates an environment where achieving equity in both health and wealth is problematic, where redistributive ambitions such as the Sustainable Development Goals (SDGs) become unachievable when the maintenance of power and dominance have primacy (Labonté and Schrecker, 2004):

> A social and economic system that accelerates capital accumulation and results in extreme wealth concentration is inconsistent with achieving equity goals.
>
> The Curitiba Declaration on Health Promotion, 2016 (Akerman *et al.*, 2019a).

Who Makes Policy?

Policy actors and stakeholders

Policy actors are individuals, groups or organizations involved in policy making. The term 'stakeholders' is used to refer to groups or individuals with an interest in, or those who are likely to be affected by, policy. The study of policy actors is important to gain an understanding of how policy is formed and implemented.

Spicker (2014) gives three categories of stakeholders:

- organizations, agencies and individuals directly engaged in policy making;
- individuals on the receiving end of policy (service users and also staff); and
- citizens – in a democracy, citizens have a stake in policy and are a source of political legitimacy; they might not be direct beneficiaries of a particular policy but will be affected by it as a member of society.

Key actors vary depending upon the stage of the policy process – lobby groups may be successful at getting an issue on the agenda but might be less likely to be part of the implementation process. For example, in response to the ongoing issue of gun-related violence and mass shootings in the USA, lobby groups have been successful in reaching upstream policy actors and challenging the dominant cultural norms by engaging consumers and citizens directly. However, such attempts have not yet resulted in significant changes to the law (Huff, 2017).

There are a number of policy actors with differential levels of power. There are global policy makers who are concerned with international policies made between nations and national-level policy from individual governments. Policy is also made locally, for example at a regional level, within defined communities or organizations and enacted through local agencies. The following list shows the diverse range of actors who participate within the policy-making process:

- international agencies/policy-making bodies, e.g. the WHO, the United Nations (UN);
- government, local, federal or national;
- civil servants and local government officers, e.g. those who work in the department/ministry of health;
- professional bodies, e.g. doctors' organizations like the General Medical Council within the UK;
- trades unions, e.g. those who act on behalf of workers (in the UK, Unison is a trade union that acts for public sector workers);
- experts/advisory groups, e.g. the UK EAGA, the Expert Advisory Group on AIDS, which is a non-statutory public body that provides advice within policy circles about HIV/AIDS;
- interest or lobby groups, e.g. environmental groups such as Greenpeace, women's rights groups and anti-abortion campaigners;
- user groups, e.g. disability rights campaigners and mental health service users;
- non-governmental organizations (NGOs); and media.

Analysing the power that actors hold is necessary in relation to understanding both agenda setting and policy making. For example, Dean (2011) argues that the media in the UK has enjoyed an extent of power that has led to distortion of policy making and has actually undermined the democratic process. Similar claims have been emerging more recently regarding the influence of social media on health and social policy (Fast et al., 2015; Bou-Karroum et al., 2017). Professional lobbyists in many industrialized countries enjoy a level of access to policy makers and government officials that arguably has gotten out of hand. A 'revolving door' approach where key political and scientific figures are recruited by industry to lobby for commercial interests has proved to be an effective tactic, often at the expense of public health policy (McKee and Stuckler, 2018; Robertson et al., 2019).

It is useful to look at who is excluded as well as included in the policy process. Barrett et al. (2003) provide a fascinating case study of how the needs of people with disabilities were taken into account (or not!) in Leeds City Council's transport policy. The case study shows how people living with disability are marginalized and excluded from policy making. The authors call for urgent changes given that policy making is dominated by large funded agencies and pays inadequate attention to the voices of those experiencing disability.

The role of the state/government

The state or government is an important player in the policy-making process; they deal with the provision of services, laws and regulations and distribution of resources.

> The modern state is a set of institutions comprising of the legislature, executive, central and local administration, judiciary, police and armed forces. Its crucial characteristic is that it acts as the institutional system of political domination and has a monopoly on the legitimate use of violence.
>
> (Abercrombie et al., 2006)

Once elected, national governments can alter the direction of policy. The US and UK governments for example, previously embraced the idea of 'nudging' as a policy directive. Nudging is discussed in more detail in Chapter 4, but, briefly here, it can include a variety of approaches that aim to prod or gently move social and physical environments to make certain healthier behaviours more likely (Thaler and Sunstein, 2009). Despite there being no precise definition of nudging and minimal evidence to support it as a means to improve population health, it appeals to policy makers because it is low cost and does not require legislation. However, 'nudging' as a policy measure remains contentious and it would have to take place across many policy sectors to achieve health improvements (Arno and Thomas, 2016).

As we can see from Table 3.3, minimal state intervention is an ideological aspiration and can be plotted along a continuum on the Nuffield Ladder of Intervention (Nuffield Bioethics Council, 2007, p. 128). This model provides a useful analytical tool when considering policy options that range from libertarian to authoritarian. For example, the UK Conservative government 'Responsibility Deal' eschewed more powerful legislative tools for softer, industry voluntary self-regulation, adopting measures lower down on the ladder. Gilmore *et al.*, (2011) provide an interesting critique of this approach.

Policy sectors and inter-sectoral collaboration

We have seen that public health issues invariably come into a number of sectors outside of the health care policy sector. For example, the education, environment and employment sectors all affect health outcomes. Early policy analysis tended to focus on studies of public administration within specific ministries. Current policy analysis literature reflects interest in the horizontal dimension of policy making and the activities with and between different policy sectors because policy can support health in a number of ways, across a variety of sectors. In terms of analysis, the complex inter-relationship of numerous factors within different policy sectors (Tesh, 1988) and the development of inter-sectoral collaboration is what is of interest. Leeds Beckett played a leading role in early research on what makes inter-sectoral collaboration work well (Delaney, 1994). Attempts were made, for example, in Zambia to show how inter-sectoral collaboration can help to develop alliances and advocacy to enhance maternal survival (Manandhar *et al.*, 2008).

Policy networks are another key part of the picture in terms of policy actors and stakeholders. They develop and exist due to interdependence between different organizations in order to meet mutual goals. A typology of networks is presented by Hudson and Lowe (2004, p. 131, adapting Marsh and Rhodes, 1992; Box 3.3).

Policy networks, organizations and communities vary in their ability to influence the policy process and this is context dependent, with more liberal democracies in theory facilitating more opportunities for participation within the policy process, compared with more authoritarian regimes (Walt, 1994).

What Makes Policy Happen?

Given the complexities of the policy process, an important question is: what makes policy happen? Sutton (1999) draws together an extensive list of factors that facilitate the development of a policy innovation:

- new research, which clarifies the issues and the course of required action;
- the existence of good linkages between organizations and a history of lessons learned;
- a powerful person in authority becomes interested in a specific issue, influencing policy development in the area;
- the timing being right, for example with those in authority interested and new research being published at the same time;
- a crisis situation, which requires an immediate response;
- a dominant epistemic community that is an influential group, closely linked to policy makers able to get an issue onto the policy agenda;
- a general consensus within networks or organizations that change needs to be facilitated;

Box 3.3. A typology of networks.

Type	Characteristics
Policy community	Stable, restricted membership, vertical interdependence, limited horizontal dimension
Professional network	As above but with shared goals of serving the profession
Intergovernmental network	Limited membership, limited vertical interdependence, extensive horizontal dimension
Producer network	Fluctuating membership, limited vertical interdependence, serves interest of the producer
Issue network	Unstable and large membership, limited vertical interdependence

- a change in discourse resulting in different priorities and therefore a shift in policy direction; and
- change agents or networks of change drive forward new policy directions.

All of these demonstrate the complexity of the policy process at the development stage prior to the consideration of how any policy is to be implemented.

Implementation

Implementation is an essential stage of the policy process. Policies are not always implemented fully, often creating concern over the 'implementation gap'. Barriers to implementation include:

- practitioners – levels of commitment, experience, attitudes to change, time and perceived incentives act as barriers;
- resources – financial, staffing, facilities;
- policy overload and contradiction;
- policy not based on sound theory and understanding;
- organizational structures and reorganization;
- uncooperative partners who undermine implementation;
- lack of political will or leadership support;
- poor project management;
- lack of community consultation and engagement;
- insufficient lead in time and unrealistic expectations; and
- poor communication and coordination.

More simply, Hogwood and Gunn (1984) identify barriers to policy implementation:

- bad execution: non-cooperation or ineffectiveness of those implementing policy;
- bad luck: external factors intervene to prevent implementation, e.g. funding withdrawn; and
- bad policy: based on faulty information, poor reasoning and unrealistic assumptions.

Policy outcomes frequently differ from intentions and some policies result in unexpected consequences, both negative and positive. Policy analysts have attempted to understand implementation processes and offer solutions (see Hill and Hupe (2009) for a thorough discussion) and there are some interesting empirical studies in this area.

Theories of implementation can be broadly divided into three types:

1. Top-down models – for example, legislation such as taxation of unhealthy products in order to reduce consumption.
2. Bottom-up models – for example, community-led campaigns for speed restrictions in specific areas in order to reduce road deaths and injuries.
3. Models that seek to integrate both approaches – for example, community campaigns resulting in changes in legislation.

Top-down implementation

Analysts looking at implementation from a top-down approach focus on the policy inputs and the extent to which organizational or policy goals are achieved. Top-down implementation is strongly associated with rational models of policy making and the aspiration of better organizational structures and project management to improve implementation. However, there are many criticisms of rational approaches to policy making – in practice, it is rather messy and its outcomes are complicated social, institutional and political processes (Smith, 2013). The same author suggests that policy is a chaotic series of accidents and this argument certainly hold weight when the implementation of policy is examined. Gunn (1978) asks the question: why is implementation so difficult? He argues that there are ten conditions required for 'perfect implementation', as follows:

- the circumstances external to the implementing agency do not impose crippling constraints;
- adequate time and sufficient resources are made available;
- the required combination of resources is actually available;
- the policy is based on a valid theory of cause and effect;
- the relationship between cause and effect is direct and there are few, if any, intervening factors;
- dependency relationships are minimal;
- there is understanding of, and agreement on, the objectives;
- tasks are fully specified in correct sequence;
- there is perfect communication and coordination; and
- those in authority can demand and obtain perfect compliance.

These perfect conditions rarely exist within the real world and implementation does not simply follow a top-down direction.

Bottom-up approaches to implementation

Bottom-up approaches are concerned with administrators and professionals who actually implement the policy and less with policy-making bodies. Emphasis is less on a failure to comply or implementation gap and more on the role of professionals and others in shaping policy. There is a focus on the study of professional power bases and the use of professional discretion. For example, Lipsky (1980) discusses 'street-level bureaucracy' and describes this as the decisions made by operational professionals. His analysis suggests that their routine and coping mechanisms to deal with both work pressures and uncertainties mean that policies may not be implemented as intended but according to the interpretation of those on the 'front line'. Hudson and Lowe (2004) suggest that policy outcomes are shaped at the point of final delivery, where individual workers have agency to direct policy at the point of implementation. In our work on the implementation of policy regarding health-promoting prisons, prison staff are 'street-level bureaucrats' and, according to their inclinations, can block or enhance the implementation of a 'whole-prison approach' to health promotion (Dixey and Woodall, 2012). Studies have shown, too, that prison staff disregard health promotion, frequently perceiving it as constituting additional work or something that is outside their professional remit (Bird *et al.*, 1999; Caraher *et al.*, 2002). This shows that public policy is not just about those in power administrating from the top down – implementation requires a range of players. Wells (2007) found that workers in a mental health team when implementing policy had to balance four tensions: political imperatives with local management agendas, professional and peer cultures in which they worked, and finally their perceptions of perceived advantages that may result from implementing the policy. Wells (2007) provides a useful analysis in explaining why implementation is so complex and does not necessarily happen as the original architects envisage. Both managers and policy makers may not scrutinize local-level implementation too deeply because of these complexities, as a way of deflecting any blame associated with negative outcomes (Wells, 2007).

Policy or Social Entrepreneurs

Bornstein (2007) has argued the need for social entrepreneurs to facilitate change. Social entrepreneurs share the same characteristics as commercial entrepreneurs but use their enterprise skills in the social arena. They have focus on vision and opportunity, the ability to convince and facilitate empowerment, but this is coupled with a desire for social justice. The concept of social entrepreneurs has been linked to Kingdon's notion of a windows of opportunity. Kingdon (1995) characterized the policy-making process as having three streams – policy streams, problem streams and political streams. Issues are placed on the policy agenda when all three streams come together. Policy entrepreneurs are needed to capitalize on such opportunities and are involved in complex, interrelated social processes including the generation of ideas, problem framing, dissemination, strategic activities, lobbying and evaluation (Guldbrandsson and Fossum, 2009). Policy entrepreneurs when interviewed felt that, whilst they were able to influence the flow of events, there were other factors and players who remained important (Roberts and King, 1991). Perkmann (2002) also analysed policy entrepreneurs in the context of the European Commission and argued that grassroots actors can engage in policy entrepreneurship and this is a necessary governance challenge. Craig *et al.* (2010) document how public health professionals can act as policy entrepreneurs to advance health-related goals when windows of opportunities open, with an analysis that focuses upon the development of a childhood obesity strategy in Arkansas. Health promoters, in practice, then are able to use their knowledge within given windows of opportunities to facilitate policy change and the development of healthy public policy.

Strategies for Building Healthy Public Policy

Advocacy

A key strategy for building healthy public policy is that of advocacy (WHO, 1986). Advocacy can be defined in a number of ways and is used as a term in judicial systems, in individual casework, for example in mental health and in policy making. Smithies and Webster (1998, p. 105) define advocacy as:

Advocacy is about people speaking up for or acting on behalf of themselves, possibly with the support of another person/group or 'advocate'. It is also about taking action to get something changed, in order to take more control over our lives.

Advocacy may be taken at an individual or group level to create living conditions more conducive to health and healthier lifestyles (Nutbeam, 1993). Advocacy for health therefore is about empowerment, protecting those who are considered vulnerable and tackling inequalities. Health advocacy in the context of public health and health promotion is used to describe a process of support for health programmes and healthy public policy. Different types of advocacy can be seen in practice. For example, advocacy can be confrontational by challenging powerful commercial anti-health interests such as the tobacco lobby (Givel, 2007) or it can be about mediating and negotiating between opposing groups and positions to try to achieve positive health (Nutbeam, 1993). Advocacy may also be capacity building, enabling individuals and groups to gain control over their lives and to improve their health by becoming effective policy advocates (Shilton *et al.*, 2013). Ultimately, advocacy in relation to policy is about trying to influence the policy-making process so that healthier legislation and healthy public policies are introduced and implemented. For example, the Bill & Melinda Gates Foundation advocates to raise awareness of less well-known and neglected diseases affecting lower-income countries because there is already much more political attention directed towards HIV/AIDS, TB and malaria. Smithies and Webster (1998) present a typology of advocacy to outline the different levels of advocacy that can occur. Table 3.4 outlines these types of advocacy levels and provides some health-related examples.

Carlisle (2000) also identifies four advocacy models: first, representational in which work is carried out on behalf of people; secondly, facilitational in which people are helped to represent their own needs; thirdly, confrontational in which powerful interests are challenged; and finally, advocacy can be in the form of acting as a conduit in order to mediate and negotiate between interests. She uses a conceptual framework to categorize advocacy based on two dimensions, whether the goals are empowerment oriented or protection/prevention oriented and whether the level is policy that addresses structural or individual-level issues. Advocacy is also associated with campaigning and

Table 3.4. Types of advocacy (adapted from Smithies and Webster, 1998).

Type of advocacy	Explanation	Example
Citizen advocacy	People in the same community establish supportive relationships; this can be about addressing a specific problem or about protecting the vulnerable and giving them a voice	Local community volunteers ensuring that young people in the community are not ignored when large decisions are being made
Peer advocacy	This is support from individuals who have undergone similar experiences	Mental health service users working on behalf of other similar service users
Self-advocacy	This is about speaking up for yourself and making your views and wishes clear	Individual right-to-die campaigners try to challenge existing rules about assisted suicide within countries where this is illegal
Legal advocacy	People with specialist knowledge and training often represent others in a paid capacity within a formal setting such as a court or tribunal	The rights of patients to decide to refuse life-saving treatment can be legally agreed
Professional advocacy	People are paid, trained and employed to advocate on behalf of others	Paid organizations support people with learning disabilities in understanding the medical treatment that they are receiving
Staff advocacy	Workers in a specific organization advocate for each other as well as broader groups including service users	Accident and emergency staff may advocate for changes in traffic speeds to reduce accident admissions
Campaigning advocacy	This is often from issue-based groups who unite to raise awareness of specific problems	A community group forms to challenge the creation of a new waste disposal facility that is causing health concerns

includes a variety of methods such as individual casework, the use of the mass media/media advocacy, political lobbying, community mobilization and coalition building.

Advocacy in the policy process

Advocacy is often associated with agenda setting but can occur at different stages of the policy-making process, from international to micro-level policy making.

- Getting issues on the agenda. This can be through using the media or by directly lobbying politicians. The media is a useful tool in advocacy campaigns. For example, in Canada, the Manitoba Public Insurance campaigns demonstrate that media advocacy can be used to deal with alcohol- and tobacco-related health issues (Asbridge, 2004).
- Changing public or policy makers' perceptions of issues. This is called issue framing. For example, advocates for the benefits of breastfeeding using the evidence to reframe support and facilitation as a matter of equity and basic human rights and therefore the responsibility of governments and legislators (Griswold, 2017).
- Presenting and lobbying for alternative options for policies (selection of options). This would involve presenting a number of solutions and options for how the problem could be tackled.
- Making sure policies are legitimized in order to move to the implementation stage.
- Mobilization and allocation of resources to implement policies. Who will implement a policy and at what levels is implementation required? This is where gaps are often recognized as existing.
- Lobbying for improved implementation.

Involvement in advocacy – lobby groups

Many individuals and groups participate in the policy process by advocating for a specific policy outcome. Parsons (1995) contrasts policy communities with stable and restricted memberships that are highly integrated into the policy process and issue networks that have dynamic, non-exclusive memberships and weaker points of entry to the policy process. There are many different lobby and interest groups, some known across the world such as Greenpeace and Black Lives Matter. Others work on a more national level, for example the British Medical Association, which operates in the UK to lobby on behalf of doctors and medical students. There are also many lobby groups funded by commercial industry that are well-funded, well-coordinated and influential. This is cited as problematic by many because governmental regulations on lobbying are weak. For example, in the USA, the pharmaceutical industry has promoted profitable drugs deemed unsafe by their own research (Angell, 2004). The UK-based Portman Group is supported by drinks producers despite it being concerned with the social responsibility issues surrounding alcohol. The group is well placed to lobby, which it does effectively, leading many to suggest that it is not independent of industry and that UK policy is too heavily influenced by alcohol manufacturers (Harkins, 2010). In 2004, the alcohol strategy for England and Wales was produced, which ignored independent evidence calling for changes in alcohol pricing and availability. The Portman Group was cited in the final report as an 'alcohol misuse' group – an example of successful pressure on the government from a powerful commercial group that ultimately influenced how evidence was used to decide policy (Stevens, 2007). Similarly, in 2003 the sugar industry demanded that the WHO remove its planned healthy-eating guidelines when they were about to be published. The guidelines were to recommend that sugar should not make up more than 10% of a healthy diet. The industry had the power to demand that the US Congress would no longer fund the WHO if the guidelines were published (Boseley, 2003). The guidelines were not published at that time but have since been updated (WHO, 2014).

There have also been successful health-benefiting changes made to the law despite heavy lobbying by industry, with health advocates and various other policy players mobilizing and campaigning for changes in corporate behaviour in order to improve population health (Freudenberg, 2005). Indeed, Wilson-Clay *et al.* (2005, p. 196) state that 'we have learned that a small group of committed individuals can gain access to lawmakers, participate successfully in the democratic process, and influence public health policy'.

Lobby and interest groups can differ on a number of dimensions. Their effectiveness can vary with issues and campaign tactics. Some key dimensions of interest groups are highlighted below.

- insider groups versus outsider groups;
- consensus building versus conflict generating;
- focus on a single issue versus involvement in a number of issues;
- covert lobbying versus open participation;
- formal mechanisms of involvement in decision making versus informal mechanisms of involvement; and
- use of legal methods versus the use of illegal methods.

Advocacy is also carried out through social movements, which have been a focus of much academic interest and are a prominent feature of 21st-century policy making. Some of the current social movements, such as anti-capitalist and environmental movements, have clear links to both health promotion and public health issues. For example, environmental lobbying capacity has been enhanced, reaching a wider and younger audience with the emergence of a charismatic figurehead, Greta Thunberg, and more effective use of social media.

Barry and Doherty (2001) suggest that social movements have a collective identity but one that is fluid and provisional, are made up of groups and individuals linked in a loose network with a mix of formal and informal ties, protest and use (direct) action and pose a challenge to power bases.

Activism around health issues conducted through health-related social movements has been important in achieving social change. For example, in the USA, women's health activists have changed conceptualizations around women in gender, reproductive rights and treatments (Morgen, 2002). More recently the 'Me Too' movement has expanded globally to successfully challenge sexual abuse and exploitation of women. Furthermore, self-care and disability activists have broadened awareness of the capacity of lay people to be involved in their own health (Barnes, 2007). However, within the literature, there are debates about how positive advocacy actually is, with several criticisms of the process. For example, Seedhouse (1997) argues that whilst health promotion and associated advocacy may be done on request, it is also carried out without prompt from intended recipients. Other critics of advocacy suggest that there is a contrast between the health promotion discourse of community participation and empowerment and the paternalistic construction of people as uneducated and requiring help from those who 'know better' (Wenzel, 1999, cited in Carlisle, 2000). Nevertheless, with health seen as an increasingly global issue and the influence of globalization described as important, advocacy at a global level by health promoters is important to influence the global policy-making environment.

Health promoters – a role in advocacy?

Advocacy has been identified as a key strategy for health promoters working in practice (see Sharma (no date) for a useful guide). There are, however, different models of advocacy, so as a practitioner, how do you decide to advocate? Using a rationalist approach, Maycock *et al.* (2001) propose an advocacy model to guide practitioners to make decisions about whether to advocate for a public health policy. The public health decision-making model has five questions:

1. What is the problem and is it significant?
2. Is it amenable for change?
3. Are the intervention benefits greater than costs?
4. Is there acceptance of the interventions?
5. What actions are recommended?

The reluctance of some professionals to become involved in advocacy is discussed within the literature. Galer-Unti *et al.* (2004) identify some common barriers including workers feeling that they were not 'activist', did not have time, did not know enough about advocacy, felt it would not make a difference or that the advocacy be ineffective.

In addition, values and ideological perspectives influence and underpin our professional practice. Fraser's (2005) four approaches to community participation summarize some of the positions held:

- anti-/reluctant communitarians and economic conservative approaches:
  o self-reliance and support for individual freedom;
- technical-functionalist communitarians and managerialist approaches:
  o pluralists – not challenging the status quo;
- progressive communitarians and empowerment approaches:
  o focus on social justice and reform. Egalitarian, democratic and inclusive in orientation; and
- radical/activist communitarians and transformative approaches:
  o reject reform agenda; argue for redistribution of power/ resources.

Despite these complexities, Labonté and Laverack (2010) still argue for health promoters to become advocates for a new global governance system and say that, although there are no blueprints for health promoters, there are steps that they can take and many strategies already exist within health promotion practice kits. Indeed, this is true of advocacy in general. Such steps include aligning with organizations and networks for the global movement for health and justice to develop a more powerful campaign for health promotion principles within the international arena; building partnerships that are empowering for health promotion, which use bottom-up approaches; entering current policy debates, either as individuals or via social movements; and practising optimism as an act of political resistance.

Power, Policy and Partnerships

Given the range of actors involved in policy making and the number of sectors that influence health, inter-sectoral collaboration has been called for to achieve better health outcomes. Inter-sectoral collaboration refers to 'the collective actions involving more than one specialized agency, performing different roles for a common purpose' (Adeleye and Ofili, 2010, p. 1). Indeed, the SDGs require input from a variety of sectors in order for targets to be achieved, showing the importance of such strategies for the delivery of improved health outcomes. However, there are numerous problems with such approaches: Adeleye and Ofili (2010) suggest a tripod of neglect when describing how inter-sectoral collaborations affect primary health care: often the non-health strategies are outside of the statutory control of the health sector, for example the provision of clean water; primary health care is not seen as significant in other sectors and health benefits tend to result by coincidence rather than as planned. For example, policy decisions are driven by politics rather than any perceived health benefits; collaboration projects between the health and non-health sectors are uncommon.

Despite this, partnership working and inter-sectoral collaboration do have the potential to bring about improvements in health and partnerships have been increasingly emphasized as a tool to deliver policy effectively within contemporary discourses.

Partnerships in policy

Partnerships can exist at any level of policy making from international alliances to groups working together at neighbourhood level. Partnerships can be inter-sectoral, inter-organizational and inter-professional (joint working). Some national governments have been keen to support partnership working, again demonstrating the importance of context for policy development. The previous UK New Labour government, 1997–2010, supported partnership working to develop policy in order to tackle cross-cutting issues, with the view that complex problems require multi-dimensional solutions, with this approach continuing to be encouraged by successive governments (NHS, 2014). Indeed, there are many rationales for partnership working because it attracts and pools resources, can reduce policy conflicts through common goals, can reduce competition, and break down barriers to implementation.

Despite these rationales, Dowling et al. (2004, p. 315) point to a dearth of evidence on partnership approaches saying:

> Current policies advocate partnerships, rather than markets or bureaucratic hierarchies, as the preferred mode of coordinating organisations, services and teams. Although it might be assumed that this preference rests upon clear evidence of the superiority of partnerships in delivering welfare over other types of relationships, this does not appear to be the case.

Cook (2015) reviewed the evidence on partnership working in the UK and was unable to document partnership working within public services with improved outcomes, although he does outline the features that contribute to effective partnerships as including transparency, inclusivity, flexibility and responsiveness to the needs of those involved (partners and service users alike). Therefore, many problems remain within partnership approaches. Hudson (2002) identifies the 'Achilles heel' of partnership working, discussing barriers including professional identity, professional status and professional discretion and accountability. Despite the focus on sustainable 'partnerships' in the discourse of development, and its emphasis in funding calls suggesting that donor agencies value partnerships, there is little literature on the processes and operationalization of such types of collaboration (Jentsch, 2004). In terms of 'North/South' partnerships, Brehm (2001) suggests that whilst the financial power is held by the 'Northern' partner, there is little hope that a partnership can mean true equality and the sharing of responsibilities.

In relation to health promotion practice, partnerships are often termed 'healthy alliances' in which the notion of a coalition is often used, where policy actors come together to advance a shared goal. Douglas (1998) points out that healthy alliances are not 'natural alliances' but are driven by needs of health agenda. Larkin *et al.* (2017) developed a framework for global health partnerships and argue that they can work if all of those involved agree to a common minimum programme from the design stage, and have adequate resources specifically allocated. Within the literature, questions remain about who holds the power within alliances and the processes of participation remain similarly debated. Despite this, participation within the policy process has been cited as increasingly important within recent discourses.

Participation and power

In recent years, citizen participation within the policy process has been labelled as positive and increasingly important. Participation was discussed in Chapter 2, and the role of active citizens will be taken up again in Chapter 5 but is discussed here in relation to participation in policy making.

Taylor (2003) defines four types of approaches to public involvement including consumerist approaches, representative approaches, interest group approaches and network approaches. Furthermore, involvement within both partnerships and the policy process is based upon a number of assumptions. First, participation is assumed to be a good thing. Some of the reasons advanced for public participation in policy making are that it:

- assists in targeting disadvantaged groups;
- widens inputs into policy and therefore results in more creative and innovative solutions;
- results in more responsive services targeted at needs;
- creates more ownership and involvement leading to more sustainable solutions;
- requires greater engagement for individuals to accept changes and support health improvement;
- brings benefits for individuals, communities and organizations; and
- is about democratic renewal in the sense that individuals have the right to be consulted.

The second assumption is that people want to be involved. However, involvement is complex and can be understood in different ways. Four categories of public involvement are identified by Taylor (2003): community leaders; initiators of activities and groups who are committed to and active in an issue or cause; participators in activities – individuals who join activities and support causes and events; and non-participators.

The third assumption is that community organizations and leaders represent the community. Some form of collective representation is necessary if participation is to be more than consultation. However, the structures in communities may reflect and support established power relations, for example in relation to gender. Carlisle (2010) carried out research on community engagement in policy making in Scotland and found a mismatch between the ideology of participation and practical constraints. OECD (2017) discourse states that effective participation of citizens in policy making remains central to government reform, yet the wider political context in many countries makes this difficult (Akerman *et al.*, 2019b).

The fourth assumption is that power sharing can take place. Barnes and Walker (1996), in discussing the principles of empowerment, argue that power is not a zero sum, and partnership models exist where the empowerment of one group is not at the expense of another. However, there are more complex descriptions of how power operates within policy partnerships. Lukes (2005) describes three dimensions of power. First, the pluralist view of power where conflicts of (subjective) interest exist within policy making. This is associated with liberal ideology and moves to improve the quality of participatory processes with little critique of structural interests. Secondly, the inclusion of groups in policy making termed the 'mobilization of bias'. This is associated with reformist ideologies, with a focus on combating social exclusion and bringing disadvantaged groups into policy making. Thirdly, power is seen as an all-encompassing control that determines and shapes public wants, and therefore demands, in a political system. Powerful interests may not be visible in policy arenas as they remain hidden. This perspective is linked to radical ideologies and arguments to seize control and radically change the system.

These perspectives make for interesting debates given the centrality of advocacy and partnership working to health promotion practice, and they have ramifications for the skills of health promoters, which will be taken up in Chapter 5. One aspect of the policy process that health promoters have become involved in is health impact assessment, which is a process of assessing the impact of a policy on health. The WHO (2020) provides useful discussion and practical guidance on how to carry out health impact assessments.

Global Health Policy

The final section of this chapter will consider the need for globally focused policy making to benefit health, arguably much needed given the impacts associated with the processes of globalization. The concept of globalization is often debated, as are its impacts upon health and the environment – it can be both positive and negative. Globalization for some increases global demand and production, leading to environmental exploitation and the depletion of natural resources (Afesorgbor and Demena, 2018). As health is increasingly conditioned and determined by both global processes and relationships (Yuill et al., 2010), there are consequently global health problems and issues, which require tackling on a worldwide scale. Global health challenges identified in the literature, include HIV/AIDS, malnutrition and lack of resources (*Grand Challenges in Global Health*, 2012). The need for global solutions has resulted in the development of global health policy organized through an increasing number of global actors (Davies, 2010). A number of large international organizations have made attempts to combat global health issues (Kaufmann, 2009), with many agencies working together through alliances to deliver health-related programmes (Walt and Buse, 2006). Governmental organizations and NGOs including the WHO, the World Bank, charities such as Oxfam, private foundations such as the Bill & Melinda Gates Foundation and large corporations such as pharmaceutical companies work globally to deal with numerous health problems and to define global health priorities (Table 3.5; Ollilia, 2005).

Table 3.5 provides a brief overview of the types of organizations that are working in the global policy arena and influencing policy. There has been a plethora of criticisms about the work that these organizations do and the overall impact that they have in relation to global health outcomes (Fidler, 2007). The huge growth of NGOs in the 1990s led to them being seen as a 'magic bullet' for resource-poor countries in terms of development, health and governance problems (Vivian, 1994), especially in contexts such as Africa (Fowler, 1998). Criticisms emerged, however, that NGOs gained too much influence on policy making, especially where they are based in the global North and working in the global South (Manji, 2006). Nevertheless, NGOs often operate in challenging and complex policy environments, sometimes at odds with state intentions, for example when supporting the health and wellbeing of unwanted migrants (Pursch et al., 2020).

The ideological underpinnings of some global organizations have been questioned (Macdonald, 2007), as have their priorities and interests (Ollilia, 2005). McNeill and Ottersen (2015) report power differences across the organizations involved in global policy making and the dominance of specific social norms, leading to negative side-effects and increased health inequalities from some policy implementation. Some criticisms also need to be revisited; Markel (2014) criticized the WHO for being too focused upon infectious diseases rather than tackling more chronic health and environmental concerns, yet, in the wake of the Covid-19 pandemic, this focus is incredibly relevant. More recent criticisms of the WHO focused on its inadequate response to the 2014/15 Ebola epidemic (Kickbusch and Reddy, 2015), and similar criticisms have been levied in relation to Covid-19.

Despite these issues, the role of global policy actors and associated governance has led to some health improvements. For example, the Millennium Development Goals were created as a set of global targets related to poverty and inequalities and health as an effort to promote global collective responsibility for health threats (Davies, 2010). Many practical challenges were experienced in achieving the goals, which have now been replaced by the SDGs. These are again a universal set of goals, targets and indicators that United Nation member states are expected to draw upon in order to shape, frame and inform their own policy and practice until 2030. They were established from consultation and the Rio+20 summit in 2012. The SDGs are cited as being more inclusive and better focused upon the environment and sustainability (Melamed and Ladd, 2013), but again encompass ambitious targets. Despite attempts at global improvements through such targets, national interests remain central to policy making and can thus challenge efforts to improve global health. For example, the UK's Brexit (exit from European

Table 3.5. Overview of global policy actors.

Organization	Remit
Membership-based organizations of the poor (see Chen *et al.*, 2007)	• Organizations that attempt to promote the representation and inclusion, rather than exclusion, of informal workers (and most resource-poor countries are dominated by the informal sector) in policy-making structures • The People's Health Movement is an example of marginalized and indigenous people coming together to represent their own interests (Baum, 2001; People's Health Movement, 2012)
The UN	• A collective of several countries who formed an international organization to promote human rights and social progress; it has many specialist agencies including the WHO • Established 1948 • UN's specialist agency for health • Has the aim of attaining the highest possible level of health for all people • Has implemented many vertical programmes such as immunization • Implemented mass eradication programmes such as the successful smallpox campaign and the unsuccessful malaria eradication campaign • Has emphasized the importance of primary health care • Produces an annual report about global health
The World Bank	• Works like a bank in the traditional sense • Provides low-interest loans to low-income countries • Imposes policy conditions for repayment, thus public sector reform is encouraged • 'Invests in people' • Has described health as an investment • Has encouraged the privatization of health care
The World Trade Organization	• Established in 1995, its role is to regulate trade • Promotes free trade • Has no specific health remit but trade of course affects health in many ways
International Monetary Fund	• Shaped the global economy since the 1940s • Encourages economic growth and stability • Stabilizes economies and reduces poverty • Responsible for much criticized structural adjustment programmes, which have resulted in less investment in health care in several lower income countries
Charities, NGOs and not-for-profit organizations	• Charities are funded via private donations • Each have their own remit and goals: for example, Oxfam helps people in crisis and aims to help reduce global poverty, whereas Save the Children has a focus upon saving children, protecting them from harm and educating them • Aid agencies are dedicated organizations aiming to distribute aid, which comes from a variety of sources • Many are governmental such as USAID, SIDA, EUROPEAID, and donate bilaterally from country to country • Aid is either humanitarian and used to respond to specific crises or developmental to help countries achieve economic improvements • Legal organizations set up for philanthropic purposes • The Bill & Melinda Gates Foundation is the largest in the USA and is dedicated to finding innovative solutions to global health and development problems • Started the Global Alliance for Vaccines and Immunisation (GAVI), an independently governed initiative (Yamey, 2002)
Aid agencies	Private foundations

Union membership), and the USA's suspension of funding to the WHO in April 2020 do not align positively with global goals.

An example of how policy analysis can be used to understand how a particular policy came about is provided in Box 3.4.

> **Box 3.4. An example of policy making – smoke-free legislation**
>
> The 2007 UK Health Act resulted in all enclosed public places and workplaces becoming smoke free. The Act became law on 1 July 2007, marking the end of a decade of politicking about this issue.
>
> Walt and Gilson's (1994) policy triangle framework, where 'actors' are placed in the centre, can be used to analyse the way in which this policy came to fruition. The key actor in this case were the tobacco industry, which used its wealth to fund an organization called Forest, which campaigns for smokers' rights. It also mobilized the hospitality trade to make an economic argument that smoke-free legislation would cause huge losses for bars, restaurants and pubs. Other actors included the anti-smoking group ASH, which does not have large financial backing, the BMA (British Medical Association), Cancer Research UK, the British Lung Foundation, the Royal College of Physicians, the Trades Union Congress, the Charted Institute of Environmental Health, scientists and various government ministers and politicians. Arnott *et al.* (2007) show how this broad alliance, the Smokefree Action Coalition, lobbied the Labour government, illustrating how the various actors who are in agreement on an issue need to form strong alliances. Arguably, it was scientists who consolidated the argument by laying down strong evidence bases for legislation. Previous attempts to encourage a voluntary approach to smoking reduction remained ineffective in terms of compliance (DOH, 2004, p. 12). Opposition to the ban was strongly evident even amongst politicians, illustrating the importance of individual actors with immense power both blocking or progressing policy which chimes with Parsons' (1995) point that the role of personalities and of actual people is a missing ingredient from policy analysis. Arnott *et al.* (2007) suggest that what really led to successful implementation of the legislation was the role of the health lobby, which managed to convince the public and media of the risks of second-hand smoke, and of the greater pleasure afforded by smoke-free leisure spaces. Cairney (2009), in addition, suggests that 'policy transfer', where policy makers are influenced by what is happening in other countries, was a key feature. This, together with the mounting 'hard' scientific evidence of the dangers to health, which began to outweigh the evidence on economic harm to industry, shifted the balance of power, enabling the window of opportunity (Kingdon, 1995) to be seized.
>
> Many other countries have passed smoke-free legislation: Ireland, 2004; Canada, 2007; and Spain and Saudi Arabia 2012. The WHO (2019) reports that progress is still being made, with more countries implementing legislation, so that 65% of the world's population are now covered by tobacco control policies. However, implementation remains hugely variable in terms of how these bans are enacted, with some covering all public places (others not) and variance in terms of the age at which cigarettes can be purchased. Evidence shows that where successful implementation is achieved, health outcomes such as reduced exposure to second-hand smoke are abundantly clear, yet political and social obstacles remain evident in many countries, and the tobacco industry continues to lobby hard against legislative changes (Gruer *et al.*, 2012). Gonzalez-Salgado *et al.* (2020) argues that policy in this area has not accounted for inequalities in attitudes, and health behaviours across communities and therefore call for a public health inequalities perspective in future. Furthermore, legislation also needs to be accompanied with health promotion services in the form of smoking cessation support to enable individuals to quit.

In terms of moving on in the 21st century, health promoters have become more sophisticated in borrowing ideas from political science and using policy analysis in developing their policy work (Cairney and Weible, 2017). Rutten *et al.* (2011) developed a model for health promotion policy called ADEPT in their attempt to move theory into practical steps. The model identifies the causal drivers that influence policy making and then explains the logic of events that can determine policy impacts. They claim that the model is of practical value to health promotion as 'it actually aids actors to influence the policy process' (Rutten *et al.*, 2011, p. 328), which of course is what it's all about, because understanding the policy process remains crucial to the success and sustainability of health promotion initiatives, in all contexts (Robertson-James *et al.*, 2017).

Summary

This chapter has established that policy is crucial to health and more particularly that health in all policies is a central aspect of health promotion. Every sector of policy making, and all policies, therefore need to give consideration to health and how it might potentially impact upon health outcomes.

Divergent views remain about how policy is, and should be, developed, enacted and implemented, and how the impacts of policy on health should be measured, as this chapter has illustrated. Debates about power and whose interests are served within the policy-making process remain ongoing. All of these debates have implications for health promotion practitioners and therefore health promotion practice involves advocating and becoming involved within the policy-making process.

The centrality of policy to health promotion thinking can result in those working on the ground feeling disempowered, as they are often not in positions where they *can* influence policy. They may be working in what is really a health education role. This does lead some to move jobs, and to seek a position where it is more possible to effect policy change. But what also could help is a shift in thinking, adoption of advocacy roles and developing a more holistic approach which *could* incorporate a contribution to health in all policies.

Note

[1] The previous version of this chapter entitled 'Healthy Public Policy' was written by Louise Warwick-Booth, Rachael Dixey and Jane South.

Further Reading

Farmer, P., Kleinman, A., Young, K. and Basilicio, M. (eds) (2013) *Reimagining Global Health: An Introduction*. University of California Press, Berkeley, California.

Hill, M. and Irving, Z. (2020) *Exploring the World of Social Policy: An International Approach*. Policy Press, Bristol, UK.

McInnes, C., Lee, K. and Youde, J. (2020) *The Oxford Handbook of Global Health Politics*. Oxford University Press, Oxford, UK.

Schrecker, T. and Bambra, C. (2015) *How Politics Makes Us Sick: Neoliberal Epidemics*. Palgrave Macmillan, Basingstoke, UK.

References

Abercrombie, N., Hill, S. and Turner, B.S. (2006) *Penguin Dictionary of Sociology*. Penguin Books Ltd, London.

Adeleye, O.A. and Ofili, A.N. (2010) Strengthening intersectoral collaboration for primary health care in developing countries: can the health sector play broader roles? *Journal of Environmental and Public Health*, article ID 272896, doi: 10.115/2010/272896

Afesorgbor, S.K. and Demena, B.A. (2018) Globalization may actually be better for the environment. *The Conversation*, 24 April 2018. Available at: http://theconversation.com/globalization-may-actually-be-better-for-the-environment-95406 (accessed 20 May 2019).

Akerman, M., Mercer, R., Franceschini, M.C., Penaherrera, E., Rochja, D., Weiss, V.P.A. and Moyses, S.T. (2019a) Curitiba Statement on Health Promotion and Equity: voices from people concerned with global inequities. *Health Promotion International* 34, i4–i10.

Akerman, M., Moyses, S.T., Franco de Sa, R.N.P., Mendes, R., Nogueira, J.A.D., Zancan, L., Manoncourt, E. and Wallerstein, N. (2019b) Democracy and health promotion. *Health Promotion International* 34, S1 i1–i3 doi: 10.1093/heapro/daz016

Alston, P. (2018) Statement on Visit to the United Kingdom, by Professor Philip Alston, United Nations Special Rapporteur on extreme poverty and human rights. Available at: https://www.ohchr.org/EN/NewsEvents/Pages/DisplayNews.aspx?NewsID=23881&LangID=E (accessed 2 October 2019).

Angell, M. (2004) *The Truth about the Drug Companies: How They Deceive Us and What to Do About It*. Random House, New York.

Arno, A. and Thomas, S. (2016) The efficacy of nudge theory strategies in influencing adult dietary behaviour: a systematic review and meta-analysis. *BMC Public Health* 16, 1–11.

Arnott, D., Dockrell, M., Sandford, A. and Willmore, I. (2007) Comprehensive smoke free legislation in England: how advocacy won the day. *Tobacco Control* 16, 423–428.

Asbridge, M. (2004) Public place restrictions on smoking in Canada: assessing the role of the state, media, science and public health advocacy. *Social Science & Medicine* 58, 13–24.

Bambra, C., Fox, D. and Scott-Samuel, A. (2005) Towards a politics of health. *Health Promotion International* 20, 187–193.

Barnes, C. (2007) Disability activism and the struggle for change: disability, policy and politics in the UK. *Education, Citizenship and Social Justice* 2, 203–221.

Barnes, M. and Walker, A. (1996) Consumerism versus empowerment: a principled approach to the involvement of older service users. *Policy and Politics* 24, 375–393.

Barrett, E., Heycock, M., Hick, D. and Judge, E. (2003) Issues in access for disabled people: the case of the Leeds transport strategy. *Policy Studies* 4, 227–242.

Barry, J. and Doherty, B. (2001) The Greens and social policy. *Social Policy and Administration* 35, 387–609.

Basu, L. (2019) Living within our means: the UK news construction of the austerity frame over time. *Journalism: Theory, Practice, and Criticism* 20(2), 313–330.

Baum, F. (2001) Health, equity, justice and globalisation: some lessons from the People's Health Assembly.

Journal of Epidemiology and Community Health 55, 613–616.

Baum, F., Lawless, A., Delany, T., Macdougall, C., Williams, C., Broderick, D., Wildgoose, D., Harris, D., McDermott, D., Kickbush, I. and Marmot, M. (2016) Evaluation of Health in All Policies: concept, theory and application. *Health Promotion International* 29, S1.

Bird, L., Hayton, P., Caraher, M., McGough, H. and Tobutt, C. (1999) Mental health promotion and prison health-care staff in young offenders' institutions in England. *The International Journal of Mental Health Promotion* 1, 16–24.

Blakemore, K. and Griggs, E. (2007) *Social Policy. An Introduction*. Open University Press, Maidenhead, UK.

Bornstein, D. (2007) *How to Change the World*. Updated edn. Oxford University Press, New York.

Boseley, S. (2003) Sugar industry threatens to scupper WHO. *The Guardian*, 21 April.

Bou-Karroum, L., El-Jardali, F., Hemadi, N., Faraj, Y., Ojha, U., Shahrour, M., Darzi, A., Ali, M., Doumit, C., Langlois, E.V., Melki, J. Haidar, A. and Akl, E.A. (2017) Using media to impact health policy-making: an integrative systematic review. *Implementation Science* 12, 1.

Brand, H., Rosenkitter, N., Clemens, T. and Michelsen, K. (2013) Austerity policies in Europe – bad for health. *British Medical Journal* 346, 7.

Brehm, M.V. (2001) *Promoting Effective North–South NGO Partnerships*. Occasional paper series 35. INTRAC, Oxford, UK.

Brown, R.C. (2018) Resisting moralisation in health promotion *Ethical Theory and Moral Practice* 21, 997–1011.

Buck, D. (2018) The NHS should redefine its role to tackle health inequalities. *Health Services Journal*. Available at: https://www.hsj.co.uk/health-inequalities/the-nhs-should-redefine-its-role-to-tackle-health-inequalities-/7022029.article (accessed 10 May 2020).

Cairney, P. (2009) The role of ideas in policy transfer: the case of UK smoking bans since devolution. *Journal of European Public Policy* 11, 57–77.

Cairney, P. and Weible, C.M. (2017) The new policy sciences: combining the cognitive sciences of choice, multiple theories of context, and basic and applied analysis. *Policy Sciences* 50, 619–627.

Caraher, M., Dixon, P., Hayton, P., Carr-Hill, R., McGough, H. and Bird, L. (2002) Are health-promoting prisons an impossibility? Lessons from England and Wales. *Health Education* 102, 219–229.

Carlisle, S. (2010) Tackling health inequalities and social exclusion through partnership and community engagement? A reality check for policy and practice aspirations from a Social Inclusion Partnership in Scotland. *Critical Public Health* 20(1), 117–127.

Carlisle, S. (2000) Health promotion, advocacy and health inequalities. *Health Promotion International* 15, 369–376.

Castano J., Ospina, J.E., Cayla, J.A. and Greer, S.L. (2016) Restricting access to health care to immigrants in Barcelona: a mixed-methods study with immigrants who have experienced an infectious disease. *International Journal of Health Services* 46(2), 241.

Chapman, J., Edwards, C. and Hampson, S. (2009) *Connecting the dots*. Demos, London. Available at: http://www.demos.co.uk/publications/connecting-the-dots (accessed 6 November 2012).

Chastin, S., De Clecq, B. and Van Cauwenberg, J. (2018) In tackling our physical inactivity pandemic, we risk ignoring those who need the most help. *The Conversation*, 8 November 2018. Available at: https://theconversation.com/in-tackling-our-physical-inactivity-pandemic-we-risk-ignoring-those-who-need-the-most-help-106456 (accessed 10 May 2020).

Cheetham, M., Moffat, S. and Addison, M. (2018) 'It's hitting people that can least afford it the hardest': the impact of the roll out of Universal Credit in two North East England localities: a qualitative study. Teesside University, Middlesborough, UK. Available at: https://www.gateshead.gov.uk/media/10665/The-impact-of-the-roll-out-of-Universal-Credit-in-two-North-East-England-localities-a-qualitative-study-November-2018/pdf/Universal_Credit_Report_2018pdf.pdf?m=636778831081630000 (accessed 17 August 2020).

Chen, M., Jhabvala, R., Kanbur, R. and Richards, C. (eds) (2007) *Membership-based Organisations of the Poor*. Routledge, New York.

Colebatch, H.K. (2002) *Policy*, 2nd edn. Open University Press, Philadelphia, Pennsylvania.

Cook, A. (2015) Partnership working across UK public services: evidence review. What Works Scotland, Scotland.

Craig, R.L., Felix, H.C., Walker, J.F. and Phillips, M.M. (2010) Public health professionals as policy entrepreneurs: Arkansas's childhood obesity policy experience. *American Journal of Public Health* 100, 2047–2052.

Crammond, B.R. and Carey, G. (2017) Policy change for the social determinants of health: the strange irrelevance of social epidemiology. *Evidence & Policy* 13, 365–374.

Crow, D. and Jones, M. (2018) Narratives as tools for influencing policy change. *Policy and Politics* 46, 217–234.

Dahlgren, G. and Whitehead, M. (1991) *Policies and Strategies to Promote Social Equity in Health*. Institute of Futures Studies, Stockholm.

Davies, S.E. (2010) *Global Politics of Health*. Polity, Cambridge, UK.

Dean, M. (2011) *Democracy Under Attack – How the Media Distort Policy and Politics*. The Policy Press, Bristol, UK.

Delaney, F. (1994) Muddling through the middle ground: theoretical concerns in intersectoral collaboration and health promotion. *Health Promotion International* 9, 217–225.

Dixey, R. and Woodall, J. (2012) The significance of 'the visit' in an English category-B prison: views from prisoners, prisoners' families and prison staff. *Community, Work and Family* 15, 29–48.

DOH (2004) *Choosing Health: Making Healthier Choices Easier*. The Stationery Office, London.

Douglas, R. (1998) A framework for healthy alliances. In: Scriven, A. (eds) *Alliances in Health Promotion. Theory and Practice*. Macmillan, Basingstoke, UK, pp. 3–17.

Dowling, B., Powell, M. and Glendinning, C. (2004) Conceptualising successful partnerships. *Health and Social Care in the Community* 12, 309–317.

Easterly, W. (2003) MF and World Bank structural adjustment programs and poverty. In: Frankel, J.A. and Dooley, M.P. (eds) *Managing Currency Crises in Emerging Markets*. University of Chicago Press, Chicago, Illinois.

Esping-Anderson, G. (1990) *The Three Worlds of Welfare Capitalism*. Polity Press, Cambridge, UK.

Fast, I., Sorensen, K., Brand, H. and Suggs, L.S. (2015) Social media for public health: an exploratory policy analysis. *European Journal of Public Health* 25(1), pp. 162–166.

Fidler, D.P. (2007) Architecture amidst anarchy: global health's quest for governance. *Global Health Governance* 1, 1–17.

Fowler, A. (1998) NGOs in Africa: achieving comparative advantage in relief and micro development, IDS Discussion Paper 249. Institute of Development Studies, Brighton, UK.

Fraser, H. (2005) Four different approaches to community participation. *Community Development Journal* 40, 286–300.

Freudenberg, N. (2005) Public health advocacy to change corporate practices: implications for health education, practice and research. *Health Education and Behaviour* 32, 298–319.

Gagliani, M. (2019) Smoking ban in the United Kingdom. Available at: https://www.centreforpublicimpact.org/case-study/smoking-ban-united-kingdom/ (accessed 2 October 2019).

Galer-Unti, R.A., Tappe, M.J.K. and Lachenmayr, S. (2004) Advocacy 101: getting started in health education advocacy. *Health Promotion Practice* 5, 280–288.

Gardiner, B. (2019) *Choked: The Age of Air Pollution and the Fight for a Cleaner Future*. Granta, London.

Gavens, I., Holmes, J., Buykx, P., de Vocht, F., Egan, M., Grace, D., Lock, K., Mooney, J.D. and Brennan, A. (2019) Processes of local alcohol policy-making in England: does the theory of policy transfer provide useful insights into public health decision-making? *Health and Place* 59, 358–364.

Gilmore, A.B., Savell, E. and Collin, J. (2011) Public health, corporations and the New Responsibility Deal: promoting partnerships with vectors of disease? *Journal of Public Health* 33(1), 2–4.

Givel, M. (2007) Consent and counter-mobilization the case of the national smokers alliance. *Journal of Health Communication* 12(4), 339–357.

Gonzalez-Salgado, I., Rivera-Navarro, J., Sureda, X. and Franco, M. (2020) Qualitative examination of the perceived effects of a comprehensive smoke-free law according to neighborhood socioeconomic status in a large city. *SSM Population Health* 11, 100597.

Grand Challenges in Global Health (2012) Available at: http://gcgh.grandchallenges.org/about (accessed 13 September 2016).

Green, C.P., Heywood, J.S and Navarro, M. (2018) *Did the London Congestion Charge Reduce Pollution?* Economics Working Paper Series 2018/007. Lancaster University, Lancaster, UK.

Griswold, M.K. (2017) Reframing the context of the breastfeeding narrative: a critical opportunity for health equity through evidence-based advocacy. *Journal of Human Lactation* 33, 415–418.

Gruer, L., d'Espaignet, T., Haw, S., Fernández, E. and Mackay, J. (2012) Smoke-free legislation: global reach, impact and remaining challenges *Public Health* 126, 227–229.

Guldbrandsson, K. and Fossum, B. (2009) An exploration of the theoretical concepts policy windows and policy entrepreneurs at the Swedish public health arena. *Health Promotion International* 4, 434.

Gunn, L.A. (1978) Why is implementation so difficult? *Management Services in Government* 33, 169–176.

Hallsworth, M. with Parker, S. and Rutter, J. (2011) *Policy Making in the Real World: Evidence and Analysis*. Institute for Government, London.

Harkins, C. (2010) The Portman Group – Lobby Watch column. *British Medical Journal* 340, b5659.

Hill, M. (1997) *The Policy Process in the Modern Society*, 3rd edn. Prentice Hall, London.

Hill, M and Hupe, P. (2009) *Implementing Public Policy*, 2nd edn. Sage, London.

Hogwood, B. (1987) *From Crisis to Complacency? Shaping Public Policy in Britain*. Clarendon, Oxford, UK.

Hogwood, B. and Gunn, L. (1984) *Policy Analysis for the Real World*. Oxford University Press, Oxford.

Horton, R. (2020) Offline: CoHERE: a call for a post-pandemic health strategy. *The Lancet* 395(10232), 1242.

Hudson, B. (2002) Interprofessionality in health and social care: the Achilles' heel of partnership? *Journal of Interprofessional Care* 16, 7–17.

Hudson, J. and Lowe, S. (2004) *Understanding the Policy Process. Analysing Welfare Policy and Practice*. The Policy Press, Bristol, UK.

Hudson, J., Kuhner, S. and Lowe, S. (2008) *The Short Guide to Social Policy*. The Policy Press, Bristol, UK.

Huff, A.D. (2017) Addressing the wicked problem of American gun violence. *Journal of Macromarketing* 37(4), 393.

Jentsch, B. (2004) Making Southern realities count: research agendas and design in North-South collaborations. *International Journal of Social Research Methodology* 7, 259–269.

Joffe, M. and Mindell, J. (2004) A tentative step towards health public policy. *Journal of Epidemiology and Community Health* 58, 966–968.

Johnston, R. and Deeming, C. (2016) British political values, attitudes to climate change, and travel behavior. *Policy and Politics* 44, 191–213.

Karanikolos, M., Mladovsky, P., Cylus, J., Thomson, S., Basu, S., Stuckler, D., Mackenbach, J.P. and McKee, M. (2013) Financial crisis, austerity, and health in Europe. *Lancet* 381(9874), 1323–1331.

Karger, H., Midgley, J. and Risal, S. (2014) Austerity versus stimulus. *Journal of Sociology and Social Welfare* 41(2), 3–10.

Kaufmann, S. (2009) *The New Plagues. Pandemics and Poverty in a Globalised World*. Haus Publishing, London.

Kemm, J. (2001) Health impact assessment: a tool for healthy public policy. *Health Promotion International* 16, 79–85.

Kerasidou, A. and Cribb, A. (2019) Austerity, health and ethics. *Health Care Analysis: An International Journal of Health, Philosophy and Policy* 27(3), 153.

Kickbusch, I. and Reddy, K.S. (2015) Global health governance – the next political revolution. *Public Health* 129, 838–842.

Kickbusch, I., Draper, R. and O'Neill, M. (1990) Healthy public policy: a strategy to implement the Health for All philosophy at various governmental levels. In: Evers, A., Farrant, W. and Trojon, A. (eds) *Healthy Public Policy at the Local Level*. European Centre for Social Welfare Policy and Research, Vienna, 1–6.

Kingdon, J.W. (1995) *Agendas, Alternatives and Public Policy*. Harper, New York.

Krieger, N. (2011) *Epidemiology and the People's Health : Theory and Context*. Oxford University Press, Oxford, UK.

Kuye, R., Donham, K., Marquez, S., Sanderson, W., Fuortes, L., Rautiainen, R., Jones, M. and Culp, K. (2007) Pesticide handling and exposures among cotton farmers in The Gambia. *Journal of Agromedicine* 12, 57–69.

Labonté, R. and Schrecker, T. (2004) Committed to health for all? How the G7/G8 rate. *Social Science & Medicine* 59(8), 1661–1676.

Labonté, R. and Laverack, G. (2010) Capacity building in health promotion, Part 1: For whom? And for what purpose? *Critical Public Health* 11, 111–127.

Larkin, F., Uduma, O., Akinmayọwa, S.A. and van Bavel, B. (2017) Developing a framework for successful research partnerships in global health. *Globalization and Health* 12, 17, doi: 10.1186/s12992-016-0152-1

Lipsky, M. (1980) Street level bureaucracy: dilemmas of the individual in public services. Russell Sage. In: Hill, M. (ed.) *(1993) The Policy Process: A Reader*. Prentice Hall, London.

Lukes, S. (2005) *Power: A Radical View*. Palgrave Macmillan, Basingstoke, UK.

Macdonald, T. (2007) *The Global Human Right to Health: Dream or Possibility?* Radcliffe Publishing, Oxford, UK.

Manandhar, M., Maimbolwa, M., Muulu, E., Mulenga, M.M. and O'Donovan, D. (2008) Intersectoral debate on social research strengthens alliances, advocacy and action for maternal survival in Zambia. *Health Promotion International* 24, 58–67.

Manji, F. (2006) Collaboration with the South: agents of aid or solidarity? In: Eade, D. (ed.) *Development, NGOs and Civil Society*. Oxfam, Oxford, UK.

Mantoura, P. and Morrison, V. (2016) *Policy approaches to reducing health inequalities*. National Collaborating Centre for Healthy Public Policy, Canada.

Markel, H. (2014) Worldly approaches to global health: 1851 to the present. *Public Health* 128, 124–128.

Marmot M. (2010) *Fair Society, Healthy Lives: Strategic Review of Health Inequalities in England Post-2010*. Institute of Health Equity, London.

Marmot, M. (2015) *The Health Gap: The Challenge of an Unequal World*. Bloomsbury, London.

Marmot, M., Allen, J., Boyce, T., Goldblatt, P. and Morrison, J. (2020) *Health Equity in England: The Marmot Review Ten Years On*. Institute of Health Equity, London.

Marsh, D. and Rhodes, R.A.W. (1992) *Policy Networks in British Government*. Clarendon Press, Oxford, UK.

Maycock, B., Howat, P. and Levin, T. (2001) A decision-making model for health promotion advocacy: the case of drunk driving control measures. *Promotion and Education* 8, 59–64.

McKee, M. and Stuckler, D. (2018) Revisiting the corporate and commercial determinants of health. *American Journal of Public Health* 108(9), 1167–1170.

McKeown, T. (1979) *The Role of Medicine: Dream, Mirage or Nemesis?* Blackwell, Oxford, UK.

McNeill, D., and Ottersen, O.P. (2015) Global governance for health; how to motivate political change? *Public Health* 129, 833–837.

Melamed, C. and Ladd, P. (2013) How to build sustainable development goals: integrating human development and environmental sustainability in a new global agenda. ODI, London.

Mills, C. Wright (1959) *The Sociological Imagination*. Oxford University Press, New York.

Mohindra, K.S. (2007) Healthy public policy in poor countries: tackling macro-economic policies. *Health Promotion International* 22, 163–169.

Monks, P. (2020) Coronavirus: lockdown's effect on air pollution provides rare glimpse of low-carbon future. *The Conversation*, 15 April. Available at: https://theconversation.com/coronavirus-lockdowns-effect-

Morgen, S. (2002) *Into Our Own Hands: The Women's Health Movement in the United States, 1969–1990*. Rutgers University Press, New Brunswick, New Jersey.

NHS (2014) *Five Year Forward View*. Available at: https://www.england.nhs.uk/wp-content/uploads/2014/10/5yfv-web.pdf (accessed 3 June 2020).

Nuffield Bioethics Council (2007) Public health: ethical issues. Available at: https://www.nuffieldbioethics.org/publications/public-health (accessed 20 May 2020).

Nunes, J. (2020) The COVID-19 pandemic: securitization, neoliberal crisis, and global vulnerabilization. *Cadernos de Saude Publica* 36(5), doi: 10.1590/0102-311x00063120

Nutbeam, D. (1993) Advocacy and mediation in creating supportive environments for health. *Health Promotion International* 8, 165–166.

Nutbeam, D. (1998) Health Promotion Glossary. *Health Promotion International* 13, 349–364.

OECD (2017) *Government at a Glance 2017*. OECD Publishing, Paris. Available at: http://dx.doi.org/10.1787/gov_glance-2017-en

Ollilia, E. (2005) Global health priorities – priorities of the wealthy? *Globalisation and Health* 1, 1–6.

Parsons, W. (1995) *Public Policy: An Introduction to the Theory and Practice of Policy Analysis*. Edward Elgar, London.

People's Health Movement (2012) Available at: http://www.phmovement.org/ (accessed 30 January 2012).

Perkmann, M. (2002) *Policy entrepreneurs, multilevel governance and policy networks in the European Polity: The case of the EUREGIO*. Department of Sociology, Lancaster University. Available at: http://www.lancs.ac.uk/fass/sociology/papers/perkmann-policy-entrepreneurs.pdf (accessed 3 November 2012).

Platt, L. (2019) What is social policy? International, interdisciplinary and applied. Available at: http://www.lse.ac.uk/social-policy/about-us/What-is-social-policy (accessed 1 October 2019).

Potts, L., Dixey, R. and Nettleton, S. (2007) Bridging differential understanding of environmental risk of breast cancer: why so hard? *Critical Public Health* 17, 337–350.

Potts, L., Dixey, R. and Nettleton, S. (2008) Precautionary tales: exploring the obstacles to debating the primary prevention of breast cancer. *Critical Social Policy* 28, 115–135.

Pursch, B., Tate, A., Legido-Quigley, H. and Howard, N. (2020) Health for all? A qualitative study of NGO support to migrants affected by structural violence in northern France. *Social Science and Medicine* 248, https://doi.org/10.1016/j.socscimed.2020.112838

Reilly, R.G. and McKee, M. (2012) 'Decipio': examining Virchow in the context of modern democracy. *Public Health* 126, 303–307.

Roberts, I. with Edwards, P. (2010) *The Energy Glut. The Politics of Fatness in an Overheating World*. Zed Books, London and New York.

Roberts, N.C. and King, P.J. (1991) Policy entrepreneurs: their activity structure and function in the policy process. *Journal of Public Administration Research and Theory* 2, 147–175.

Robertson, N.M., Sacks, G. and Miller, P.G. (2019) The revolving door between government and the alcohol, food and gambling industries in Australia. *Public Health Research & Practice,* 29(3).

Robertson-James, C., Sawyer, L., Nunez, A., Campoli, B., Robertson, D., Devilliers, A., Congleton, S. and Alexander, S. (2017). Promoting policy development through community participatory approaches to health promotion: the Philadelphia Ujima experience. *Women's Health Issues* Suppl 1, S29–S37.

Roderick, P. and Pollock, A. (2018) Rights that protect against socioeconomic disadvantage are long overdue – the UK is already paying the price. *The Conversation*, 7 December. Available at: https://theconversation.com/rights-that-protect-against-socioeconomic-disadvantage-are-long-overdue-the-uk-is-already-paying-the-price-108439 (accessed 10 May 2020).

Ruckert, A. and Labonté, R. (2017) Health inequities in the age of austerity: the need for social protection policies. *Social Science & Medicine* 187, 306–311.

Rutten, A., Gelius, P. and Abu-Omar, K. (2011) Policy development and implementation in health promotion – from theory to practice: the ADEPT model. *Health Promotion International* 26, 322–329.

Salajan, A., Tsolova, S., Ciotti, M. and Suk, J.E. (2020) To what extent does evidence support decision making during infectious disease outbreaks? A scoping literature review. *Evidence and Policy* 1–23, doi: https://doi.org/10.1332/174426420X15808913064302

Seedhouse, D. (1997) *Health Promotion: Philosophy, Prejudice and Practice*. John Wiley & Sons, Chichester, UK.

Sharma, R. (no date) *An Introduction to Advocacy: A Training Guide*. Office of Sustainable Development, USAID, Africa Bureau.

Shilton, T., Champagne, B., Blanchard, C., Ibarra, L. and Kasesmup, V. (2013) Towards a global framework for capacity building for non-communicable disease advocacy in low- and middle-income countries. *Global Health Promotion* 20(4 Suppl), pp. 6–19.

Smith, K.E. (2013) *Beyond Evidence Based Policy in Public Health: The Interplay of Ideas*. [ebook] Palgrave Macmillan, UK

Smithies, J. and Webster, G. (1998) *Community Involvement in Health: From Passive Recipients to Active Participants*. Ashgate Publishing, Aldershot, UK.

Spicker, P. (2014) *Social Policy: Theory and Practice*, 3rd edn. Policy Press, Bristol, UK.

Stenning, A. and Hall, S.M. (2018) On the frontline: loneliness and the politics of austerity. *Discover Society*. Available at: https://discoversociety.org/2018/11/06/on-the-frontline-loneliness-and-the-politics-of-austerity/ (accessed 10 May 2020).

Stevens, A. (2007) Survival of the ideas that fit: an evolutionary analogy for the use of evidence in policy. *Social Policy and Society* 6, 25–35.

Stuckler, D., Reeves, A., Loopstra, R., Karanikolos, M. and McKee, M. (2017) Austerity and health: the impact in the UK and Europe. *European Journal of Public Health* 27, 18–21. Available at: https://doi.org/10.1093/eurpub/ckx16

Sutton, R. (1999) *The Policy Process: An Overview*. Working paper 118. Overseas Development Agency, London.

Taylor, P. (2003) The lay contribution to public health. In: Orme, J., Powell, J., Taylor, P., Harrison, T. and Grey, M. (eds) *Public Health for the 21st Century: New Perspectives on Policy, Participation and Practice*. Open University Press, Maidenhead, UK, pp. 128–144.

Tesh, S. (1988) *Hidden Arguments: Political Ideology and Disease Prevention Policy*. Rutgers University Press, New Brunswick, New Jersey.

Thaler, R.H. and Sunstein, C.R. (2009) *Nudge: Improving Decisions about Health, Wealth and Happiness*. New International edn. Penguin, London.

Tones, K. and Green, J. (2004) *Health Promotion: Planning and Strategies*. Sage, London.

United Nations (2011) High Level Meeting on the Prevention and Control of Non-communicable Diseases. Available at: http://www.un.org/en/ga/ncd-meeting2011/ (accessed 1 May 2020).

United Nations (UN) (2020) *The Paris Agreement*. Available at: https://unfccc.int/process-and-meetings/the-paris-agreement/the-paris-agreement (accessed 19 May 2020).

Vivian, J. (1994) NGOs and sustainable development in Zimbabwe: no magic bullets. *Development and Change* 25, 181–209.

Walt, G. (1994) *Health Policy: An Introduction to Process and Power*. Zed Books, London.

Walt, G. and Buse, K. (2006) Global cooperation in international public health. In: Merson, M.H., Black, R.E. and Mills, A.J. (eds) *International Public Health: Diseases, Programs, Systems and Policies*. Jones and Bartlett Publishers, Boston, Massachusetts, pp. 649–680.

Walt, G. and Gilson, L. (1994) Reforming the health sector in developing countries: the central role of policy analysis. *Health Policy and Planning* 9, 353–370.

Walt, G., Shiffman, J., Schneider, H., Murray, S.F., Brugha, R. and Gilson, L. (2002) Doing health policy analysis: methodological and conceptual reflections and challenges. *Health Policy Planning* 23, 300–317.

Warwick-Booth, L., Cross, R. and Lowcock, D. (2021) *Contemporary Health Studies: An Introduction*, 2nd edn. Polity Press, Cambridge, UK.

Wells, J.S.G. (2007) Priorities, 'street level bureaucracy' and the community mental health team. *Health and Social Care in the Community* 5, 333–342.

WHO (1986) Ottawa Charter for health promotion. *Health Promotion* 1, iii–v.

WHO (1997) *Jakarta Declaration on Leading Health Promotion into the 21st Century*. WHO, Geneva. Available at: http://www.who.int/healthpromotion/conferences/previous/jakarta/declaration/en/index1.html (accessed 12 October 2012).

WHO (2000) *Mexico Ministerial Statement for the Promotion of Health: From Ideas to Action*. Fifth Global Conference on Health Promotion: Bridging the Equity Gap, Mexico, 5–9 June. WHO, Geneva.

WHO (2005) *The Bangkok Charter for Health Promotion in a Globalised World*. WHO, Geneva. Available at: www.who.int/healthpromotion/conferences/6gchp/bangkok_charter/en/index.html (accessed 12 October 2012).

WHO (2011) *Rio Political Declaration on Social Determinants of Health*. Available at: http://www.who.int/sdhconference/declaration/en/ (accessed 1 May 2020).

WHO (2013) *The Helsinki Statement on Health in All Policies. The 8th Global Conference on Health Promotion*, Helsinki, Finland, 10-14 June.

WHO (2014) WHO calls on countries to reduce sugars intake among adults and children. Available at https://www.who.int/mediacentre/news/releases/2015/sugar-guideline/en/ (accessed 7 June 2020).

WHO (2019) *WHO Report on the Global Tobacco Epidemic* 2019. Available at https://www.who.int/tobacco/global_report/en/ (accessed 7 June 2020).

WHO (2020) *Health Topics. Health Impact Assessment*. Available at: https://www.who.int/topics/health_impact_assessment/en/ (accessed 7 June 2020).

Wilkinson, R. (1996) *Unhealthy Societies: The Afflictions of Inequality*. Routledge, London.

Wilkinson, R. and Pickett, K. (2009) *The Spirit Level: Why More Equal Societies Almost Always Do Better*. Allen Lane, London.

Williams, O. and Fullagar, S. (2019) Lifestyle drift and the phenomenon of 'citizen shift' in contemporary UK health policy. *Sociology of Health and Illness* 41, 20–35.

Wilson-Clay, B., Rourke, J.W., Bolduc, M.B., Stagg, J.D., Flatau, G. and Vagh, B. (2005) Learning to lobby for probreastfeeding legislation: the story of a

Texas bill to create a breastfeeding-friendly physician designation. *Journal of Human Lactation* 21, 191–198.

Wren-Lewis, S. (2016) What Brexit and austerity tell us about economics, policy and the media. Sheffield Political Economy Research Institute, 36. Available at: http://speri.dept.shef.ac.uk/wp-content/uploads/2018/11/SPERI-Paper-36-What-Brexit-and-austerity-tell-us-about-economics-policy-and-the-media.pdf (accessed 14 May 2020)

Yamey, G. (2002) Why does the world still need WHO? *British Medical Journal* 325, 1294–1298.

Yuill, C., Crinson, I. and Duncan, E. (2010) *Key Concepts in Health Studies*. Sage, London.

4 Health Communication

RUTH CROSS AND IVY O'NEIL[1]

> This chapter aims to:
> - consider models of communication and assess their relevance to health communication;
> - suggest that health promotion must adopt participatory means of communication;
> - critique top-down 'banking' approaches to communication and education;
> - discuss the implications of digital technology development on health communication;
> - assert the importance of health education and consider the idea of health literacy;
> - explore and critique social marketing; and
> - explore and critique psychological models of behaviour change.

Introduction

We asserted in the previous chapters that our view of health promotion is that of a social movement aimed at bringing social justice in health, and that it contains three broad areas of activity – working with communities, influencing policy and communicating about health. This chapter takes up the last of those three areas. The chapter first considers some of the models of communication that are now regarded as being too simplistic to understand the process of communication, but which were products of their time. Although they are now dated, they continue to influence the way that communication is perceived – as a one-way, top-down process of information transfer. Use of the latter has gained health education a bad name, as victim blaming and ineffective. Humanistic models of education are therefore explored, in an attempt to outline which ideas of education are truly helpful in bringing about empowered communities. Useful ideas from the counselling and psycho-analytic literature are also presented. This chapter thus explores the importance of health communication in promoting health and attempts to address some of the issues in communicating health messages including the impact, and implications, of developing digital technology. It will also critically look at theories about health behaviour, and how messages can be translated into behaviour changes. It covers social marketing and health literacy in relation to communicating health messages, as these have become part of the modern public health discourse. Following the themes of the book, we assert that methods that involve communities and individuals, which are 'bottom-up', are essential in enabling people to take control of their own health.

Given the importance of health communication, the understanding of effective communication within health promotion has not really received the same attention as other health promotion theories and models. This is surprising, as communication plays a critical role in the promotion of health (Cross *et al.*, 2017). Health communication is about communicating health messages that hopefully will help people to think about their health and the determinants of their health, and to change their behaviour if that is appropriate. The issue is not because there is a lack of health information (there might in fact be too much at times) but that health messages are inconsistent, uncoordinated and out of step with the way people live their lives (Blue *et al.*, 2016; Brown, 2018) – see the case study on Covid-19 later in this chapter for illustration. Health messages are often communicated in a top-down manner, which is not always appropriate, is culturally insensitive or simply does not seem relevant to the people for whom the information is intended. It is clear through the philosophy of this book that we adopt an asset-based view of people, seeing people as resourceful. However, there are situations where people do need information from an expert, and there are examples where people do not have basic, correct information. How health promoters can provide such information in ways that are empowering is a conundrum that this chapter hopes to address. Moreover, there are obvious links between communication and some of the other key values outlined previously, such as participation. This chapter, more than others, crosses over into issues of health care, as well as of health promotion. Often one-to-one communication is with patients, and the need for patient education can be described as a neglected area within health promotion (Hubley, 2006).

The advance of digital technology in the past few decades has also had an impact on health communication. Through the development of Web 1.0 to the interactive Web 2.0 and now the Internet of Things era, there is no doubt that the development of digital technology has facilitated and improved the communication of health messages, enhancing health service provision, increasing accessibility, effectiveness and efficiency as well as the management of healthcare services. The increase of global connectivity also gives rise to the Big Data phenomenon and a concern on the quality and accuracy of information as well as data security (O'Neil, 2019). In the latter part of this section on communication, we will explore the implications of digital technology on public health and health promotion and critically consider the impact of it on health inequality and health equity.

Communication

Basic communication theories

Early health education assumed that a change in people's knowledge and beliefs would translate to a change in their behaviour. This perspective suggests that communication is unidirectional, uncomplicated, involving a linear flow of information from experts to individuals (Lee and Garvin, 2003).

Health practitioners often ask 'Why don't they listen?' 'They' are the 'public' and health promotion has tended to have an obsessive emphasis on changing 'their' behaviour. Health messages are only considered effective when the audience has acted or responded to a message in some way (Corcoran, 2013). The focus of effective intervention is often placed on the intended recipients – Did they get the message? Have they changed their behaviour? Evaluation tends to focus on the outcomes, or the impact, rather than on the process of intervention. The latter would involve asking searching questions: Am I an effective communicator? Have I chosen the right communication method? Was the design of the health messages appropriate? *Why* are our health messages not effective? Successful intervention is of course about the health promoters as much as the intervention itself. Having good communication skills as well as understanding the factors that influence the effectiveness of health messages are seen as essential to health educators and promoters. Later in this chapter, some of these skills at an interpersonal level are considered in more detail. First, we discuss theories of communication.

'In health education, communication is a planned process which is effective when the client attains certain goals' (Kiger, 2004, p. 84). This two-way communication concerns the exchange of meanings through a common set of symbols, a process that involves the transmission of a 'coded' message between a source and an audience, 'a process in which participants create and share information with one another to reach a mutual understanding' (Rogers, 1995, p. 17). Lee and Garvin (2003) argue that we should move beyond the traditional practices, the one-way information transfer, toward a more useful and appropriate concept of information exchange – a two-way communication (Fig. 4.1). This is, of course, more consistent with participatory ways of working and with dialogue, rather than simply telling people what to do.

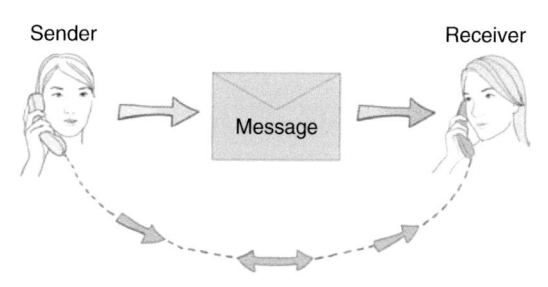

Fig. 4.1. Messages sent from the health promoter to the individual. It then goes forward and backward between the two.

The development of communication theories

In its conventional wisdom about communication, health promotion has borrowed ideas from the long-standing study of communication as a discipline. At the beginning of the 'mass media' period, Lasswell (1948) developed the classic formula for communication (Box 4.1) – 'who says what to whom in which channel with what effect'. This formula is well known to those who subscribe to the transmission model of communication where communication is about the transfer of information from the source to the recipients.

This traditional linear model of communication is a one-way process where the main purpose is to transmit a message; the purpose of effecting a change within the recipient is implicit. An historical perspective is essential here, as Lasswell was developing his ideas at a point when the power of fascist regimes was at its height, and the power of propaganda machines appeared terrifying. The persuasive power of the top-down communication message symbolized the power of mass communication.

The Shannon–Weaver model of communication (1949) (Box 4.2), another linear transmission model of the same period, included a further element – 'noise', meaning anything that could interfere with the effective transmission of the message.

Traditional linear models of communication do not reflect the richness and dynamics of the process of human communication (Rogers, 1986). We now see communication more as a cyclical process (Corcoran, 2013), or at least a two-way process (Kiger, 2004), as theorized by Osgood and Schramm's model of communication (Steinberg, 2006) (Fig. 4.2). They saw communication as a circular process where messages are passed between coders and encoders (senders and receivers). The communication process is endless – the sender can become the receiver, and the receiver becomes the sender, both giving and receiving feedback and interpreting each other's messages. The interpretation of the message is the 'noise' in their model where messages can be misinterpreted by different coders and encoders. The meaning of the messages thus changes depending on who is decoding and encoding those messages.

Within health promotion, Green *et al.* (2019) present a communication model (Fig. 4.3) that clearly shows the communication process and the reciprocal relationship between the sender and the receiver. The model shows how messages are encoded by the sender and decoded by the receiver. The message can be transmitted through a symbolic means such as a picture; iconic means such as a pink ribbon for breast cancer or red ribbon for HIV/AIDS; or through an 'enactive code' such as an exercise involving participation. It also shows that memory and motivation have an influence on the interpretation of messages.

These models tend to view communication as a rational and technical process, and they are widely used in planning and developing health campaigns. McGuire's communication/persuasion model (1989), for example, suggests five 'input variables' – source, message, channel, receiver and destination – and there are many texts that elaborate on the most effective ways of manipulating these variables to maximize impact (e.g. Kreuter and McClure, 2004). Looking at this critically, two questions can be posed. First, is the process of communication a rational and technical process or an emotional, 'messy', complex set of processes? Secondly, is the idea of developing persuasive messages potentially dangerous and when does it become manipulation? The latter question is even more complex in a situation where knowledge needs are quite legitimate and where, in addition, health promoters *do* have an agenda – that is, we *would* prefer people to make healthy choices, not to smoke and so on. In other words, health promoters

---

Box 4.1. The Lasswell Formula (1948).

Who (communicator) → Says what (message) → How (medium or channel) → To whom (receiver) → With what effect (impact).

Box 4.2. Shannon–Weaver model of communication (1949).

Transmitter (information source – giving a signal) → Noise (some kind of interference) → Receiver (message reaches destination).

are interested in getting the message across, and in methods that result in people changing their health for the better. (Some of the ethical issues raised by communication methods are explored in more detail in Chapter 5.) So the whole area of what are appropriate and effective means of communicating about health is complex and difficult.

Educating 'the public' and communicating health messages

Many health care practitioners and indeed members of the general public, and view health promotion as providing information, or advice giving – a health education approach to health promotion (Naidoo and Wills, 2016). Gambling (2003, p. 68) writes, 'The aims of any health education programme are to improve knowledge about the [health] condition, increase health-promoting behaviours and enhance compliance with medication and treatment regimens'. The medical model thus sees the importance of information-giving, adherence to advice and, in particular, tends to assume that change in an individual's knowledge, attitudes and beliefs results in the change of that person's behaviour. If the evidence is reliable enough, then the individual will act rationally and change should follow, as in the diagram in Fig. 4.4.

The assumption is that provision of information should be enough to 'empower' people, enabling them to make healthy choices and improve their health regardless of their social and environmental context. Thus telling someone to always sleep under an insecticide-treated bed net, or giving someone a diet sheet at a doctor's surgery, will inevitably produce changes. This is clearly fatuous. Evidence suggests that people do often know how to protect their health but cannot, due to their material circumstances, or they have taken deliberate decisions not to act on the advice provided, or they do intend to act on the information but other factors intervene.

The one-way transfer of knowledge in health education, however, remains prevalent, and according to Lee and Garvin's view (2003) can be closely linked to the transmission of knowledge perspective in education (Pratt and Associates, 2005), where education is about imparting or acquiring knowledge from one person to another. Effective transmission of knowledge is content focused, based on the sender's expertise in the subject matter and their skills in delivering that content (Pratt and Associates, 2005). Using the acquisition metaphor as described by Sfard (1998),

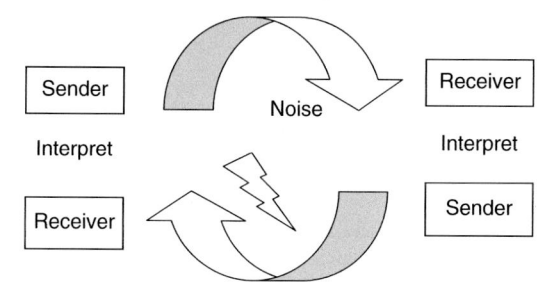

Fig. 4.2. Adapted from Osgood and Schramm's model of communication.

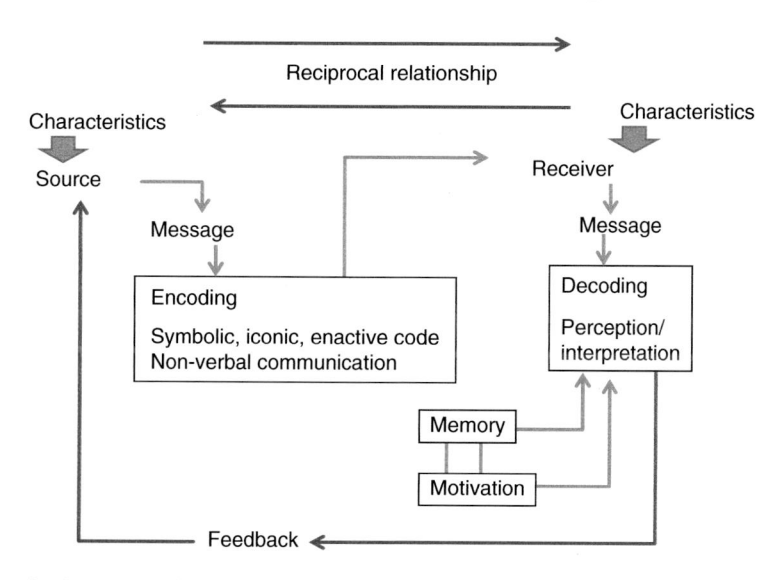

Fig. 4.3. A communication model (Green *et al.*, 2019, p. 345).

Information → Increased knowledge → Change in attitude → Change in behaviour → Better health outcomes

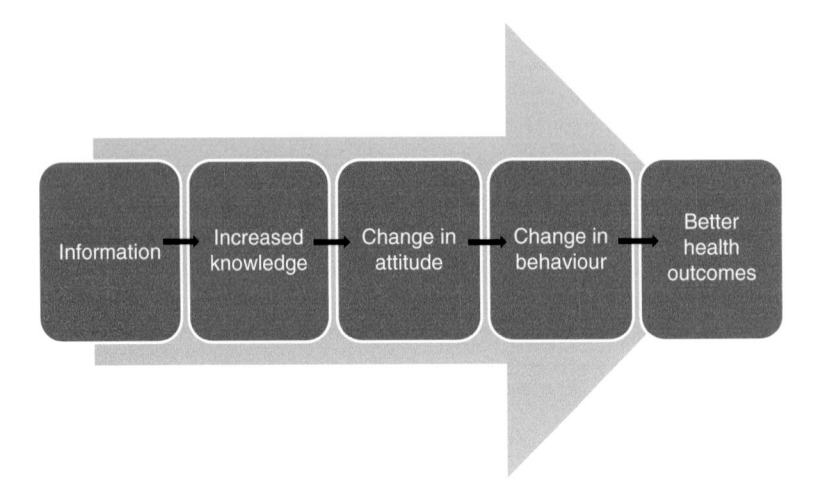

Fig. 4.4. Key assumptions underpinning health education approaches.

human learning is conceived of as an acquisition of something, gaining ownership over a body of knowledge. Knowledge is seen as a commodity, which can be applied, transferred and shared with others. The owner of that knowledge becomes privileged in some way, possessing something which others do not have (Sfard, 1998). This encompasses a 'deficit' model whereby the non-expert recipient of the knowledge is viewed as deficient in some way, which may, in turn, be described as a paternalistic perspective.

This one-way transfer of knowledge focuses on the individual message recipient and the scientific knowledge of the expert (Lee and Garvin, 2003); the health promoter is the expert who gives advice and information to the people. Many health practitioners do align themselves with this top-down approach to health promotion, but it is one of the reasons why health education began to be seen as victim blaming, resulting in the paradigm shift to 'health promotion'. If health promotion is about empowerment, then we clearly have to reject this approach to education. And if 'knowledge is power' then we clearly have to think through what approaches to education, knowledge-transfer and health communication will truly empower individuals and communities. We also need to recapture the important place of education within health promotion. Health education is an integral part of health promotion and, arguably, there is an educative element in *all* efforts to promote health.

Moving to two-way, transformational education methods

Lee and Garvin (2003) argue that health practitioners must move from a monologue information *transfer* model of practice to a dialogue information *exchange* in order to reorient health communication practice. Likewise, Campbell and Cornish (2010, p. 1)

> …distinguish between technical communication (the transfer of health-related knowledge and skills from experts to communities) and transformative communication (a more politicised process, where marginalised groups develop critical understandings of the social roots of their ill-health, and the confidence and capacity to tackle these).

The latter addresses the balance of power and control assumed by the 'expert'. This is particularly needed in public health where health communications tend to be firmly rooted in individual behaviour, ignoring the social context and the adaptive power of the people (Lee and Garvin, 2003). This way of 'doing' health promotion can be seen as similar to Freire's (2000) 'banking approach' to education, where the experts have a body of knowledge that they transmit to learners. Freire believed that 'banking' approaches to education serve only to mould oppressed people to fit into the roles expected of them by society; the aim is to immobilize people. He believed education should be dialogical, similar to the social reform perspective we see in education (Pratt and Associates, 2005).

Earlier, Dewey (1916) argued that the purpose of education should not revolve around the acquisition of a pre-determined set of skills, but rather the realization of one's full potential and the ability to use those skills for the greater good. He believed that education provides a catalyst for personal and social change and development. Education is a problem-solving activity and it facilitates democracy. He considered education to be the key to empower people. Hence education would raise people's consciousness of health issues, so that they are able to make choices and eventually create pressure for healthy public policies (Naidoo and Wills, 2016), transforming society.

Dewey's humanistic and liberal approach shows that education can ultimately facilitate social change (Purdy, 1997). He challenged the authoritarian relationship between teachers and learners, arguing that schools should be run along democratic lines, which was a major challenge at the time to the hierarchical nature of schools, where children had little or no power. The teacher's role is not to transmit knowledge to passive students; rather, s/he should be a facilitator and guide, a partner in the learning process. Carl Rogers' humanistic view of education (Rogers, 1969; Kirschenbaum and Henderson, 1989) carries on this theme, asserting that we cannot teach another person directly, we can only facilitate his or her learning. Rogers is perhaps more well known for developing person-centred counselling, but his views on education have been equally influential, placing the learner in the centre of the learning process and promoting the dignity and self-efficacy of learners. These ideas have now been mainstreamed to a greater or larger extent in different parts of the world, but they were revolutionary when Rogers first introduced them.

Education and learning are social and interactive processes with the potential to bring about social reform, building a society of mutual respect (Freire, 2000). Freire was, of course, writing at a time when there was a dictatorship in his native Brazil and his 'pedagogy of the oppressed' aimed to give a voice to those who had no choice but to be silent. He started by developing a system of teaching literacy, not merely teaching people to read and write, but at the same time developing their political consciousness, an awareness of their true position in the world. The main purpose of education is therefore to develop skills of enquiry in our social world, not merely to transmit what is known.

Dewey believed that education should strike a balance between delivering knowledge while also taking into account the interests and experiences of the student. This can be related to the participatory metaphor of Sfard (1998), which emphasizes togetherness, solidarity, collaboration and people in action in a constant flux. Thus, in educational contexts, in order for education to be effective, content must be presented in a way that allows students to relate the information to prior experiences, thus deepening the connection with the new knowledge.

In health promotion, many of our learners are adults, implying that the principles of adult learning and of informal learning need to be understood. Adult learners are motivated to learn what they need to know, bringing with them their experience and knowledge; they tend to be problem-centred self-directed learners, driven internally to learn (Bach *et al.*, 2007). In adult education, according to Knowles (1980), the purpose is to enhance adult learners' ability to be self-directed in their learning. The educator's task is to facilitate learning, and prepare and share sufficient information and knowledge to help the learners participate in the learning process.

The humanistic view is that every human being is capable of looking at the world critically, in a 'dialogical encounter' with others. Education therefore needs to be based on dialogue, not curricula where people act *on* one another, but on people working *with* each other – a problem-posing education, a process of consciousness raising (Freire, 2000). Freire believed that through education, people can be liberated, see their oppression and act to change it. Through education, the learners' world is being 'decoded' so that they become aware of the oppressive forces that shape their lives; they would be able to gain power to transform these forces, to reflect on their situation, enabling them to take some control over their lives. Discussion and sharing experience help learners to explore diverse perspectives, recognize and investigate their assumptions, develop new appreciation for continuing differences, encourage attentive respectful listening, increase intellectual agility, help learners to learn the process and habits of democratic discourse, leading to transformation where we assimilate knowledge in a critical manner to become responsible decision makers (Mezirow, 1981). Unlike Dewey, Rogers and Knowles, Freire's view relates education even further to the social dimension of the education process and challenges the individualism of the humanistic perspective. Health promotion is therefore much more than educating the individual. It is about empowering, building skills, making conscious decisions and ultimately changing society.

The aim of education is thus to bring about social change in a collective manner, producing a better society. Health promotion teaching relates closely to the social reform perspective in education, learners are encouraged to look at the principles and values of promoting health. Probing questions are asked to provoke thinking. Learners are encouraged to question their practice. They are asked to critically discuss, analyse the literature and their practice, synthesize and apply their learning in practice.

Empowerment is central to health promotion, as is social change. If students are empowered to learn, to understand critically the beliefs and values of society, it is possible to bring about social change. Social reform is based on a constructivist approach to the understanding of the world (Pratt and Associates, 2005). Critical approaches in questioning the truth help to challenge the assumptions of knowledge and realities. Students learn through the reconstruction of knowledge and incorporating it into the social realities of their lives. The acquisition metaphor (Sfard, 1998), the one-way transfer of knowledge (Lee and Garvin, 2003) or the transmission perspective in education (Pratt and Associates, 2005) alone do not give power to the individual. As in health promotion, the top-down medical, educational or behavioural approach (Naidoo and Wills, 2016) to health promotion does not empower the people as we aspire to do in practice. Teaching based on the social change perspective enables learner engagement, encourages learners to critically look at their learning, and relate their learning to their social context, and thus helps learners to take action to change their lives.

Transformative or profound learning is where a 'shift' in the horizons of one's life world is experienced to the extent that it causes questioning of self-identity and has an impact on how the world is perceived, interpreted and acted on. Mezirow, a key thinker in understanding transformative educational experiences, asserts that in order for transformational learning to take place, learners have to intentionally want to learn from an experience; thus willingness to learn is a key aspect – transformational learning will not take place 'by accident' – the learner has to want learning to happen (Mezirow, 2003). This implies something about the 'attitude' that learners need to bring with them to the educational encounter. Earlier, Rogers pondered on the nature of 'significant' learning, whereby experiential learning can lead to self-actualization, where learners want to become more than they are. A related idea, of 'threshold concepts' (Meyer and Land, 2005), suggests that crossing a threshold can transform one's world view and/or cause a 'shift in perspective (that) may lead to a transformation of personal identity, a reconstruction of subjectivity' (Meyer and Land, 2005, p. 376). Whereas most learning is not *that* transformational or profound, it can provide learning that is transferable, enabling the release of capacity for action in a range of spheres or new situations. This transferable learning may have transformative power. (Standing up and giving a talk in a village meeting *could* lead to having the confidence to stand up in the corridors of power such as a national assembly.)

In contrast to some of these ideas, Appiah (2006, p. 73) argues that the way that people 'move' is through 'just a gradually acquired new way of seeing things'. Whether people learn and develop through sudden leaps of transformation or more gradually over time, profound learning can take them to a crossroads, which Baxter Magolda (2001), as noted above in Chapter 1 on empowerment, says is essential in terms of 'becoming the author of one's own life'. This notion clearly links with empowerment and has implications for the way that health promoters need to work to facilitate 'profound learning'. Health promoters can help people change their lives in less transformational ways, and a common phrase in health promotion is 'small steps', i.e. helping people to make small but significant changes, which are accumulative. We now turn attention to the characteristics of the messengers or educators.

The Communication Process as Conventionally Applied in Health Promotion

Hubley *et al.* (2021) present a model that clearly illustrates the characteristics of the four key components of the communication process – senders, messages, channels and receivers – with many factors within each component that could affect the effectiveness of health messages. They also include the feedback loop within their model to demonstrate the importance of feedback within the communication process. Conventionally, each of these components in the journey of messages from the senders through to the receivers need to be scrutinized in turn in order to improve the effectiveness of health communication. The discussion below

Table 4.1. The components within the communication process.

Senders	Who we are and how we communicate
	Our communication skills – verbal, non-verbal, written
	Interpersonal communication skills
	Do we listen to the message receivers?
Messages	Type of messages, simple or complicated, its appropriateness
Channels	Communication methods, vehicle used
	The environment where the messages were transmitted
Receivers	Who are the audience – their literacy level, their state of mind, their views, their beliefs and their attitudes?

(Table 4.1) uses the four components (senders, messages, channels and receivers) to frame an exploration and critique.

The senders

In any communication, the sender often assumes that they are a credible source and that they are doing everything correctly. However, humanistic education (which challenges the power dynamic between teachers and learners) and the newer models of communication (which stress the role of the relationship between senders and receivers of messages) have facilitated a move to understanding the role, credibility, motives and skills of the communicator or teacher. In simple terms, the focus has shifted from seeing the 'problem' as residing in the receiver (or learner) to seeing failures of communication as residing in the sender (or teacher). For example, Fraser and Restrepo-Estrada (1998) cited experiences from Bolivia, Uganda and Algeria where a range of workers in health and agriculture had such poor communication styles, were condescending, did not listen and were too theoretical, that their work could not be effective. Effective, reflective practitioners clearly will take time to reflect on their own communication styles, methods and effectiveness, though in practice, practitioners do not always take this time. Here are some useful ideas, which help to illuminate the processes of human interaction.

Communication is a necessary process in any human relationship, and certainly is essential in the relationship between health promoters and the individuals and communities they work with. It is transactional, inevitable, purposeful, multi-dimensional and irreversible (Hargie *et al.*, 1994). It takes place within (and is influenced by) the context, e.g. geographical location, time, relationships. Interpersonal communication is about face-to-face interaction that involves few people – a process by which information, meanings and feelings are shared by persons through the exchange of verbal and non-verbal messages in a social interaction (Cross *et al.*, 2017).

Credibility of the source of information is very important in health communication, with the perceived authority of the message source affecting the receivers' acceptance of the message; for example, on a superficial level, gender and age can be an influence. The communication skills and style are also important, highlighting the need for communicators to be self-aware and to design and communicate messages in a way acceptable to the audience.

The Johari window (Luft and Ingham, 1955), is a useful tool in interpersonal communication, helpful for both community members to question their status in the process of conscientization, and also for health professionals needing to consider how they come across to the community they are working with. Created by Joseph Luft and Harry Ingham in 1955, it consists of a four-paned 'window' (Box 4.3) representing open, hidden, blind and unknown areas. The lines dividing the four panes are like window shades, which can move as an interaction progresses. If you know yourself well and others know you, you are in a more open relationship with others. Through feedback from others and self-disclosure, you learn more about yourself. Being aware of your own strengths and weaknesses helps you to know more about yourself and your actions when you communicate.

The Johari window challenges the usual power relationship between health promoters and the groups or individuals they are working with. The top-down expert would not be expected necessarily to share their own thoughts, feelings and insecurities with their 'client' groups; a health promoter working in an open, dialogical way would need to do this if they were truly being transparent and honest in their dealing with the community.

Transactional analysis (Berne, 1964) is another approach to understanding the psychological

> **Box 4.3. Johari Window, adapted from Luft and Ingham (1955).**
>
> | | Known to self | Unknown to self |
> |---|---|---|
> | Known to others | Free and open, known to others and self – the impression you know you are giving | Blind self – the impression you may be giving, unknown to yourself |
> | Unknown to others | Hidden self – you know, but others don't, the part of you that you hide | Unknown self – both you and others don't know |

> **Box 4.4. Transactional analysis, adapted from Berne (1964).**
>
> | Parent | Nurturing, controlling | Feel and behave in ways learnt from mother, father, teacher, etc. It concerns taking responsibility or taking charge. |
> |---|---|---|
> | Adult | Rational | Observe, collect data, think, weigh probable outcomes of alternate course, make decisions. |
> | Child | Feeling, intuiting, adapting | Feel and behave typically as a child; you experience strong feelings and emotions, create, have fun, adapt to or feel bad about the demands of more powerful people. |

> **Box 4.5. I'm OK – you're OK, adapted from Harris (2004).**
>
> | | |
> |---|---|
> | I'm OK – You're OK | Fine with yourself and accept others |
> | I'm OK – You're not OK | Uncomfortable with yourself but disown it and reflect on other |
> | I'm not OK – You're OK | Feel sorry for yourself and think others doing better |
> | I'm not OK – You're not OK | Unhappy about yourself and negative towards others |

interpretation of how and why we act as we do when we interact with others (Box 4.4). It is useful to understand and be aware of the way we act when we are communicating with others. It draws on Freudian psychodynamic theory and was developed by Eric Berne. Berne identifies three observable changes in personalities – parent, adult, child – the three ego states within every individual's personality. At any given moment, each individual in a social situation will exhibit a parent, adult or child ego state. In each one of us, one state is more dominant than the others. We use these three states when interacting with others. Do we present ourselves as a parent when we deliver our health message, taking a paternalistic approach in imparting our knowledge, a top-down, medical or educational approach? Or do we present our health messages in an emotional manner – behave like a child when we discuss important issues with clients? It is important that we know how we communicate with others, behave as an adult and treat others as adults when we communicate, taking a dialogical approach that empowers the learner, an empowerment approach.

Within transactional analysis, it is suggested that we adopt four orientations towards other people and the world around us when we communicate (Harris, 2004). Health educators working from a top-down perspective can adopt the position of a controlling parent telling a child what to do, and implicitly from a 'deficit' position of 'I'm OK – you're not OK' (Box 4.5). Using these kinds of ideas to reflect critically on the communication process may help to increase understanding of why so many messages appear to 'fail'.

In terms of moving towards more empowering encounters between health workers and patients or people in the community, a number of attempts have been made to capture what creates that empowerment (Feste and Anderson, 1995; Kettunen et al., 2001, 2003). Attention has also been given to the non-verbal communication of workers, which can communicate a clear and strong message – more than the message sender realizes (Kiger, 2004). Non-verbal communication such as body language, facial expressions, eye contact, tone of voice and personal space can transmit messages that we did not intend to pass on – the blind self. Studies show that during interpersonal communication, 7% of the message is verbally communicated while 93% is transmitted non-verbally. Out of the 93% non-verbal communication, 38% is through vocal tones and 55% is through facial expressions (British Institute of Learning Disability, 2005). Often we communicate our feelings about our views and attitudes via our body language, sometimes in conflict with our verbal message, a non-verbal leakage such as lack of genuineness or empathy (Green et al., 2019). Active listening is regarded as an essential skill of health promoters (Hubley et al., 2021). It demonstrates genuine understanding and empathy of the other's point of view, whilst the ability to show respect can help to build rapport and establish trust.

The channel and the message

Marshall McLuhan's famous dictum, 'The medium is the message', was coined in 1967. He argued that 'societies have always been shaped more by the nature of the media by which men communicate than by the content of the communication' (McLuhan and Fiore, 1967, p. 1). The meaning for us is that the choice of medium used is more important than the message itself. He was writing at a time when mass media had arrived in the developed world. He wrote:

> The medium, or process, of our time – electric technology – is reshaping and restructuring patterns of social interdependence and every aspect of our personal life. It is forcing us to reconsider and re-evaluate practically every thought, every action, and every institution formerly taken for granted. Everything is changing – you, your family, your neighbourhood, your education, your job, your government, your relation to 'the others'. And they're changing dramatically.
> (McLuhan and Fiore, 1967, p. 1)

Clearly, these points are echoed in the 21st century with the arrival of electronic media, but whereas he wrote that the 'television generation is a grim bunch' (p. 126), the arrival of electronic technology is seen by many as allowing new forms of expression, a new pluralism and greater democracy. We will revisit this later in the chapter.

A wide range of methods and channels is used to communicate health messages ranging from interpersonal, to groups and mass media, and at the individual, local, national and international levels. Examples are: face-to-face discussion or forms of counselling; written communication such as leaflets and posters; participatory arts such as drama, role play, storytelling, games and songs; and mass communication through television, film, radio, newspaper, mail shots, billboards and digital communication such as the internet, podcast, YouTube and mobile phone. This list is by no means exhaustive. Studies of successful health communication suggest that a combination of channels contributes to success (Laverack and Dap, 2003).

Health communication is a goal-orientated activity – the designer's goal is to prompt active thought in what they presume is a passive audience. Well-designed messages can motivate people, who then will actively seek, attend and process messages. For example, unexpected or discrepant content can trigger active thought in a passive audience, such as outlining fat content on the menu in a restaurant (Maibach and Parrott, 1995). For education to be effective, participatory learning is needed to promote learner engagement and enhance the understanding and acceptance of health messages, enabling people to internalize and act on the message to suit their needs and make changes according to their situation. Thus, although a great deal of energy and resources have gone into mass audience campaigns, their effectiveness can be questioned. Recently, the use of celebrities by the mass media has become a popular and useful way of attracting attention, encouraging people to be actively involved in health activities, doing what their admired personalities want them to do. Many examples have shown how celebrities raise the profile of health issues. For example, Bob Geldof seriously shamed world leaders over their neglect of world hunger through his 'Feed the World' campaigns in 1984 and 1991 and, in the UK, the celebrity chef Jamie Oliver led a crucial campaign not only highlighting the need for healthier food in schools but also showing how it could be achieved. Whether these campaigns do effect sustainable change is a moot point.

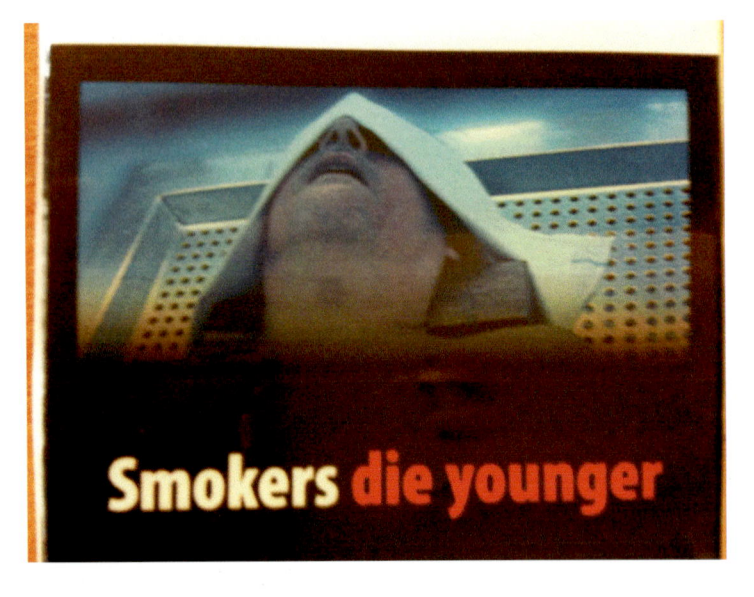

How effective are health warnings? ('Unscary health warnings' by renaissancechambara is licensed under CC BY 2.0)

The receivers

As health communicators, it is essential to understand the 'audience' – the individuals and communities worked with – to understand their knowledge levels, their beliefs and, more importantly, their constraints – the barriers they are facing when making health choices. The design of the messages and the methods in communicating the messages need to be acceptable, bearing in mind the characteristics of the audience, the situation they are in, their demographics as well as psychographics. For example, people often want information when they have become ill, but how can health messages be designed to suit patients' needs in hospital, and is it a good time to promote health when they are ill? Is it unrealistic to expect people in poverty to be able to act on healthy eating advice and to choose 'healthy' food? Their age, gender, cultural background, their ability and disability, their mental health state, literacy levels, their living and work environment all need to be taken into consideration.

It is generally agreed that health care provision should be culturally appropriate, and so should health communication. It is worth unpicking the wide-ranging label of 'culture'. Culture can be defined as: 'the learned, shared, and transmitted knowledge of values, beliefs, norms and life ways of a particular group that guides their thinking, decisions, and actions in a patterned way' (Leininger, 1991, p. 47). However, 'culture' is a complex concept, more often assumed than assessed (Kreuter *et al.*, 2003). Health promotion materials that are designed for a population-based health education programme may not always be culturally appropriate for the numerous possible cultural groups and sub-groups in any given society. Often health promotion materials are translated and adapted to different cultural groups from the mainstream health promotion materials rather than specifically developed for a particular group or population (Larkey and Hecht, 2010). Further, individuals within 'cultures' are not all alike.

Messages cannot be 'free' of cultural perspectives, but it is obviously important to understand what cultural perspectives are shown. Reflecting the values and norms of a particular audience, specifically designed narrative-based health promotion programmes such as storytelling, drama, soap operas and radio broadcasts can be used to produce culturally grounded health messages (Larkey and Hecht, 2010). Kreuter *et al.* (2003) discuss the five strategies often used to ensure culturally appropriate health education material. These are: (i) peripheral strategies where materials are packaged to appeal to a given group; (ii) evidential strategies where the relevance of the health issues is directed to a particular group; (iii) linguistic strategies where materials are translated to the group's language; (iv) constituent-involving strategies where experiences are drawn directly from members of the group; and (v) sociocultural strategies where health issues are discussed in the context of the broader social and cultural values and characteristics of the intended audience. Targeting the needs of the audience can also be seen in 'audience segmentation' as in social marketing strategies as discussed later in this chapter.

The theme of lay knowledge, which runs through this book, is also pertinent here. People's experiences and beliefs can impact on their health-seeking behaviour. Some may wonder if the knowledge from one individual's experience can be generalized in health care. However, privileging expert, scientific knowledge over lay knowledge can undermine clinical practice (Henderson, 2010), impacting on the health communication process and health promotion practice. For a detailed discussion of lay beliefs and knowledge, please see Chapter 1.

Mass Media Communication

The growth in the use of mass media to influence people rose to prominence in the propaganda campaigns of the Second World War (Grant, 1994). It has since been widely used as a method in transmitting health messages to the public particularly to promote behaviour change. Ours is a media-driven society and mass media is a powerful agent of communication. It can be argued the media has a medicalized approach to health. Coverage is about the prevention of ill health rather than the promotion of good health. It relates health promotion to lifestyle problems and unhealthy influences, e.g. tobacco, alcohol, fast food, selling health rather than giving choices to the people. It is a 'tragedy' or sensationalist model with interests focused on newsworthy topics that will attract public attention.

In general, mass communication media for health promotion can be categorized into four different types (Corcoran, 2013). They are:

- audio-visual broadcast media such as television and, radio;
- audio-visual non-broadcast media such as video, CD, DVD and self-help packages;
- print media such as newspaper, magazine, leaflets, mail shots and billboards; and
- digital media such as internet, YouTube and mobile phones.

Mass media is one-way communication with messages transferred from the source to a presumed receptive audience. The message is impersonal. Direct feedback from the audience can be difficult to obtain. Mass media can have a strong influence on the public's perception of health issues (e.g. the perception in 1998 in the UK that the MMR injection can cause autism and irritable bowel syndrome). Once the message is broadcast, the interpretation is left to the receivers. The communicators have no control. Conventionally, health promoters see many advantages in the use of mass media, and are influenced by the putative success of commercial advertisers. Mass media can reach a large number of audiences in a very short space of time. However, there is no guarantee that the message will reach the target audience or that it will be understood, despite careful planning of the timing, location and type of media. Although it is expensive to produce a short media message, considering the size of audience it can reach, it could be argued that it is relatively cheap.

Mass media in itself doesn't change the structural, political and economic factors that influence health. However, it can be an effective strategy if it is supported by appropriate policies (Wakefield *et al.*, 2010). It is useful in raising awareness of health issues. It cannot provide face-to-face support or teach psychomotor skills, e.g. cooking skills, and cannot be regarded as an effective education tool. Short repeated health messages, which are reinforced regularly, can be useful as a constant reminder and have more impact, but can only convey simple information rather than complex information. It does help to place health on the public agenda, stimulate public debate and create pressure for policy changes, particularly where grassroots community organizations are involved. Evidence suggests that mass media can only be effective if used as an integral part of a campaign where multiple interventions are used (Wakefield *et al.*, 2010). The provision of supporting services to the public is an important element to support mass media health promotion. For example, when encouraging the public to stop smoking it can limit the impact if smoking cessation services are not available.

It is commonly asserted that 'mass' media is now a misnomer, as the possibility of capturing mass audiences is reduced by the proliferation of channels and outlets (Abroms and Maibach, 2008). Broadcasting can be reconceived as narrowcasting, although globalization has also produced a contraflow to this trend, with events being shown in many countries simultaneously, and the same products (TV shows, for example) being shown around the world. For example, *Shuga* was shown all over Africa in 2010; a television drama with an overt didactic element, about the lives and loves of a group of young students in Nairobi, it was seen by 60% of Kenyan youth, and 90% of these said the show had an impact on their thinking (Singh, 2011).

Communication Theories Relating to Mass Communication

One of the earliest models relating to mass media is the 'direct effect' model or the 'hypodermic needle' model, where media has a direct influence on the public, like a needle injecting a message into the people. The propaganda campaigns in the Second World War were based on this model. However, Mendelsohn (1968) saw mass media messages as an 'aerosol spray' model, where some of the spray hits the target and most of it drifts away. One of the limitations of this was demonstrated by the 'uses and gratification' theory in which it is believed that individuals interact and select messages suiting their own needs (Blumler and Katz, 1974).

Lazarsfeld and Merton (1955) identified three conditions for the effectiveness of mass media:

1. Monopolization – limited opposition of the messages in the media.
2. Canalization – messages are consistent with audience's existing motivation, it tells people what they want to hear.
3. Supplementation – it is supported by interpersonal influences, emphasizing the role of the change agent.

This links to Katz and Lazarsfeld's work on the two-step model of communication. Katz and Lazarsfeld (1955) incorporated the interpersonal aspect of communication into their work and developed the two-step flow model where mass media information is channelled to the 'masses' through opinion leaders to a wider population. The opinion leader acts as an enforcer to clarify, strengthen and enforce the importance of the message. Individuals are seen as more influential than the media: as Rogers (1983) points out, the first step is a transfer of information only, and it is the second step that provides the transfer of influences. This encourages the reception of messages showing that interpersonal communication has a superior effect on influencing changes as compared with mass media. Opinion leaders are not the only people who receive information from the mass media and they also receive information through other channels (Windahl *et al.*, 2009). This also demonstrates the lack of control in the communication process from the health communicators' point of view.

The two-step flow model laid the foundation for the study of the Diffusion of Innovations (Rogers, 2003). The principle is that an innovation (the message) can be communicated through certain channels (e.g. opinion leaders) over time among the members of a social system. The model originated from Rogers and Shoemaker's (1971) communication of innovations theory, which emphasizes the important role of the change agent and interpersonal communication. The process demonstrates a slow initial uptake of the innovation, how it then gathers momentum and slows down again when saturation is reached, creating an S-shaped curve (Green *et al.*, 2019).

The process of the adoption of any message goes through five stages (Rogers, 2003):

- knowledge – exposure to the message and developing understanding of it;
- persuasion – the forming of a favourable attitude to the message;
- decision – commitment to the adoption of the initiative;
- implementation – applying it to practice; and
- confirmation – reinforcement of the message based on positive outcomes.

The success of adoption depends on the encounter of the adopters through each stage of the process, e.g. the quality and comprehensiveness of knowledge obtained; the credibility of the information source; the acceptability of the innovation in the social system; the persuasiveness of the message; the factors influencing decision making in taking up the innovation; how easily can it be implemented; and the support provided after the implementation of the innovation. The communicator as the change agent plays an important role in the adoption process. It is acknowledged that the message becomes stronger when the adopters become the change agents themselves (Rogers, 2003). The principle of homophily also suggests that people can easily be influenced by others who are similar to themselves (Windahl *et al.*, 2009). This can be linked to peer education, where people accept health information readily from their own peers. It also reinforces the strength of interpersonal communication over the mass media channels.

Peer education

Peer education is a health promotion method used widely, particularly in programmes relating to young people's health. However, it has broader applications. Peer education has been defined as the sharing of information, attitudes or behaviours by people who are not professionally trained educators but whose goal is to educate (Finn, 1981) and where peers from the same societal group educate each other (Svenson, 1998). Peer educators can be powerful change agents, useful in promoting behaviour change (UNAIDS, 1999). Peer education can raise awareness and increase knowledge of health issues, especially in sensitive health issues such as reproductive health (Kannappan and Shanmugam, 2019; Sheidaei et al., 2019). Behaviour change theory such as social learning theory (Bandura, 1986) underpins the idea, as the peers learn through observation and modelling. It also links to the use of behaviour models, as discussed later in this chapter, as well as Diffusion of Innovation (Rogers, 2003), where health messages are passed to the target group via their peers.

Through the use of peers, the process helps to reach so-called 'hard to reach' groups in the community. Messages from peers are more acceptable and credible. Using peer education as a health education method for breast self-examination among university students, Ayran et al. (2017) found that knowledge, skills as well as self-esteem increased considerably. Similarly, in a study by Yurt et al. (2019) on the effect of peer education on health beliefs about breast cancer screening among university students, participants were highly satisfied with the programme. They were given the opportunity to ask their peers questions without feeling uncomfortable in a stress-free learning environment. Peer education helped reduce perceived barriers, increased the perception of benefits and raised levels of self-efficacy (Yurt et al., 2019).

It is also useful in increasing knowledge and skills in other areas, such as for patients receiving chemotherapy (Heydarzadeh et al., 2019), and improving the resilience of mothers of children with leukaemia (Jamali et al., 2019). The peer education process is not only beneficial for the client group, but also benefits the peer educators themselves. It can be an empowering and transformational process, building their self-confidence (Fisher and Fisher, 2018). In a systematic review of the effectiveness and cost-effectiveness of peer education and peer support in prison, Bagnall et al. (2015) found that peer interventions are effective in reducing risky behaviour, with positive effects on knowledge and behaviour. There is also evidence that peer educators are as effective as professional educators for HIV prevention outcomes and that there is strong evidence that peer delivery is more acceptable than professional delivery. In addition, there are often positive effects on the mental health of peer workers. Evidence exists to show that peers gain a lot from being engaged in this way (Green et al., 2019). Peer-to-peer interventions can take many forms. As part of a systematic review of peer interventions in prison settings, South et al. (2017) present a typology of peer interventions that includes peer education, peer support, peer mentoring and bridging roles. This provides a framework to understand peer interventions and a platform for further research in peer interventions and the development of theory.

Some caution is needed in using peer education, particularly relating to sustainability. Prisoners who operate as peers might move back to the community. In health promotion work, young people grow up and move on after a period of time. Therefore, recruitment and selection are continuous. Ongoing training as well as supervision and support are essential for effectiveness and sustainability. Complementary activities such as improved service provision, policy and structural changes are also important to provide a supportive environment for its success. If peers are not well supported through the process, it would be unacceptable from an ethical point of view (Milburn, 1995).

People's media – traditional and popular media

Methods most relevant to people themselves and which they feel most comfortable with will probably have a greater success in enabling people to think about their health in their own social context and so have the greatest chance of bringing about desired changes to people's lives. These methods are likely to be 'bottom-up', participatory and, ultimately, empowering. There is a range of methods that are close to the people who produce them – songs, stories, dramas, proverbs and oral histories – but they could also include people's attempts to produce written materials, magazines and radio broadcasts, i.e. methods that are mediated by technology. Examples abound of approaches that work alongside people, with groups or whole communities, to communicate about health. 'Community Arts for Health' projects have gained increased attention in the last 20 years or so and have been shown to increase social cohesion and community networks, thereby increasing social capital; they can attract and engage young people and other marginalized groups, and they can produce personal change (South, 2005). These methods not only enable two-way communication, but the process of producing the communication materials can also be participatory.

Mda (1993) provides a thorough analysis of the role of popular theatre in achieving development goals in a book that, though written nearly 30 years ago, is still relevant in terms of principles. The work of the Marotholi Travelling Theatre Company in Lesotho, he argues, facilitated six processes: it (i) revitalized people's own forms of cultural expression; (ii) led to intra-village and inter-village solidarity; (iii) enabled community discussion and community decision making; (iv) provided a two-way communication process with inbuilt feedback; (v) led to conscientization; and (vi) mobilized people in support of national development. Likewise, Linney's (1995) practical manual shows how people can be involved in developing materials for health communication, particularly pictorial materials, using an empowerment paradigm.

Under this heading, we could include popularly watched television programmes, or soaps, which often have a health story as a deliberate instructional means. This includes the South African *Soul City*, which has proved to be an effective multi-media initiative tackling a range of health issues. *Tribes*, a show made in Trinidad and Tobago, used social networking and word of mouth to arrange showings in homes without televisions. Although it was only seen by 8% of young people, it raised important issues about HIV testing. It is part of the Staying Alive initiative launched in 1998. To quote its publicity material,

> The Emmy Award-winning campaign consists of documentaries, public service announcements, youth forums and web content. Staying Alive provides all its television programming rights-free and at no cost to third party broadcasters globally to get crucial prevention messages out to the widest possible audience. The Staying Alive campaign has a long term partnership between MTVNI, UNICEF, UN agencies, governments and foundations. MTVNI is also an active member of the United Nations-supported Global Media AIDS Initiative (GMAI) and the Global Business Coalition on HIV/AIDS, TB and malaria (GBC).

It thus illustrates the use of multimedia and the partnership between major players in the global health arena.

At a much more local level, in The Gambia, two terms that make sense to local people and have entered the health communication discourse are *Fankanta* and *Bantaba*. Both concepts are based on traditional values and practices and have been harnessed in new ways.

The 'Fankanta' initiative originated to highlight reproductive health in a country with high rates of fertility and maternal mortality. Although family planning is a big issue in The Gambia, it cannot be discussed openly or in public, on the radio or television. Needing to clear misconceptions surrounding family planning, a nationwide survey in 1996 assessed people's perceptions and suggestions for improvement. The results led to the Fankanta initiative. *Fankanta* is a Mandinka word meaning 'planning for the future' and is an acceptable euphemism for family planning. Since 1997, Fankanta has two components – 'Support for family planning' and 'HIV/AIDS and STI control'. Traditional leaders, community health workers, women's support groups and youth associations are strongly involved with its participatory approach involving negotiating intervention principles with partners to obtain consensus. Fankanta includes culturally sensitive strategies and gains the active participation of religious leaders. As an expression that stresses the importance of thinking about the future, it has resonance with the idea of sustainability, deferred gratification and thinking about the implications of actions on others.

The 'Bantaba' approach, derived from the Mandinka word meaning a meeting ground or a

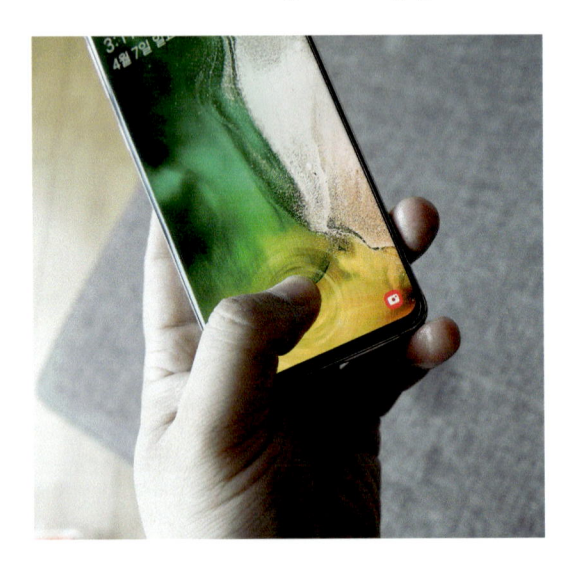

Mobile phones have spread dramatically throughout the world. (From Creative Commons source – Harbing Mobile Device by TheBetterDay licensed under CC BY-ND 2.0)

'conversation' at community level, where community members meet to discuss community issues and concerns, was initiated by a new model of health communication called 'Operation 2010' undertaken in communities by multidisciplinary health field workers. Bantaba creates a forum for community members to discuss pertinent health issues, share positive experiences and lessons, and encourage positive changes. This community forum helps to mobilize influential community leaders to take charge of promotion of health in their localities. Thus the Bantaba approach is a community-driven behaviour change strategy based on the principles of participatory appraisal and finding solutions to health problems important to communities, with health workers facilitating. It is a tool for empowerment by enhancing communication, analytical, problem-solving and health skills.

Electronic/Digital Communication

In recent decades, digital technology has progressed rapidly from Web 1.0, one-way, read only; to Web 2.0, two-way, interactive; to today's Web 3.0, 'two-way plus' communication where communication is between people and between machines with the Internet of Things or Artificial Intelligence (AI) technology (O'Neil, 2019). We are moving into the symbiotic Web 4.0 era (Almeida, 2017). Currently (April 2020), with the coronavirus pandemic, where self-isolation and social distancing are essential in preventing the spread of infection, technologies (low- or high-tech) are even more crucial for people staying at home for work, education, entertainment or social support. Technologies are valuable in public health to communicate health information to the public, particularly for strategies in infection prevention and health promotion.

New media have also been used to mobilize dissent, coordinate protest and generally bring more power to the people. In 2011's 'Arab Spring' uprising, mobile phones, social networking and other digital means were key instruments in challenging repressive governments. The radical Chinese artist Ai Wei Wei writes:

> China is at a very interesting moment. Power and the centre have suddenly disappeared in the universal sense because of the Internet, global politics, and the economy. The techniques of the Internet have become a major way of liberating humans from old values and systems, something that has never been possible until today.
>
> (Obrist, 2011, p. 6)

The capability of Information Communication Technology (ICT) in China has become huge globally and appears unstoppable as seen in the ever-expanding digital platform enterprise such as Huawei's 5G/6G network or the Alibaba group's e-commerce platform (Alibaba Group, 2019). In an era where involvement in conventional politics has waned, new media have led to a different kind of political activism, with an optimism for a different kind of democracy (Papacharissi, 2010). The vast amount of blogging and internet-based activism demonstrates that people and communities are not disinterested in current issues, politics and social affairs. The accessibility and immediacy of new media is bringing about new ways of shaping the social world. Web 2.0 interactive technology, the social web, allows users to create, collaborate and share information via virtual environments and support networks. Social media and social networking sites such as Facebook, YouTube, Instagram and Twitter, for example, are popular platforms for virtual communication and are useful 'settings' for health communication, particularly for 'hard to reach' groups (Loss *et al.*, 2014; Guo *et al.*, 2020).

At the same time, low-tech digital technology such as television, radio and telephone can still be important in health communication. These technologies can be particularly useful for people with low reading skills. Programmes such as current affairs, documentaries and debates, drama and soaps, mass media campaigns such as Don't Drink and Drive, smoking cessation and so on are popular avenues for health promotion. Radio is useful for people on the move such as professional drivers, outdoor workers, travellers, people in rural areas and those in low- and middle-income countries (O'Neil, 2019). The basic telephone is an underused technology for health care and support (Coulter and Mearns, 2016). Currently, the telephone is particularly useful during the lockdown period of coronavirus. It has become the main method for consulting with health care professionals, whilst e-prescriptions can be sent directly to the pharmacist for collection. In the UK, people suspected of having the infection can get advice over the telephone regarding actions to be taken via NHS 111.

The basic telephone has evolved to the mobile smartphone, that contains a large variety of communicative functions and health apps, providing Web 2.0 interactive communication. It can be used for simple text messaging providing tailored and personal health messages (Hazelwood, 2008; Head *et al.*, 2013); support for HIV treatment, smoking cessation, chronic illness management as well as health surveillance. Mobile phone technology is a cheap and readily available tool in healthcare. Text messaging is also useful in low resource countries (Shet *et al.*, 2010; Thirumurthy and Lester, 2012; Seidenberg *et al.*, 2012). However, the set-up costs and system maintenance can be high (Rajatonirina *et al.*, 2012). Other issues such as e-literacy and the sustainability of behaviour change also need to be considered.

Simple internet searching on digital devices is common today; for example, NHS Choices in the UK provides comprehensive health information. The ability to access information becomes an important source of social capital and aids social cohesion and communication (Bach *et al.*, 2007). There are also specific websites for long-term conditions such as diabetes and heart disease. Health apps such as those for activity tracking, management of diet and weight, smoking cessation, stress and chronic ill health can help people make informed choices and empower them to take charge of their own health (Bert *et al.*, 2014; Alghamdi *et al.*, 2015; Krebs and Duncan, 2015; Bhuyan *et al.*, 2016). The English NHS health apps library launched in 2017 provides a variety of very good health apps. However, health apps tend to lack theoretical underpinning. Evaluation on the effectiveness of behaviour change can also be inadequate (Dennison *et al.*, 2013).

Personal wearables, such as the Fitbit, have become new fashion accessories as well as empowering tools to promote health. Smart wristbands provide utilitarian purpose and aesthetic function, with a gamified element. Activity trackers help to increase physical activity levels, while data collected can help people set goals and motivate change via intrinsic or extrinsic rewards (Karapanos *et al.*, 2016). Etkin (2016) has argued, however, that counting steps may decrease people's enjoyment of walking and undermine intrinsic motivation, making physical activity a chore. They are also more likely to be used by people who are already healthy and want to quantify their progress (Piwek *et al.*, 2016). The effectiveness of technology-enhanced solutions such as wearables to reduce sedentary behaviour is clear in the short term, but can lessen over time (Stephenson *et al.*, 2017). Studies have also shown 32% of users stop wearing devices after 6 months and 50% after a year (Ledger, 2014). In addition, measuring and monitoring can turn the human body into a set of measurable data – the 'Quantified Self' (Barrett *et al.*, 2013).

Young people are 'digital residents' (White and Le Cornu, 2011) and natural internet users. The use of social media can promote self-esteem, a sense of power and control, help strengthen identity, build resilience and increase self-efficacy for young people. However, there are many unhealthy influences online, such as those from food and drink advertising. A meta-analysis by Vannucci *et al.* (2020) found a link between social media use and adolescents' risk-taking behaviour. There are also debates on screen-time usage versus levels of physical activity. Cyberbullying and abuse, cyber-racism and sexting are also important issues (Rice *et al.*, 2016), illustrating the potentially negative impact that social media can have, particularly on mental health. Online health promotion is well suited for taboo topics such as sexual health and substance misuse. However, the use of social networking sites for sexual health promotion has been limited (Gold *et al.*, 2011). Most sexual health programmes are about the problems and risky behaviour associated with sexuality and sexual habits rather than addressing positive sexual health (Lupton, 2015a). Widespread implementation is also problematic because of, for example, technical issues, reservations from teachers and parents, and blocks to websites. In addition, health education sites are generally unregulated (Mann and Bailey, 2016; Abroms, 2019).

Mental health promotion is important for keeping people mentally healthy. Globally, young people face challenges and barriers to mental health care facilities particularly in low-and middle-income countries with a high proportion of young people, both with poor health profiles and poor access to health care (Saraceno *et al.*, 2007; Hampshire *et al.*, 2015). New technology has also been used constructively for issues such as eating disorders, schizophrenia, obsessive compulsive disorder, addictive behaviour, insomnia and depression. It can also be useful for displaced populations and people in conflict zones, refugees and asylum seekers. Mental health online services are useful in providing privacy, accessibility, anonymity and confidentiality. However, access by young people is low (Lawrence *et al.*, 2015; Sweeney *et al.*, 2016; Ho *et al.*, 2016), and the most common reasons for this are about stigma and poor mental health literacy. In some low- and middle-income countries, young people have themselves developed mHealth (mobile health) informally, for example, searching for health information and getting advice. However, this shifts the responsibility for health care provision from the state onto young people themselves (Hampshire *et al.*, 2015). Barriers also exist through lack of resources, guiding policy, knowledge and skills, and support from health service management.

The Centre for Health Promotion, Women's and Children's Health Network (2012) found that most health organizations don't use social media. Those who do only use it to engage clients and promote educational messages. Information overload, inaccurate and misleading information, privacy and confidentiality, data security, sustainability, cost-effectiveness and effective tools for monitoring and evaluation are some of the challenges for developing effective social media for health promotion (Korda and Itani, 2013; O'Neil, 2019). Social media providers need to have clear targets; health promotion messages need to be appropriate; platforms should encourage engagement and participation; and theory-based and evaluation for monitoring are also important (Webb *et al.*, 2010; Korda and Itani, 2013). Health promotion programmes should not just focus on behaviour change but also address the social determinants of health (Lupton, 2015b; Rice *et al.*, 2016). A more proactive involvement of governments is needed. This issue will be picked up again in Chapter 6.

Gamification (the use of game design in a non-game context) is aimed at motivating and improving user experience and engagement, taking responsibility for one's own health and promoting sustained behaviour change for good health. Computer and video games are beneficial for children in hospital both for education and for entertainment as well as for children with chronic conditions such as diabetes, asthma, mental health, disabled young people, children with developmental delay, and patients with cancer, pain and stroke, for example (Fernandez-Aranda *et al.*, 2012; Boulos *et al.*, 2015; Concepcion, 2017). Virtual reality programmes using graphics and customized avatars and face-tracking technology can help children with autism to build their confidence and skills, practising social interaction for the real world (Gregoire, 2014). Serious games are useful for educational purposes, such as in traditional subjects including maths, sciences and geography. Serious games can also help raise awareness among adolescents, for example, on dating violence and promoting healthy relationships (Bowen *et al.*, 2014). They can also be useful in mental health, stress management, confidence building and socialization (Fernandez-Aranda *et al.*, 2012); they are often perceived as more acceptable, enjoyable and engaging than traditional therapies. Exercise games (exergames) are active video games that can be useful to increase physical activity and reduce obesity (Lister *et al.*, 2014). However, console exergames might be less ideal for health promoters, replacing traditional forms of outdoor exercise such as cycling that require greater energy expenditure. There is also a need to understand the theory-base and means of effectiveness (Primack *et al.*, 2012; Boulos and Yang, 2013).

Telehealth and telecare are platforms to support the self-management of long-term conditions; provide self-care advice; and to allow remote monitoring of patients cared for at home (Coulter and Mearns, 2016; Honeyman *et al.*, 2016). Wearables can be used to aid rehabilitation and relay adverse events such as falls, helping older people to live independently (Godfrey, 2017). Telehealth is the remote exchange of data between individuals and health care professionals, whereas telecare is the remote monitoring of an individual's condition or lifestyle in their home environment aiming to manage risk in independent living. However, most of these give users limited involvement. Control remains with health professionals who monitor results and make decisions. Technology cannot replace human contact and people can feel isolated in their own home (Sanders *et al.*, 2012; Weymann *et al.*, 2014; Coulter and Mearns, 2016). Some also argue that these services invade people's privacy – care becomes technocratic and medicalized. In addition, such technology might not help people with memory loss, such as those with dementia, or people with hearing or sight impairment (Milligan *et al.*, 2011).

Alignment of digital communication to health promotion principles

As we have outlined, the normative ideal of health promotion is about equity, equality and social justice, a value-based, political and ethical activity. Internet interconnectiveness aids collaboration, participation and co-production, which can lead to personal and societal empowerment and stimulate critical thinking/bottom-up information processing and therefore aligns with health promotion principles. However, digital health promotion focuses on a behaviour- and lifestyle-change approach, shaped by a neoliberal environment. This, combined with traditional education and medical approaches to health, distances health promotion practice from its normative ideal (O'Neil, 2019). Health promotion is an anti-oppressive activity, working towards social reform and redressing imbalances of power. It is about addressing the causes of powerlessness and disempowerment. Digitalized interventions tend to focus on individual empowerment rather than collective or community empowerment. With its pathological and medicalized approach, it can be difficult for health promoters to meet the ideals of a social model approach that aligns with the principles and values of health promotion practice (O'Neil, 2019).

The principles of health promotion are also about choice and control. Digital health promotion relies on people's high self-efficacy for self-management. Control theory and social cognitive theory that underpin behaviour change health promotion activities advocate the use of feedback (Kramer and Kowatsch, 2017). Interactive personalized feedback and support can help motivate, guide, enable and empower people through the change process in the connected world. Internet-based behaviour change interventions can be effective, depending on the different combinations of design features (Mielewczyk and Willig, 2007; Michie *et al.*, 2012; Cohn, 2014; Morrison *et al.*, 2014). However, evaluation of behaviour change interventions is rare, inadequate and/or inadequately shared. The effectiveness of digital technology on patient engagement and behaviour change is also unclear (Morrison *et al.*, 2014).

The individualistic approach to health as seen in many digitalized interventions is based on freedom of choice with minimal government intervention and market fundamentalism. This has shifted the responsibility of health care from the government and health professionals to the people to become the ideal responsible citizens and ideal *digitally engaged patients* (Lupton, 2012). The burden of health shifts to the individual rather than the state (Ayo, 2010). The preoccupation of this health consciousness, facilitated by a consumer society, has become part of capitalist society in what Crawford (1980) described as *healthism*, with people taking responsibility to achieve good health, benefiting not only themselves but also the society. However, behaviour change not only depends on the person, but it also depends on the external social, economic, political and environmental factors that influence people's decision-making processes and the context of their behavioural practices (Mielewczyk and Willig, 2007; Cohn, 2014). Focusing on health practice would help health promoters design appropriate interventions (for example, through building an online community on social-networking sites that incorporates discussion where people can share experience and support each other).

The health of a nation is both personal and collective. It requires change at individual *and* societal levels. Health promotion needs *both* individualist and structuralist approaches to health (Bandura, 2004). It is therefore argued that a multi-pronged behaviour approach, together with an empowerment approach and a strong policy framework creating a supportive environment, would be more effective (Laverack, 2017). Theory and evidence are important, as well as collaborative approaches to web design with practitioners, web developers and, crucially, citizens (Michie *et al.*, 2012; Winter *et al.*, 2016). According to Webb *et al.* (2010), more extensive use of behaviour change theory and techniques such as those in stress management and general communication skill training were associated with a bigger impact. It is unclear, however, whether and how theory can influence intervention effectiveness with digital health promotion. The success of individualistic behavioural and lifestyle approaches by itself is limited, even with the development of innovative technology. There is a need to research feasibility, acceptability and effectiveness. Practitioners also need to understand the use of different theories and models as they all have different strengths and weaknesses. Behaviour theory will be discussed in more depth later in this chapter.

Health service management in the digital era

The use of digital technology in health service management is also apparent. Electronic medical records are widely used in Denmark, the Netherlands, Sweden and the UK (Piette *et al.*, 2012). In low- and middle-income countries, electronic medical records are available in large specialist hospitals; electronic tools are used to support clinical decisions and laboratory information, as well as being successfully implemented in disease surveillance systems. Information on health outcomes is, however, generally lacking (Piette *et al.*, 2012). In England, *The Next Step on the NHS Five Year Forward View in England* (NHS, 2017) builds on the recommendation of the Wachter review (2016), demonstrating the government's commitment to digitizing the NHS. Digital technology can improve health surveillance and support behavioural changes, and improve health system management for health education and clinical decision making. In May 2015, 97% of GPs in England offered online services such as appointment booking, prescription requests and accessing health record summaries (Ipsos MORI, 2015). As mentioned, given the current Covid-19 pandemic, digital access to health services is even more important.

As digital technology use has expanded, Rice and Sara (2019) suggest that another layer of influence, ICT, should be added onto the Dahlgren and Whitehead (1991) Social Determinants of Health Model to reflect societal change. This can co-ordinate policy and ensure interventions to improve our health in an integrated manner – the Determinants of Health Model 2.0 – meeting the challenge of public health in the digital age. In England, the government has acknowledged the social determinants of health with Public Health moving to local authority control in 2013. However, the organizational structure is complex; the fragmentation of services is evident, even with the advance of digital technology, and data access and sharing are surprisingly problematic (House of Commons Health Committee, 2016). Problems can also arise when system failures occur, emphasizing the importance of staff training in coping with IT failures and the use of technology at work (Johnson, 2010), as seen in the May 2017 cyber-attack on the UK's NHS when many health service computers were locked by a ransomware program.

The Big Data effect

The increased use of digital technology results in the expansion of web traffic and a huge amount of data in cyberspace. This is the Big Data era. We share information freely about ourselves in cyberspace, intentionally through personal communication and unintentionally through e-commerce transactions and our use of search engines, etc. These data are mined, analysed, repackaged and re-purposed as part of data assemblage, whereby data is constantly disassembled and reassembled to provide insights into our health/commercial behaviour for secondary uses (Kitchin and Lauriault, 2014). Crowdsourcing as a method in participatory public health research is particularly useful for monitoring the spread of infectious diseases in real time. In a panopticon world, a Foucauldian concept, the panoptical gaze in a surveillance society has power over us and we voluntarily and willingly become self-managers of our own health (Lupton, 2012). Through online crowd surveillance, as in Medicine 2.0/Health 2.0 or in 'infodemiology' and 'infoveillance', population-level information can be used to study health status and behaviour (Hill *et al.*, 2013). Big datasets can be used to assess health needs, identify risks and develop health promotion strategies. Quantified Self data, such as Fitbit information, can be accumulated and aggregated to a population level, becoming a Quantified Community. Electronic health records and health apps also provide rich data about people over longer periods of time (Barrett *et al.*, 2013; Hill *et al.*, 2013). Social media information can also reflect public opinion and concerns, providing fast and cheap updates about real-world events (Dredze, 2012). Non-health data on the environment, for example, climate, pollution levels, traffic patterns, socio-economic data, crime data and so on, can also be useful in terms of social, economic and environmental determinants of health within locational contexts, such as identifying local asthma hotspots and providing information on environmental factors influencing health conditions.

Big Data is difficult to manage and is often incomplete and inaccurate, yet huge amounts of data are often easily and continuously available leading to system security as well as information security issues (Baig *et al.*, 2015). Data in the cloud are also difficult to erase (Lupton, 2015b). We live in the 'end of forgetting' era (Bossewitch and Sinnreich, 2013). The secondary use of datasets also presents problems linking to privacy, confidentiality and identity, as well as ethical concerns (Lafferty, 2013), as seen in the use of Facebook personal data by Cambridge Analytica in 2018. Mittelstadt and Floridi (2016) cite five ethical themes that cover informed consent, privacy issues, ownership, research validity and 'objectivity'. The Big Data divide, created when the huge volumes of data are collected and managed by large organizations, can cause difficulties for individuals, researchers and small organizations who lack access. There is therefore a power imbalance between the self-serving interests of social media corporations and the interests of often powerless and uninformed individuals. Vast amounts of unstructured data can also lead to misinformation. Thus the self-governance of social media privacy and data security is a concern (Hunter *et al.*, 2018) and the globalized nature of internet data also gives rise to confusion as to which country's data-protection legislation applies.

The digital divide

The constraints of people's circumstances and their accumulated dispositions over their life course can be a barrier for behaviour change. Reducing health inequalities is a global agenda. Health service providers are turning to eHealth technologies for solutions (WHO, 2011; Lewis *et al.*, 2012). According to Laverack (2017), however, the modest successes of behavioural strategy have been for those at the top of the social gradient. This could exacerbate health inequalities. While electronic and mobile devices are widely available and competitively priced, studies from the US Department of Commerce (2013) showed that there is a stubbornly persistent digital divide by socio-economic status, race/ethnicity and urbanization. Improving health and life chances might favour the very people with abilities and resources, not those without these advantages, for example, lower-income groups, older people with chronic ill-health, those with poor mental health, housebound, disabled people, technophobes, as well as those with poor internet-network access and those generally lacking self-efficacy. Engagement in eHealth is also a concern (Chou *et al.*, 2013). There are some people who like human contact and do not want to use online services as 'empowered consumers' of healthcare, the so-called self-excluded groups (Coulter and Mearns, 2016). Inequality of access to internet or electronic devices is a key issue. Rather than providing a solution, new technologies might actually exacerbate inequality gaps.

Norman (2012) suggested that social media can reduce inequities created by organizations and social position as everyone functions equally, with an equal voice on the internet and opportunities to act on issues on the same platform. New media can provide a voice and visibility, allowing the non-powerful and marginalized a space in which to counter the dominant media culture (Lievrouw, 2009). However, Lupton (2012, 2013, 2015b) has argued that existing social inequities and poor health can be increased by lack of knowledge or access to digital technology. The barrier is not just about access. It is also about the skills in using, or aspiring to benefit from, the technologies. For example, almost a quarter of UK adults (23%) lack basic digital skills and 11% have never used the internet (Good Things Foundation, 2016). Digital divide is at the level of information use and aspiration not just information access (Zach *et al.*, 2011; Marschang, 2014). Navigating through complex health care systems can also be a challenge even for well-educated groups. Web-based information is generally designed for aesthetic appearance rather than usefulness. Measures of health literacy need to be based on sound theory, able to measure the health literacy of individuals as well as of health systems and health professionals, both information-seekers and information-givers (Pleasant *et al.*, 2011). There is also a need to promote eHealth literacy skills (Norman and Skinner 2006; WHO 2013).

The uncontrollable, non-moderated and viral nature of the social web can lead to misinformation and disinformation, for example, social bots and malicious actors (Jamison *et al.*, 2019). People need to learn to access, critically assess and appraise Web information. People who are digitally excluded also tend to be those with greater health needs (Honeyman *et al.*, 2016). As more advantaged groups continue to have good digital access and skills, disadvantaged groups are left behind, leading to a steeper social and health gradient. eHealth development should not be technology driven. Using Bourdieu's concept of capital and field, Baum *et al.* (2012) conceptualize the digital world as a societal field where there is struggle for resources and where power is unevenly distributed. They found people who are already disadvantaged are further excluded and lack power in the digital field. Maintaining equity is therefore as important as improving access. Support should be provided on the basis of people's needs; for example, non-digital forms of communication may need to continue. Other support might include financial support and education, and better computer/software design that can help people with severe disabilities. Studies of inequality also need to move from studying the inequality of health outcomes to studying the inequity of opportunities that lead to health inequalities (Frohlich and Abel, 2013).

Challenges of digital technology for health

In the Health 4.0 era of digital transformation of health and medicine (Kickbusch, 2019), the use of digital technology can no doubt improve health for many individuals and communities, enhancing health services provision, and supporting independent living through empowerment, research and better decision-making processes. With Web 3.0, the Semantic Web or the Intelligent Web era with the development of Internet of Things (IoT) enables people and things to be connected not only anytime, anywhere, but with anyone and anything, as well as with any network and any service (Borgia, 2014), as can be seen in artificial intelligence (AI) development. Technologies such as wearable body sensors for monitoring bodily functions and activating any medical interventions mean that tracking daily activities to provide suggestions for health improvements is no longer a dream. Using interactive personalized AI technology, health messages can be made personal, social and contextual for specific individuals, customized to individual health needs (Neuhauser *et al.*, 2013). In the middle of learning the use of Web 2.0 and 3.0, we are moving into Web 4.0 (the Pervasive or Ubiquitous Computing era) that covers a set of multiple dimensions, offering a distinct, simultaneous and comprehensive view of the Web world (Almeida, 2017). However, digitizing health services needs time and resources. Careful design and comprehensive evaluation may deliver efficiencies only in the longer term. The Montreal Declaration for responsible development of AI identifies ten key ethical principles and eight recommendations (Montreal Declaration, 2018). A collaborative approach among all stakeholders is needed at the global level as technologies develop into the future.

For a comprehensive review of the use of digital technologies and the implications for health promotion, see O'Neil (2019).

Summary

So far, we have looked at the process of communication and woven in aspects of educational theory. We have attempted to challenge the conventional wisdom of the communication theories so readily adopted in health promotion, and to show how they have very often be top-down. Health education doesn't have to be 'victim blaming' and is an essential part of health promotion. People do have needs for information and for knowledge and learning. However, given past limitations of health education to achieve health gains, more recently there have been other approaches in communicating about health. The development of digital technologies has refocused ideas about successful health communication methods but also raised concerns about health inequality and inequity and, therefore, social justice as we have discussed.

Moving on, social marketing has been prominent as an alternative to health education, and more recently the concept of 'nudge' has gained attention. We would argue that it is not health education *per se* that is failing. Rather, it is unrealistic to expect educational methods to achieve health gains without supporting measures such as healthy public policy and the other 'planks' of the Ottawa Charter. 'Health literacy', and indeed eHealth literacy, has also risen as a 'new' concept which some see as an important aspect of health education. Health literacy and motivational interviewing will be discussed as two current terms within health promotion, and we also include a consideration of the more dominant theories of individual behaviour change. Conventionally, it is held that 'successful' communication strategies need to be underpinned by theory, so these theories are now explored and their utility assessed.

Social Marketing and Health Promotion

The rise of 'social marketing' – the use of marketing principles to sell social goods – within health promotion has received mixed reviews. Its chief proponent, Richard Manoff, applied marketing techniques to family planning, nutrition and other health practices back in 1965 (Manoff, 1985). Since then, social marketing has been used in many 'health' areas; however, this has been with mixed results and certain types of health behaviours are more amenable to this approach. Certainly there is some evidence of the effectiveness of social marketing in promoting better nutrition, for example Blitstein *et al.* (2016). However, Chau *et al.* (2018) argue that not all health campaigns purporting to use social marketing are actually doing so, which indicates that adherence to the key characteristics of social marketing is not consistent in practice. The ethno-centric nature of social marketing in published research and literature has been acknowledged in terms of the dominance of the global North (Gordon, 2016). In the UK context, French (2017), like others, argues that social marketing provides a valid alternative to expert-led, top-down approaches to population health improvement which have tended to characterize health promotion efforts. Alternatively, Werner and Sanders (1997, p. 29) assert that social marketing 'often comes closer to brainwashing than awareness-raising' and 'does not give people the opportunity to make their own decisions and take autonomous action'. It is, of course, diametrically opposed to Freire's open-ended, problem-solving approach and thus resembles his 'banking' approach to education; social marketing does not enable people to make the first, crucial decisions about what types of communication activities could be useful for them (Linney, 1995). In addition, Langford and Panter-Brick (2013) argue that social marketing approaches can actually worsen health inequities because they focus on individual agency rather than on the structural conditions in which behaviour takes place. Green et al. (2019), like Griffiths et al. (2008), take a more pragmatic approach to social marketing and conclude that health promotion and social marketing remain distinct, with social marketing having an important place within health promotion but that the two working together increases the potential for effectiveness.

Arguably, a key aim of both health promotion and social marketing is behaviour change and the encouragement of healthier choices. Each also takes into account people's circumstances and attempts to gain insights into what people need and want. Like other approaches to health communication social marketing is prone to using messages based on harm to health rather than more positively framed messages (Djian et al., 2019) and it tends to neglect factors such as pleasure, which can drive behaviour (Pettigrew, 2015). Green et al. (2019) argue that social marketing, like health promotion, is also concerned with tackling the wider determinants of health. A key question for Green et al. (2019), then, is 'is social marketing an alternative to health promotion?' (p. 438). This raises a further question about what, if anything, are the differences between the two? For this, we return to the underpinning values of health promotion. Here we see a clear contrast between the emphasis on empowerment in health promotion and on the achievement of behavioural goals in social marketing. There is also, arguably, a difference in approaches – health promotion being committed to bottom-up ways of working and social marketing, arguably, working in more prescriptive, top-down, directive ways – although Lefebvre (1997) contends that if people are kept at the centre then the result is bottom-up ways of working. In addition, Naidoo and Wills (2016) claim that health promotion faces a dilemma when employing social marketing techniques because using advertising strategies necessarily means using images that are most likely to be effective and these tend to be those associated with consumer culture. They propose that the difficulty is that consumer culture promotes stereotypical ideas, many of which are inherently 'unhealthy'.

The cost–benefit analysis that takes place in social marketing is the same as that described within certain behaviour change models (for example the Health Belief Model), which refer to a value-expectancy mechanism. These models (described later in this chapter) are often used to plan, implement and evaluate health promotion programmes (Wills and Earle, 2007).

The advocacy mechanism within social marketing is employed differently to that in health promotion. Green et al. (2019) argue that in social marketing, advocacy is more likely to be done on *behalf* of people rather than involving them in the process. Further challenges to health promotion values are the strong persuasive element in social marketing and the ultimate focus on the individual, which emphasizes personal responsibility for health (Naidoo and Wills, 2016). However, supporters of social marketing would counter this and highlight the 'voluntary' nature of our consumer behaviour (Hastings and Stead, 2006), the implication being that power and control about decision making ultimately lie with the individual. This claim becomes tenuous if we consider the powerful influences of marketing and advertising processes on our subconscious decision making; after all, for example, how often do we end up buying things that we don't really need?

A final point about social marketing relates to upstream approaches. As previously noted, social marketing can be criticized for its downstream focus on individual actions at the expense of wider determinants of health. However, Gordon (2013) distinguishes between downstream and upstream social marketing and highlights how upstream social marketing focuses at the policy level, or on influencing the decision makers. Upstream social marketing would therefore 'target individuals at the organisation, industry or governmental level… those in key policy decision positions for mitigating wicked problems' (Kennedy et al., 2018, p. 262). Upstream social marketing necessitates influencing those in powerful positions, those with the might to effect significant change at policy, regulatory and structural levels (Strategic Direction, 2018).

For a comprehensive overview of social marketing and public health please see French et al. (2017).

The notion of 'nudge'

Nudging people is an idea that also has parallels in marketing approaches, and has individualistic,

Western origins. The notion of 'nudge' is becoming more and more influential in the UK and, specifically, its influence on public health policy is increasingly evident alongside a lean towards behavioural economics approaches (Lodge and Wegrich, 2016). In 2008, a book was published about the concept of 'nudge', written by two professors from Chicago (Thaler and Sunstein, 2008). Underpinning the concept of 'nudge' is a set of assumptions essentially to do with making whole populations change or modify their behaviour (Marteau et al., 2011). These include the idea that small changes in our immediate environment or context can 'nudge' (or encourage) us to behave in different ways and/or make different choices. Thaler and Sunstein (2008) argue that relatively small changes can have a large impact on the way in which people behave and the choices that they make. Consequently, 'nudges comprise a key component of the regulatory toolbox' (Nahmias et al., 2019, p. 43).

'Choice architecture' is a related term and is about designing environments and contexts (even situations) in order to alter people's decision making and behaviours. Choice architects are therefore people who have 'responsibility for organizing the context in which people make decisions' (Thaler and Sunstein, 2008, p. 3). Choice architecture is altering environments so that people make healthier choices rather than restricting individual freedom (Cross et al., 2017). The label 'choice architect' can be applied to many different people in different types of roles. This idea can also be applied to public health and health promotion. The premise is that we can design environments with the aim being to 'nudge' people to make the healthier choice by default, 'steer(ing) people in certain directions but maintain(ing) freedom of [...] choice' (Loibl et al., 2018, p. 655).

Nudge and choice architecture are about unconscious processes for the most part. Marteau et al. (2011, p. 263) state that this is to do with an 'automatic, affective system that requires little or no cognitive engagement and is driven by immediate feelings and triggered by our environments'. As Marteau et al. (2011) argue, this strategy is one that is widely used by the advertising industry. As a result, 'subtle changes to the context or environment in which individuals make decisions may have powerful implications for behaviour change' (Martin et al., 2020, p. 53).

There are several difficulties with nudge as a concept, however. First, it lacks a clear definition (Marteau et al., 2011). Secondly, it is difficult to find evidence in health to support 'nudge', although intuitively it appears to make a lot of sense and we do know, from marketing for example, that it does work. It is also difficult to isolate 'nudge' as a single causative agent in behaviour change and some raise methodological concerns which lead to an inability to draw firm conclusions from the research (Lin et al., 2017). As Marcano-Olivier et al. (2020) argue, in relation to using nudges to promote healthier eating in schools, many different types of nudges are often used in tandem so it can be difficult to isolate an effect. Thirdly, there are conceptual and philosophical challenges. Thaler and Sunstein (2008) argue that the concept of nudge (nudging people towards making decisions that are better for them) is 'libertarian paternalism' – 'libertarian' to do with the position that people should be free to do what they like. The meaning of the word 'paternalism', they argue, becomes different when it is preceded by the word 'libertarian'. This, they argue, modifies it to mean 'liberty-preserving' (p. 5). A paternalistic position is justified from the point of view that it is 'legitimate ... to try to influence people's behaviour in order to ... make their lives healthier' (p. 5). The question here then is: does the means justify the end? The notion of 'liberty' (freedom of choice) is undermined by the inherent contradiction in the manipulation of the unconscious mind. If we are being nudged to behave in certain ways and make decisions that we otherwise would not have made, then we aren't really free to do as we 'want'. This whole idea brings us back to a fundamental foundational principle in health promotion – that health is something to be highly valued and something to attain or strive towards. The direct implication of this is that there is a set of behaviours and choices that are deemed to be either 'good for us' or 'bad for us' (right or wrong) (Crossley, 2002) and that there are people that know better than us about what we should be doing (Chriss, 2015). 'Nudging' people towards changing behaviour is based on the premise that we know what people want and that this is 'better health and longer life' (Hastings and Stead, 2006, p. 141). This is paternalism in action. It is also evidence of 'healthism', which is another general critique of health promotion. Fourthly, as well as being an infringement on individual liberty, some may even go as far as to argue that 'nudge' is an infringement on human rights and the manifestation of a nanny state (Chriss, 2015). By definition, it takes away rights to behave in certain ways assuming inherent flaws in human judgement. Fifthly, in terms of health promotion, nudge also raises questions to do with empowerment. Arguably, rather than enabling people to take control of their health and their lives, choice architecture takes control away and puts control in the hands of the architects. And finally, the ethics of nudging may also be questioned (Lin et al., 2017). 'Nudge' appears to align itself with manipulative, coercive and persuasive ways of working, which are contrary to some of the underlying principles of health promotion that would suggest that using such approaches is unethical.

Health Literacy

'Health literacy' has become an increasingly important concept in health promotion and is positively linked to a number of valued outcomes such as more healthy decisions, healthier behaviours, management of ill-health and even social action (IUHPE, 2018). It is therefore considered as a key asset for promoting health and wellbeing, and for sustainable development (Sørensen et al., 2019). There appears to be general agreement in the literature that health literacy concerns the level of understanding required to make sense of health information, as well as an ability to subsequently act 'correctly' on that information (i.e. make the right decision as a result of understanding it). In the *Health Promotion Glossary*, Nutbeam (1998) links health literacy to participation and argues that access to education and information is key to empowering individuals and communities. Nutbeam (1998, 2000) clearly links health literacy to health education, highlighting the importance of it for promoting health, and argues that it is a key outcome of health education. Nutbeam defines health literacy as representing 'the cognitive and social skills which determine the motivation and ability of individuals to gain access to, understanding, and use information in ways which promote and maintain good health' (p. 10). So, for Nutbeam, health literacy isn't merely about being knowledgeable about health but it is also about being able to put that knowledge into positive effect for health gain. However, a person may be fully cognisant about an aspect of their health yet still choose to make unhealthy choices – does this then render them 'health illiterate'?

Nutbeam (2000, p. 263) proposed three levels of health literacy:

- **Functional (or basic) Literacy**: sufficient basic skills in reading and writing to be able to function effectively in everyday situations.
- **Interactive (or communicative) Literacy**: more advanced cognitive and literacy skills, which together with social skills, can be actively used to participate in everyday activities, extract information and derive meaning from different forms of communication as well as to apply new information to changing circumstances.
- **Critical Literacy**: more advanced cognitive skills, which, together with social skills, can be applied to critically analyse information and to use this information to exert greater control over life events and situations.

These different levels highlight the empowering nature of health literacy as they give a clear indication of what someone who is health literate has the capacity to *do* as a result. This typology also emphasizes the need for basic levels of literacy as a basis for developing *health* literacy, which is an extremely important factor given that low levels of literacy remain a global issue, especially for women in poorer countries, although literacy rates have vastly improved during the past 50 years (Roser and Ortiz-Ospina, 2018). It is also a key factor in inequalities in health. In his paper, Nutbeam (2000) makes reference to the fact that health literacy has been around for some time (albeit under the umbrella of 'health education') and he uses the phrase 'new oil into old lanterns' in recognition of the 'repackaging' within health literacy of familiar terms such as health education and empowerment. However, Tones (2002) argues that additional theorizing around the term 'health literacy' is unnecessary and that the various ways in which it is used within the health promotion literature increases the confusion surrounding it. Nevertheless, it seems that the term health literacy is here to stay and it could be argued that it provides a practical shorthand way in which to refer to the more complex ideas that are being discussed here. Certainly, health literacy has received increasing attention globally and in health policy and practice, and there is strong evidence of the need for higher levels of health literacy (Baldwin and Fleming, 2020).

In a paper revisiting the concept of health literacy, Peerson and Saunders (2009) argue that health literacy remains a confusing concept, not least because it is hard to define and therefore to measure. Yet there still appears to be a number of studies that have tried to do both. Various different scales have been produced in order to try to measure health literacy but it is argued that these need further testing and refinement (see Peerson and Saunders, 2009, for a summary). In addition, Peerson and Saunders (2009) argue that we need to better understand the role of motivation and activation in health literacy and use this to inform health promotion.

Corcoran (2011, p. 160) defines health literacy as 'the ability to locate and understand and act upon basic health information'. By definition, then, health literacy is linked to general levels of literacy (the ability to read and write), which can help or hinder people's health (Nutbeam, 1998). This is very important for the way in which messages about health are communicated. Corcoran (2011) argues that there are several ways in which written health information might be designed to make it more readable, understandable and more likely to be acted upon.

eHealth literacy (Neter and Brainin, 2019) is also increasing important. Rapid increases in technology and the ever-expanding internet and social media mean that the way in which information is presented and accessed is undergoing huge changes, resulting in a move away from a reliance on paper-based sources of health information. Arguably, this means that 'health literacy' is necessarily becoming an expanded concept. Skills in finding accurate, reliable and up-to-date information using information technology are just as important as knowing what to do with it once it has been accessed. Ishikawa *et al.* (2008) highlight the importance of this in their research on health literacy among Japanese office workers. They found that workers with higher levels of health literacy were more likely to report better health-related and coping behaviours than those with lower levels. Robinson and Robertson (2010) also demonstrate that this is an issue that will need to be further considered as technology advances and impacts on the way in which information is communicated. This requires the 'user' to possess and hone certain IT skills, which are becoming increasingly important to health literacy.

There are many studies that demonstrate the disadvantages and potential negative effects of a lack of health literacy, however it is defined and measured. This is a key argument for its significance in promoting health. However, there appears to be some further distinction in the literature about the nature of health literacy. Pleasant and Kuruvilla (2008) argue that it is possible to differentiate between two different approaches to health literacy – the 'clinical' approach and the 'public health' approach. The 'clinical' approach has historically focused on promoting better communication between patients and health care professionals

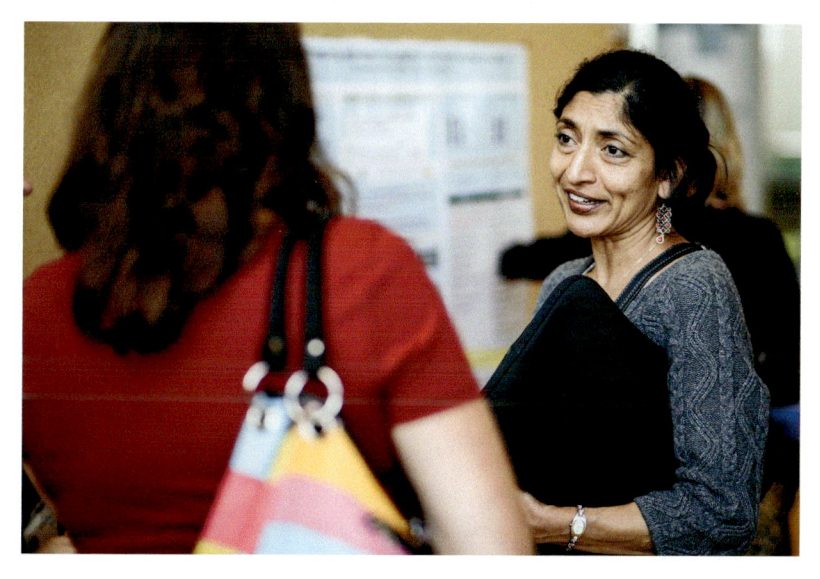

Learning from others ('2014 CTLT Institute - Flexible Learning Open House events' by UBC_CTLT is licensed under CC BY 2.0).

in order to promote compliancy, imposing a deficit model on the patient (lack of knowledge or understanding as being primarily problematic). The 'public health' approach, in contrast, connects health literacy to health promotion, education and empowerment. Pleasant and Kuruvilla (2008) conclude that a combination of both approaches is needed to be fully effective in promoting public health. However, both approaches have implications for research and practice. For example, a more clinical approach will lead to more diagnostic ways of trying to measure health literacy.

Zarcadoolas *et al.* (2005) define health literacy as 'the wide range of skills and competencies that people develop to seek out, comprehend, evaluate and use health information and concepts to make informed choices, reduce health risks and increase quality of life' (pp. 196–197). This covers many different things, from being able to listen effectively to being able to access information through mobile technology. One of the key features would appear to be the ability to adapt to changes over time – changes in the ways in which information is communicated and reproduced as well as the ability to discern what is most important at any given time. Definitions of health literacy continue to evolve (Rudd, 2015), which can be problematic; however, they tend to cohere around the functional, rather than the critical, aspects of it (Cross *et al.*, 2017). Nevertheless, health literacy is viewed as a key global priority for health promotion (WHO, 2016). For a more detailed critical discussion about health literacy please see Cross *et al.* (2017).

Central Components in Behaviour Change

A number of models of behaviour change have been developed over the years, which can aid our understanding of health behaviour and behavioural choices at an individual level. The purpose of this section of the chapter is not to go into great depth about these types of models but instead to provide an overview of them within the context of health communication. (Individual models of behaviour change have been explored in detail in the wider literature, so the reader is encouraged to look elsewhere for this.) One of the most important roles that behaviour change theory plays in health communication is to provide a theoretical foundation for the design, implementation and evaluation of public health and health promotion activities. In addition, theory can be useful in determining what works, or is effective, in health communication and behaviour change (as well as what does not work).

A number of different factors influence health behaviour and behavioural choices. Some of these exist at the individual level. The philosophical underpinnings and value base of health promotion exhort us to examine wider social determinants and factors in order to account for health-related behaviour. Nonetheless, behaviour change models can be useful and they may enable us to take account of individual factors when planning health promotion interventions and communicating for health. The roots of behaviour change theory are within a number of different fields, most notably psychology but also ecology and philosophy. Behaviour change is complex. One of the difficulties of trying to provide a representation of it via theoretical means is that 'one size does not fit all'; however, there have been several useful attempts to capture the different variables involved in the process at an individual level. The most 'influential' models will be briefly described here in relation to the different variables identified as important in health behaviour. These have been selected on the basis that they are most frequently applied and researched within the wider literature. This discussion will therefore include reference to some of the central constructs and processes presented within key theories including the Health Belief Model (Rosenstock *et al.*, 1988), the Theory of Planned Behaviour (Ajzen, 1988, 1991), Protection Motivation Theory (Rogers, 1975, 1983), the Transtheoretical Model (Prochaska and DiClemente, 1983) and Tones's Health Action Model (Green *et al.*, 2019). The variables selected for discussion (as deemed particularly salient to the area of 'health communication') include beliefs, motivation (including a discussion of motivational interviewing), stages of change and behavioural intention.

Beliefs

The concept of beliefs (or 'perceptions') is very important to behaviour change and is a central construct in several behaviour change models, most notably the Health Belief Model, which is built primarily around a set of beliefs deemed important in influencing behavioural outcomes. Beliefs can exist about a range of different things and have a direct influence on health-related behaviour as well as whether or not someone is likely to change.

Beliefs are discussed here specifically in relation to perceptions of 'threat', perceptions of 'benefits and barriers' and perceptions of 'control'.

Beliefs about the *threat* of an illness as a mechanism for providing an incentive to act to avoid it are reflected in the Health Belief Model (labelled 'perceived susceptibility' and 'perceived severity') and Protection Motivation Theory (labelled 'severity' and 'vulnerability'). 'Threat perception' is important in communication for behaviour change. The assumption is that if a person believes themselves to be at risk of becoming unwell as a result of their current behaviour, they are more likely to want to change it. Very many health promotion messages have previously been predicated on this assumption, although this approach has had mixed results.

The Health Belief Model, developed initially to explain and predict screening behaviours (Abraham and Sheeran, 2005), also focuses on beliefs about the advantages and disadvantages of taking action (changing behaviour). These are labelled 'perceived benefits' and 'perceived barriers', respectively. This 'cost/benefit' analysis process is also reflected in the Protection Motivation Theory. The assumption here is that an individual engages in a rational and thoughtful decision-making process whereby they 'weigh-up' the pros and cons of taking action and make a decision accordingly (normally in the direction of the action that yields the greatest benefits and least costs). The Transtheoretical Model refers to this as 'decisional balance'. Health promotion and public health communication, which highlight benefits over cost, may therefore be more effective in promoting behaviour change. Many of the models presented assume that people carry out a cost/benefit analysis when they are deciding whether to change their behaviour. The adoption of an economic framework here implies that someone will take action when the advantages (or benefits) outweigh the disadvantages (or costs). This degree of rationality has been contested in the literature. Experience tells us that behaviour may result from unconscious processes, emotion and impulsivity, none of which resonates with a rational cognitive process.

Beliefs about personal capacity to take action are also important and feature (albeit in different guises) in several of the models of behaviour change under consideration. In the Theory of Planned Behaviour, beliefs about control are represented in the variable 'Perceived Behavioural Control'. 'Self-efficacy' was also later added as a variable to the Health Belief Model and, some argue, is not dissimilar from perceived behavioural control. In essence, both concepts refer to the extent to which someone believes they are capable of taking action (changing their behaviour). Self-efficacy has its roots in Social Learning Theory (Bandura, 1986) and is closely related to constructs such as self-esteem. The 'coping appraisal' variable within Protection Motivation Theory also shares some similarities with self-efficacy, and perceptions about control and self-efficacy also feature as a construct within the Transtheoretical Model (Sutton, 2005). Beliefs about control are important in health behaviour and the research shows that people with higher levels of self-esteem generally fare better health-wise, particularly when it comes to mental health (Marks *et al.*, 2018). Again, however, research on lay beliefs about control indicates that they are complex, with many aspects seen as beyond the control of individuals (as we saw in Chapter 1).

Motivation

Motivation is an important construct in behaviour change (hence the stress on motivational interviewing as a technique). Many different factors can impact on motivation to change behaviour. These may be crudely separated into two main areas – 'internal' motivation (from *within* the individual) and external (from *outside* of the individual, or existing within the wider socio-politico-economic environment) motivation. Motivation is a central construct in Protection Motivation Theory, implied within the Health Belief Model through the variable 'cues for action' and is taken into account in the Health Action Model in relation to the construct of 'self' (personality). Regarding health communication, how messages are designed might have an impact on internal motivation in terms of changing the way in which someone thinks about something. Equally, a message about health may be viewed as 'external' motivation. Either way, we do know that, in order for change to occur, there needs to be some motivation for action at the individual level. Lack of motivation is a significant challenge for health promoters (Hardcastle *et al.*, 2015).

Motivational interviewing

Motivational interviewing is one approach trying to effect behavioural change at an individual level using a face-to-face mechanism (Hillsden, 2006). Its central purpose is to encourage exploration of reasons to change behaviour, which may not have been dwelt on before (Bennett and Murphy, 1997). Motivational interviewing, initially developed as a strategy for working with people with addictions, was first described by William Miller, and has been further developed by Miller and Rollnick (Hillsden, 2006). It is increasingly used within health promotion as a strategy designed to influence behaviour at the individual level in relation to 'problematic' health behaviours. Miller defined motivational interviewing as follows: 'a client-centred, directive method for enhancing intrinsic motivation to change by exploring and resolving ambivalence' (Miller and Rollnick, 2002, cited in Hillsden, 2006, p. 75).

It is apparent from this definition that the concept of ambivalence is central to motivational interviewing. Ambivalence has only relatively recently come into play in contemporary health promotion. Hillsden (2006) argues that it is this that distinguishes motivational interviewing from other types of approaches to behaviour change, based on more traditionally medically or disease-focused approaches. Maio *et al.* (2007) highlight the importance of ambivalence as an obstacle to healthier behaviour. Different factors such as freedom of choice, stress and habit formation influence feelings of ambivalence towards health behaviour change. The challenge is therefore in designing health promotion activities that tackle ambivalence and encourage change.

What is significant about motivational interviewing (and consistent with the underpinning principles of health promotion) is that the 'client' is seen as an autonomous person with the right to choose to change or not and so it promotes autonomy and collaboration (Day *et al.*, 2017). The concept of motivation is central to motivational interviewing. Motivation is to do with what makes us take certain actions or behave in a certain way (or not). Different types of motivation have been identified in the literature. The importance of the concept of motivation is highlighted by Green *et al.* (2019, p. 140) in the Health Action Model where the 'motivation system' is depicted as one of four interacting systems determining health behaviour. The motivation system consists of four kinds of motivation – values, attitudes, drives and emotional states (affect) (Green *et al.*, 2019). Motivation may also be defined as being 'intrinsic' – 'based on feeling of pleasure, pride or enjoyment brought about by participating in an activity' – or 'extrinsic' – 'based on external factors such as appearance, conformity or norms' (Marks *et al.*, 2018, p. 439). Hillsden (2006) identifies three essential components of motivation as conceived within motivational interviewing – readiness to change, the importance or value placed in change and confidence in the ability to change. Hillsden also outlines a set of principles for motivational interviewing (as detailed in Box 4.6) and states that a key strategy in motivational interviewing is 'change talk'. 'Change talk involves the client expressing personal advantage of changing behaviour, optimism for change, intention to change and the disadvantages of change' (Hillsden, 2006, p. 78).

Motivational interviewing has similarities with 'brief behavioural counselling' (which might also be referred to as 'brief behavioural intervention'; Steptoe *et al.*, 2003) and 'health coaching' (Palmer *et al.*, 2003). Although some may argue that motivational interviewing and health coaching differ, there are many similarities and it is gaining in popularity (Palmer *et al.*, 2003). Palmer *et al.* (2003, p. 93) offer a 'tentative definition' – 'health coaching is the practice of health education and health promotion within a coaching context, to enhance the well-being of individuals and to facilitate the achievement of their health-related goals'. The similarities with motivational interviewing are evident here. Either can take place face to face or via the telephone (Dejonghe *et al.*, 2020). Palmer *et al.* (2003) emphasize the links between health

---

Box 4.6. Principles of motivational interviewing.

1. Expressing empathy – this refers to showing acceptance of where a person is.
2. Developing a discrepancy – this is about establishing the difference between where a person is and where they would like to be (or get to).
3. Rolling with resistance – this refers to accepting (on the facilitator's part) the fact that resistance is likely to occur (on the client's part) and having strategies to deal with it when it does.
4. Supporting self-efficacy – this refers to supporting the client in the belief that they have the capacity to effect change.

(Adapted from Hillsden, 2006)

coaching and more 'traditional' health education approaches. Certainly, both motivational interviewing and health coaching will involve a level of health education to some degree.

Motivational interviewing draws on a range of psychosocial theory relating to behaviour change including step change theories and Bandura's ideas about self-efficacy. It has distinct parallels with the Transtheoretical Model (Prochaska and DiClemente, 1983) and, as the Model does, motivational interviewing highlights the importance of the person's 'readiness to change' and may provide an incentive for moving through the key stages of change identified within the Transtheoretical Model (Miller and Rollnick, 2002). In terms of the underpinning principles of health promotion as outlined by the Ottawa Charter (WHO, 1986), we can see that motivational interviewing can help to build on and develop personal skills as well as enabling practitioners to work in more empowering ways with the client at the centre of the interaction (in the 'driving seat'). The focus then is away from 'telling' people what to do and much more towards facilitating the process of change if and when appropriate.

Motivational interviewing appears to have been effective in enabling behaviour change at an individual level in relation to a range of health-related issues, including nutrition and physical activity (Clifford and Curtis, 2016). However, there are a number of critiques about motivational interviewing that are worth attention. A key challenge is that motivational interviewing starts from the position that health itself provides a key motivation for change (Hillsden, 2006), but this is not always the case for everyone. The focus at the individual level fails to take into account the wider social determinants of health and the macro-factors that impact on, and influence, behaviour at an individual level.

One of the difficulties in establishing an evidence base for motivational interviewing in health promotion is that, as Hillsden (2006, p. 81) argues, it is 'quite common for people to refer to an intervention as MI because it is loosely based on MI principles'. Rubak et al. (2005) carried out a systematic review and meta-analysis to establish the effectiveness of motivational interviewing. They concluded that it was more effective in scientific settings than traditional advice giving in the treatment of a range of behavioural problems but that future research was needed, which clearly identifies exactly *how* motivational interviewing is carried out and includes direct/objective measures, as well as qualitative perspectives. Motivational interviewing may be carried out on its own, or in conjunction with, for example, a subsequent course of treatment. This also has implications for how we measure effectiveness. In addition, it may be carried out at the individual level or within groups. There are a number of studies reporting the effect of motivational interviewing in different contexts and with reference to a range of different 'health issues'. A literature review conducted by Branscum and Sharma (2010) concluded that motivational interviewing was effective in reducing alcohol use in heavy drinkers but this is not supported by findings from a meta-analysis by Lundahl et al. (2010), which failed to detect significant findings specific to motivational interviewing when used on a range of addictive behaviours including alcohol use. So, the evidence for effectiveness is not conclusive; however, a more recent systematic review did determine that 'when the balance of client ambivalence is in the direction of behaviour change' there was more likely to be a positive outcome (Magill et al., 2018, p. 140).

Stages of change

The Transtheoretical Model is probably the most well-known model that incorporates the concept of 'stages' or phases of behaviour change. Central to this idea is that people move through different stages towards changing behaviour. In the case of the Transtheoretical Model, there are five key stages: pre-contemplation, contemplation, preparation, action and maintenance. This is a more descriptive way of looking at behaviour change. In terms of communicating for health it is clear that, as Sutton (2005, p. 224) argues, 'different factors are important at different stages'. This means that the design of interventions intended to move an individual from one stage to the next may vary considerably depending on which stage they are at. The assumption is of linear progression through the stages. However, there is 'room' for relapse within this framework whereby someone may 'go back' a stage or more at any point. The acknowledgement of relapse, a very important factor in health-related behaviour change, links to a key feature in motivational interviewing discussed previously. In addition, maintenance is a key feature of this model (Green et al., 2019). The purpose of communicating health is to move people through the different stages of behaviour change towards maintenance (Cross et al., 2017) whilst recognizing the fact that people might have to make several attempts to change behaviour before they are successful (Gillespie, 2020).

Behavioural intention

Intention is another variable that features strongly in some of the behaviour change models. The focus on behavioural *intention* is often at the expense of providing an explanation for, or account of, behavioural *outcomes*. The assumption tends to be that an intention to change behaviour leads to the behavioural change, or at least that this is more likely if intention is present. A great deal of research has been done that examines the factors influencing behavioural intention. Of course, intending to behave in a certain way does not necessarily mean that the actual behaviour will occur. This is sometimes referred to as the Intention-Behaviour Gap and it reflects the fact that we are talking about a non-linear, complex process. Many different factors will impact on the point between behavioural intention and actual behaviour, including cognitive, social and structural factors (Pfeffer and Strobach, 2017). The Theory of Planned Behaviour and Protection Motivation Theory are both examples of models that include 'intention' as a key component and that assume a direct link between the two. Behavioural intention also features centrally within the Health Action Model. However, this model goes further to consider what will influence the move from intention to actual behaviour change. It therefore takes into account the wider environment, existing skills/knowledge and constructs of the 'self' (Green *et al.*, 2019) as influencing forces, which the other two models fail to do.

Critiques of behaviour change models

A number of critiques of the key behaviour change models have been offered within the literature. These are nicely summarized in Box 4.7, adapted from Warwick-Booth *et al.* (2021).

Box 4.7. General critiques of models of behaviour change.

The models tend to…

- focus at the individual level and not on the wider determinants of health (social, political, environmental, etc.) and so they tend not to account for factors outside of the individual, which influence behaviour;
- put the emphasis on the individual (a 'reductionist' approach) (Bunton *et al.*, 2000) and 'objectify' human experience in contrast to a holistic approach (Green *et al.*, 2019);
- promote individualism and individual responsibility for health (Airhihenbuwa and Obregon, 2000);
- tend to assume that people are rational decision makers (Lodge and Wegrich, 2016); and
- view individual actions or behaviour in isolation from the actions or behaviour of others (Hubley *et al.*, 2021), neglecting to consider social influences.

They tend to neglect the role of…

- past behaviour and habit (Sarafino and Smith, 2016; Upton and Thirlaway, 2014);
- affect 'emotion' (Roberts *et al.*, 2001; Lawton *et al.*, 2009); and
- culture and cultural context (Lin *et al.*, 2005).

They tend to neglect the fact that…

- processes of behaviour change take time and significant change cannot take place over a short period (Ramos and Perkins, 2006) and they also over-simplify processes of behaviour change (Abraham and Sheenan, 2005; Berry, 2007).

In terms of research, a number of difficulties have been highlighted including…

- limited predictive utility (Abraham and Sheenan, 2005);
- a weak relationship between intention and behaviour – Stevens (2008) argues that other factors should be explored, i.e. environmental factors;
- a lack of standardization across constructs in experimental design (Conner and Norman, 2015) – it is difficult to compare the results of studies that 'test' out the theories because they often use different methods and inconsistent ways of measuring the different components of the models;
- they tend to have been developed in specific contexts which can lead to a 'Western', patriarchal bias;
- much of the research using the models relies on self-report measures, which have limitations; and
- whilst many of the models draw upon aspects of sociological, psychological and anthropological theory they tend to neglect political and economic theory (Hubley *et al.*, 2021).

There are a number of things that impact on health behaviour at the individual level that are not taken into account within mainstream behaviour change theory. These include factors such as resilience, resistance and voluntary risk-taking. In addition, this whole field has come under some criticism from some at the more critical ends of health psychology and public health, where the very idea of 'health behaviour' is challenged, framing it instead as 'social practice' (Mielewcyzk and Willig, 2007) and advocating that the focus should be on the wider social, political and economic context rather than at the individual level (Cross et al., 2017). These wider factors are often seen by some branches of psychology as benign 'background factors'.

Newer paradigms of conceptualizing health behaviours will be alluded to in Chapter 6; Shove (2010, p. 3) suggests:

Much of the conventional literature supposes that behaviours are subject to external drivers like price and persuasion, or that they are obstructed by 'barriers'. This implies a linear relation between factors and effects and supposes that 'outside' forces bear down on behaviour. Although very familiar, interpretations of this kind are incapable of capturing or describing the forms of mutual adjustment, adaptation and accumulation involved in shaping and changing the repertoires of 'doings' that, in combination, constitute contemporary ways of life.

She suggests that, in terms of understanding everyday life, we need to develop radically different theories. The COM-B model (Michie et al., 2011) where C stands for capability, O for opportunity, M for motivation, and B for behaviour, is a more contemporary attempt to explain behaviour change. Whilst it contains many of the constructs of its predecessors, this is a much more complex

---

Box 4.8. Case Study: Components of health communication applied to Covid-19.

At the time of writing (April 2020), Covid-19 is having a significant impact at a global level on everyday life for most people. Governments in the majority of countries have called upon their nations to change their practices and behaviour in different ways. Compliance with government mandates without coercive measures is dependent on a range of theoretical constructs discussed within this chapter. Many people are required to comply with one of two main directives (if not both) – social distancing and self-isolation.

In the absence of martial law, compliance is not guaranteed. We can turn to the discussion in this chapter to understand how compliance might occur as follows:

1. A person must perceive that Covid-19 is a threat, either to themselves or to others. We have seen mixed responses from people who have not been categorized as high risk. Some young people, for example, do not perceive themselves to be at risk or believe that, if they do become infected, it will be mild.
2. The benefits of taking action must be clear and be seen to outweigh the barriers. The benefit in this case is staying well; the barriers will include not being able to go out of the house (bar exceptions) and not being able to socialize as normal.
3. Perceptions of control come into play, so how much control people feel they have over the situation has an impact. Some people, at the first sign of a potential lockdown, stock piled 'essential' items, which can be interpreted as a means of feeling in control of an otherwise uncontrollable situation.
4. Coping appraisal is an important factor. Coping with staying at home requires adjustments to daily life as routines are disrupted. Motivation to comply with government advice or mandates might originate from internal or external sources. Internal would be motivation to stay well or protect others; external would be motivation from those in power, for example government spokespeople.
5. The messages about Covid-19 that have been produced have not been received in the same way by different people. Some messages have been confusing, unclear and interpreted in different ways: for example, the advice to shop only for 'essential' items without a definition of what 'essential' means. What one person deems essential might not be what another person does. Advisory messages about how to prevent Covid-19 are being 'heard' within a very noisy background of contradictory, rapidly changing information.
6. Finally, lockdown periods have illuminated the importance and the usefulness of ICT. However, they have also exposed the broader implications, such as the management of Big Data and the digital divide – there are groups of people who may not have the skills to access, or access to, vital information during the pandemic.

model that is being used within the wider behavioural science literature to underpin various types of intervention (Stevely et al., 2018).

Whilst there are limitations to existing behaviour change theory, it is important to try to understand and explain behaviour change through, among other things, the development and testing of theoretical models. This is because we can then influence how we plan, implement and evaluate health promotion activities or 'communicate' with people to improve and promote health.

For further, in-depth information about the models that have been referred to here, please see the following:

- for the Health Action Model, see Green et al., (2019);
- for the Health Belief Model, Protection Motivation Theory, Transtheoretical Model and Theory of Planned Behaviour, see Conner and Norman (2015); and
- for the COM-B model, see Michie et al. (2014).

The case study (Box 4.8) illustrates some components of health communication in relation to the 2020 Coronavirus pandemic.

Summary

This chapter has attempted to take a critical look at some of the assumptions about health communication, such as that mass media is a useful means of getting health messages across, or that theories of behaviour change drawn from psychology necessarily help us to understand people's behaviour. Much of the theory about communication in health promotion relies on the 'classic' theories of one-way communication and, as such, these are out of step with the 21st century, where networking as a means of communication has taken over from hierarchical, 'expert'-led means. These one-way methods are authoritarian in that they vest the authority in the communicator, and we have suggested that methods need to be found that are interactive, empowering and helpful, rather than top-down, failing to build in feedback and serving to further the agendas of the health promoters without fully understanding the health-worlds of the individuals and communities involved. These means will be dialogical and people-centred, and thus people need to be involved in each stage of developing health messages. Furthermore, health education need not be victim blaming, and some of the attempts to rehabilitate 'health education' have only served to confuse the arena, such as by introducing 'new' concepts that are essentially the same as the old. Differing ideological perspectives inevitably lead to different views on the adoption of practices from commerce, such as social marketing, but, taking a pragmatic approach, we have shown that there are places where some of this may be appropriate. The dominance of behaviour change approaches within health promotion and the adoption of theories from psychology has been critiqued, and the fact that these are Eurocentric and provide only partial understanding is taken up again in Chapter 6.

These views present challenges for health promoters and health educators, and may cause pause for thought in terms of established ways of working. Most health education materials, for example, are produced with no involvement of the individuals and communities for which they are intended, on the assumption that the expert, whether a dietician, nurse, rehabilitation worker or any other, will 'know' what people want, and ought to know. Given the importance of knowledge, and the need for effective, evidence-based approaches, these established ways of working need to be scrutinized.

Note

[1] The previous version of this chapter entitled 'Communicating Health' was written by Ruth Cross, Ivy O'Neil and Rachael Dixey.

Further Reading

Corcoran, N. (2013) *Communicating Health: Strategies for Health Promotion*, 2nd edn. Sage, London.

Cross, R., Davis, S. and O'Neil, I. (2017) *Health Communication: Theoretical and Critical Perspectives*. Polity Press, Cambridge, UK.

O'Neil, I. (2019) *Digital Health Promotion: A Critical Introduction*. Polity Press, Cambridge, UK.

Upton, D. and Thirlaway, K. (2014) *Promoting Healthy Behaviour: A Practical Guide*. 2nd edn. Routledge, Oxford, UK.

References

Abraham, C. and Sheeran, P. (2005) The health belief model. In: Conner, M. and Norman, P. (eds) *Predicting Health Behaviours*, 2nd edition. Open University Press, Buckingham, UK, pp. 28–80.

Abroms, L.C. (2019) Public health in the era of social media. *American Journal of Public Health* S2, 109.

Abroms, L. and Maibach, E. (2008) The effectiveness of mass communication to change public behaviour. *Annual Review of Public Health* 29, 219–234.

Alghamdi, M., Gashgari, H. and Househ, M. (2015) A systematic review of mobile health technology use in developing countries. *Studies in Health Technology Informatics* 213, 223–226.

Alibaba Group (2019) *Company Overview*. Available at: https://www.alibabagroup.com/en/about/overview (accessed 22 April 2020).

Airhihenbuwa, C. and Obregon, R. (2000) A critical assessment of theories/models used in health communication for HIV/AIDS. *Journal of Health Communication* 5 (Supplement), 5–15.

Ajzen, I. (1988) *Attitudes, Personality and Behaviour*. Open University Press, Milton Keynes, UK.

Ajzen, I. (1991) The theory of planned behaviour. *Organizational Behavior and Human Decision Processes* 50, 179–211.

Almeida, F. (2017) Concept and dimensions of Web 4.0. *International Journal of Computers and Technology* 16 (7), 7040–7046.

Appiah, K.A. (2006) *Cosmopolitanism: Ethics in a World of Strangers*. Norton, New York.

Ayo, N. (2010) Understanding health promotion in a neoliberal climate and the making of health-conscious citizens. *Critical Public Health* 22 (1), 99–105.

Ayran, G., Fırat, M., Küçükakça, G., Cüneydioğlu, B., Tahta, K. and Avcı, F. (2017) The effect of peer education upon breast self examination behaviors and self-esteem among university students. *european journal of breast health* 13, 138–144.

Bach, S., Haynes, P. and Smith, J.L. (2007) *Online Learning and Teaching in Higher Education*. Open University Press, London.

Bagnall, A., South, J., Hulme, C., Woodall, J., Vinall-Collier, K., Raine, G., Kinsella, K., Dixey, R., Harris, L., and Wright, N.MJ. (2015) A systematic review of the effectiveness and cost-effectiveness of peer education and peer support in prisons. *BMC Public Health* 15, 290.

Baig, M.M., Gholam-Hosseini, H. and Connolly, M.J. (2015) Mobile healthcare applications: system design review, critical issues and challenges. *Australasian College of Physical Scientists and Engineers in Medicine* 38, 23–38.

Baldwin, L. and Fleming, M. (2020) The future for health promotion. In: Fleming, M. and Baldwin, L. (eds.) *Health Promotion in the 21st Century: New approaches to achieving health for all*. Allen & Unwin, London, pp. 263–280.

Bandura, A. (1986) *Social Foundations of Thought and Action: A Social Cognitive Theory*. Prentice Hall, Englewood Cliffs, New Jersey.

Bandura, A. (2004) Health promotion by social cognitive means. *Health Education and Behaviour*, 31(2), 143–164.

Barrett, M., Humblet, O., Hiatt, R. and Adler, N. (2013) Big data and disease prevention: from quantified self to quantified communities. *Big Data* 1, 168–175.

Baum, F., Newman, L. and Biedrzycki, K. (2012) Vicious cycles: digital technologies and determinants of health in Australia. *Health Promotion International* 29 (2), 349–360.

Baxter Magolda, M. (2001) *Making their Own Way: Narratives for Transforming Higher Education to Promote Self-development*. Stylus, Sterling, Virginia.

Bennett, P. and Murphy, S. (1997) *Psychology and Health Promotion*. Open University Press, Buckingham, UK.

Berne, E. (1964) *Games People Play*. Penguin Books, New York.

Berry, D. (2007) *Health Communication: Theory and Practice*. Open University Press, Maidenhead, UK.

Bert, F., Giacometti, M., Gualano, M. R. and Siliquini, R. (2014) Smartphones and health promotion: a review of the evidence. *Journal of Medical Systems* 38(1), 9995.

Bhuyan, S.S., Lu, N., Chandak, A., Kim, H., Wyant, D., Bhatt, J., et al. (2016) Use of mobile health applications for health-seeking behaviour among US adults. *Journal of Medical Systems* 40, 153.

Blitstein, J.L., Cates., S.C., Hersey, J., Montgomery, D., Shelley, M., Hradek., C., Kosa, K., Bell., L., Long., V., Williams, P.A., Olson, S. and Singh, A. (2016) Adding a social marketing campaign to a school-based nutrition education program improves children's dietary intake: a quasi-experimental study. *Journal of the Academy of Nutrition and Dietetics* 116 (8), 1285–1294.

Blue, S., Shove, E., Carmona, C. and Kelly, M.P. (2016) Theories of practice and public health: understanding (un)healthy practices. *Critical Public Health* 26(1), 36–50.

Blumler, J.G. and Katz, E. (eds) (1974) *The Use of Mass Communications: Current Perspectives on Uses and Gratifications Research*. Sage, Newbury Park, California.

Borgia, E. (2014) The Internet of Things vision: key features, applications and open issues. *Computer Communications* 54, 1–31.

Bossewitch, J. and Sinnreich, A. (2013) The end of forgetting: strategic agency beyond the panopticon. *New Media and Society* 15(2), 224–242.

Boulos, M.K., Gammon, S., Dixon, M.C., MacRury, S.M., Ferusson, M.J., Rodrigues, et al. (2015) Digital games for type 1 and type 2 diabetes: underpinning theory with three illustrative examples. *Journal of Medical Internet Research* 3(1), e3.

Boulos, M.K. and Yang, S. (2013) Exergames for health and fitness: the roles of GPS and geosocial apps. *International Journal of Health Geographics*, 12(18), 1–7.

Bowen, E., Walker, K., Mawer, M., Holdsworth, E., Sorbring, E. and Helsing, B. (2014) 'It's like you're actually playing as yourself': development and preliminary evaluation of 'Green Acres High'. *Psychosocial Intervention* 23, 43–55.

Branscum, P. and Sharma, M. (2010) A review of motivational interviewing-based interventions targeting problematic drinking among college students. *Alcoholism Treatment Quarterly* 28, 63–77.

British Institute of Learning Disability (2005) No need to scream: good practice made easy. *Advocacy News*, Issue 20.

Brown, R.C.H. (2018) Resisting moralisation in health promotion. *Ethical Theory and Moral Practice* 21, 997–1011.

Bunton, R., Baldwin, S., Flynn, D. and Whitelaw, S. (2000) The 'stages of change' model in health promotion: science and ideology. *Critical Public Health* 10, 55–70.

Campbell, C. and Cornish, F. (2010) How can community health programmes build enabling environments for transformative communication?: experiences from India and South Africa. Health Community and Development Group Working Papers (1). London School of Economics and Political Science, London.

Centre for Health Promotion, Women's and Children's Health Network (2012) *Where They Hang Out: Social Media Use in Youth Health Promotion*. Department of Health, Government of South Australia, Adelaide.

Chau, J.Y., McGill, B., Thomas, M.M., Carroll, T.E., Bellew, W., Bauman, A. and Grunseit, A.C. (2018) Is this health campaign really social marketing? A checklist to help you decide. *Health Promotion Journal of Australia* 29, 79–83.

Chou, W.S., Prestin, A., Lyons, C. and Wen, K.Y. (2013) Web 2.0 for health promotion: reviewing the current evidence. *American Journal of Public Health* 103, E9–E11.

Chriss, J.J. (2015) Nudging and social marketing. *Social Science and Public Policy* 52, 54–61.

Clifford, D. and Curtis, L. (2016) *Motivational Interviewing in Nutrition and Fitness*. The Guilford Press (e-book).

Cohn, S. (2014) From health behaviours to health practices: an introduction. *Sociology of Health and Illness* 36 (2), 157–162.

Concepcion, H. (2017) Video game therapy as an intervention for children with disabilities. *Therapeutic Recreation Journal* L1 (3), 221–228.

Conner, M. and Norman, P. (2015) *Predicting and Changing Health Behaviour: Research and practice with social cognition Models*. 3rd edn. Open University Press, Buckingham, UK.

Corcoran, N. (2011) *Working on Health Communication*. Sage, London.

Corcoran, N. (2013) *Communicating Health: Strategies for Health Promotion*. 2nd edn. Sage, London.

Coulter, A. and Mearns, B. (2016) *Developing Care for a Changing Population: Patient Engagement and Health Information Technology*. Nuffield Trust, London.

Crawford, R. (1980) Healthism and the medicalisation of everyday life. *International Journal of Health Services* 10 (3), 365–388.

Cross, R., Davis, S. and O'Neil, I. (2017) *Health Communication: Theoretical and Critical Perspectives*. Polity Press, Cambridge, UK.

Crossley, M.L. (2002) The perils of health promotion and the 'barebacking' backlash. *Health* 6, 47–68.

Dahlgren, G. and Whitehead, M. (1991) *Policies and Strategies to Promote Social Equity in Health*. Institute of Future Studies, Stockholm.

Day, P., Gould, J. and Hazelby, G. (2017) The use of motivational interviewing in community nursing. *Journal of Community Nursing* 31(3), 50–63.

Dejonghe, L.A.L., Rudolf, K., Becker, J., Stassen, G., Froboese, I. and Schaller, A. (2020) Health coaching for promoting physical activity in low back pain patients: a secondary analysis on the usage and acceptance. *BMC Sports Science, Medicine and Rehabilitation* 12, 2, doi: 10.1186/s13102-019-0154-4

Dennison, L., Morrison, L., Conway, G. and Yardley, L. (2013) Opportunities and challenges for smartphone applications in supporting health behavior change: qualitative study. *Journal of Medical Internet Research* 15, e86.

Dewey, J. (1916) *Democracy and Education*. Macmillan, Old Tappan, New Jersey. In: Brookfield, S.D. and Preskill, S. (1999) *Discussion as a way of Teaching – Tools and Techniques for University Teachers*. The Society for Research into Higher Education and Open University Press, London.

Djian, A., Guignard, R., Gallopel-Morvan, K., Smadja, O., Davies, J., Blanc, A., Mercier, A., Walmsley, M and Nguyen-Thanh, V. (2019) From "Stoptober" TO "Moi(S) Sans Tabac": how to import a social marketing campaign. *Journal of Social Marketing* 9(4), 345–356.

Dredze, M. (2012) How social media will change public health. *IEEE Intelligent Systems* 27, 81–84.

Etkin, J. (2016) The hidden cost of personal quantification. *Journal of Consumer Research* 42, 967–984.

Fernández-Aranda, F., Jiménez-Murcia, S., Santamaría, J.J., Gunnard, K., Soto, A., Kalapanidas, E., et al. (2012) Video games as a complementary therapy tool in mental disorders: PlayMancer, a European multicentre study. *Journal of Mental Health* 21(4), 364–374.

Feste, C. and Anderson, R.M. (1995) Empowerment: from philosophy to practice. *Patient Education and Counseling* 26, 139–144.

Finn, P. (1981) Teaching students to be lifelong peer educators. *Health Education* 12, 13–16.

Fisher, R. and Fisher, P. (2018) Peer education and empowerment: perspectives from young women working as peer educators with Home-Start. *Studies in the Education of Adults* 50 (1), 74–91.

Fraser, C. and Restrepo-Estrada, S. (1998) *Communicating for Development: Human Change for Survival*. I.B. Tauris, London.

Freire, P. (2000) *Pedagogy of the Oppressed*. 30th anniversary edition, translated by Myra Bergman Ramos, with introduction by Macedo. Continuum, London and New York.

French, J. (2017) *Social Marketing and Public Health*. 2nd edn. Oxford University Press, Oxford, UK.

Frohlich, K.L. and Abel, T. (2013) Environmental justice and health practices: understanding how health inequities arise at the local level. *Sociology of Health and Illness* 36 (2), 199–212.

Gambling, T.S. (2003) A qualitative study into the informational needs of coronary heart disease patients. *International Journal of Health Promotion and Education* 41, 68–76.

Gillespie, A. (2020) Social and behaviour change. In: Fleming, M. and Baldwin, L. (eds) *Health Promotion in the 21st Century: New approaches to achieving health for all*. Allen & Unwin, London. pp. 141–161.

Godfrey, A. (2017) Wearables for independent living in older adults: gait and falls. *Maturitas* 100, 16–26.

Gold, J., Pedrana, A. E., Sacks-Davis, R., Hellard, M. E., Chang, S., Howard, S., et al. (2011) A systematic examination of the use of online social networking sites for sexual health promotion. *BioMed Central Public Health* 11, 583.

Good Things Foundation (2016) *Health and Digital: Reducing Inequalities, Improving Society: An evaluation of the Widening Digital Participation programme*. Good Things Foundation, Sheffield, UK.

Gordon, R. (2013) Unlocking the potential of upstream social marketing. *European Journal of Marketing* 47 (9), 1525–1547.

Gordon, R. (2016) Social marketing: the state of play and brokering the way forward. *Journal of Marketing Management* 32 (11-12), 1059–1082.

Grant, M. (1994) *Propaganda and the Role of the State in Inter-war Britain*. Clarendon Press, Oxford, UK.

Green, J., Cross, R., Woodall, J. and Tones, K. (2019) *Health Promotion: Planning and Strategies*. 4th edn. Sage, London.

Gregoire, C. (2014) Why these neuroscientists are prescribing video games [online]. *The Huffington Post*. Available at: www.huffingtonpost.co.uk (accessed 22 April 2020).

Griffiths, J., Blair-Stevens, C. and Thorpe, A. (2008) Social marketing for health and specialised health promotion: stronger together – weaker apart. A paper for debate. Shaping the Future of Health Promotion. Royal Society of Public Health, National Social Marketing Centre, London.

Guo, M., Ganz, O., Cruse, B., Navarro, M., Wagner, D., Tate, B., Delahanty, J. and Benoza, G. (2020) Keeping it fresh with hip-hop teens: promising targeting strategies for delivering public health, messages to hard-to-reach audiences. *Health Promotion Practice* 21: Suppl 1, 61S–71S.

Hampshire, K., Porter, G., Owusu, S.A., Mariwah, S., Abane, A., Robson, E., et al. (2015) Informal m-health: how are young people using mobile phones to bridge healthcare gaps in sub-Saharan Africa? *Social Science and Medicine* 142, 90–99.

Hardcastle, S.J., Hancox, J., Hattar, A., Maxwell-Smith, C., ThØgersen-Ntoumani, C. and Hagger, M.S. (2015) Motivating the unmotivated: how can health behaviour be changed in those unwilling to change? *Frontiers in Psychology* 6, 835, doi: 10.3389/fpsyg.2015/00835

Hargie, O., Saunders, C. and Dickson, D. (1994) *Social Skills in Interpersonal Communication*, 3rd edition. Routledge, London and New York.

Harris, T.A. (2004) *I'm OK – You're OK*. Quill, New York.

Hastings, G. and Stead, M. (2006) Social marketing. In: MacDowall, W., Bonell, C. and Davies, M. (eds) *Health Promotion Practice*. Open University Press, Maidenhead, UK, pp. 139–151.

Hazelwood, A. (2008) Using text messaging in the treatment of eating disorders. *Nursing Times* 104 (40), 28–29.

Head, K.J., Noar, S.M., Iannarino, N.T. and Harrington, N.G. (2013) Efficacy of text messaging-based interventions for health promotion: a meta-analysis. *Social Science and Medicine* 97, 41–48.

Henderson, J. (2010) Expert and lay knowledge: a sociological perspective. *Nutrition and Dietetics* 67, 4–5.

Heydarzadeh, L., Alilu, L., Habibzadeh, H. and Rasouli, J. (2019) The effect of peer education on knowledge, comprehension, and knowledge application of patients regarding chemotherapy complications. *Iranian Journal of Nursing and Midwifery Research* 25: 40–46.

Hill, S., Merchant, R. and Ungar, L. (2013) Lessons learned about public health from online crowd surveillance. *Big Data*, 160–167.

Hillsden, M. (2006) Motivational interviewing in health promotion. In: MacDowall, W., Bonell, C. and Davies, M. (eds) *Health Promotion Practice*. Open University Press, Maidenhead, UK, pp. 74–85.

Ho, J., Cordena, M. E., Caccamoa, L., Tomasino, K. N., Duffecyb, J., Begalea, M., et al. (2016) Design and evaluation of a peer network to support adherence to a web-based intervention for adolescents. *Internet Interventions* 6, 50–56.

Honeyman, M., Dunn, P. and McKenna, H. (2016) *A Digital NHS? An Introduction to the Digital Agenda and Plans for Implementation*. The King's Fund, London.

House of Commons Health Committee (2016) *Public Health Post-2013*. House of Commons, London.

Hubley, J. (2006) Patient education in the developing world – a discipline comes of age. *Patient Education and Counselling* 61, 161–164.

Hubley, J., Copeman, J. and Woodall, J. (2021) *Practical Health Promotion.* 3rd edition Polity Press, Cambridge, UK.

Hunter, R.F., Gough, A., Kane, N.O., MsKeown, G., Fitzpatrick, A., Walker, T. et al. (2018) Ethical issues in social media research for public health. *American Journal of Public Health* 108 (3), 343–348.

Ipsos MORI (2015) *GP Patient Survey: National Summary Report.* NHS England, Leeds, UK.

Ishikawa, H., Nomura, K., Sato, M. and Yano, E. (2008) Developing a measure of communicative and critical health literacy: a pilot study of Japanese office workers. *Health Promotion International* 23, 269–274.

IUHPE (2018) *Position Statement on Health Literacy: A practical vision for a health literate world.* IUHPE, Paris.

Jamali, A. Ghaljaei, F., Keikhaei, A. and Jalalodini, A. (2019) Effect of peer education on the resilience of mothers of children with leukaemia: a clinical trial. *Medical-Surgical Nursing Journal* 8 (2), e92686.

Jamison, A.M., Broniatowski, D.A. and Crouse Quinn, S. (2019) Malicious actors on Twitter: a guide for public health researchers. *American Journal of Public Health* 109(5), 688–692.

Johnson, C.W. (2010) *Case Studies in the Failure of Healthcare Information Systems.* University of Glasgow, Department of Computing Science, Glasgow, UK.

Kannappan, S. and Shanmugam, K. (2019) Peer educators as change leaders – effectiveness of peer education process in creating awareness on reproductive health among women workers in textile industry. *Indian Journal of Community Medicine* 44, 252–255.

Karapanos, E., Gouveia, R., Hassenzahl, M. and Jodi Forlizzi, J. (2016) Wellbeing in the making: peoples' experiences with wearable activity trackers. *Psychology of Well-Being* 6 (4), 1–17.

Katz, E. and Lazarfeld, P.F. (1955) Personal influence. In: McQuail, D. and Windahl, S. (eds) (1993) *Communication Models for the Study of Mass Communications.* 2nd edn. Longman, London.

Kennedy, A., Kemper, J.A. and Parsons, A.G. (2018) Upstream social marketing strategy. *Journal of Social Marketing* 8 (3), 258–279.

Kettunen, T., Poskiparta, M. and Liimatainen, L. (2001) Empowering counselling, a case study: nurse-patient encounter in a hospital. *Health Education Research*, 16, 227–238.

Kettunen, T., Poskiparta, M. and Karhila, P. (2003) Speech practices that facilitate patient participation in health counselling – a way to empowerment? *Health Education Journal* 62, 326–340.

Kickbusch I. (2019) Health promotion 4.0. *Health Promotion International* 34, 179–181.

Kiger, A. (2004) *Teaching for Health*, 3rd edition. Churchill Livingstone, London.

Kirschenbaum, H. and Henderson, V.L. (1989) *The Carl Rogers Reader.* Houghton Mifflin, Boston, Massachusetts.

Kitchin, R. and Lauriault, T. (2014) Towards critical data studies: charting and unpacking data assemblages and their work [online]. The Programmable City Working Paper 2. Available at: www.researchgate.net/publication/267867447 (accessed 22 April 2020).

Knowles, M. (1980) *The Modern Practice of Adult Education.* Association Press, Chicago, Illinois.

Korda, H. and Itani, Z. (2013) Harnessing social media for health promotion and behaviour change. *Health Promotion Practice* 14, 15–23.

Kramer, J.N. and Kowatsch, T. (2017) Using feedback to promote physical activity: the role of the feedback sign. *Journal of Medical Internet Research* 19 (6), e192.

Krebs, P. and Duncan, D.T. (2015) Health apps use among US mobile phone owners: a national survey. *Journal of Medical Internet Research, Mhealth Ehealth* (4), e101.

Kreuter, M.T. and McClure, S.M. (2004) The role of culture in health communication.*Annual Review of Public Health* 25, 439–455.

Kreuter, M.W., Lukwago, S.N., Bucholtz, D.C., Clark, E.M. and Sanders-Thompson, V. (2003) Achieving cultural appropriateness in health promotion programs: targeted and tailored approaches. *Health Education and Behavior* 30, 133.

Lafferty, N. (2013) *NHS-HE Connectivity Project: Web 2.0 and Social Media in Education and Research.* Connectivity Best Practice Working Group of the NHS-HE Forum, Dundee, UK.

Langford, R. and Panter-Brick, C. (2013) A health equity critique of social marketing: where interventions have impact but insufficient reach. *Social Science & Medicine* 83, 113–141.

Larkey, L.K. and Hecht, M. (2010) A model of effects of narrative as culture-centric health promotion. *Journal of Health Communication* 15, 114–135.

Lasswell, H.D. (1948) The structure and function of communication in society. In: Bryson L. (ed.) *The Communication of Ideas.* Harper, New York; cited in: McQuail, D. and Windahl, S. (1993) *Communication Models: for the Study of Mass Communication*, 2nd edition. Pearson Education Limited, Harlow, UK.

Laverack, G. (2017) The challenge of behaviour change and health promotion. *Challenges* 8(25), 1–4.

Laverack, G. and Dap, D.H. (2003) Transforming information, education and communication in Vietnam. *Health Education* 103, 363–369.

Lawrence, D., Johnson, S., Hafekost, J., Boterhoven de Haan, K., Sawyer, M., Ainley, J. et al. (2015) *The Mental Health of Children and Adolescents: Report on the second Australian child and adolescent survey of health and wellbeing.* Australian Government, Canberra.

Lawton, R., Connor, M. and McEachan, R. (2009) Desire or reason: predicting health behaviour from affective and cognitive attitudes. *Health Psychology* 28, 56–65.

Lazarsfeld, P.F. and Merton, R.K. (1955) Mass communication, popular taste and organized social action. In: Schramm, W. (ed.) *Mass Communication*. University of Illinois Press, Urbana, Illinois.

Ledger, D. (2014) *Inside Wearables – Part 2*. Endeavour Partners LLC, Cambridge, Massachusetts.

Lee, R.G. and Garvin, T. (2003) Moving from information transfer to information exchange in health and health care. *Social Science & Medicine* 56, 449–464.

Lefebvre, R.C. (1997) The social marketing imbroglio in health promotion. In: Sidell, M., Jones, L., Katz, J. and Peberdy, A. (eds) *Debates and Dilemmas in Promoting Health: A Reader*. Open University Press, Basingstoke, UK, pp. 108–113.

Leininger, M. (1991) *Cultural Care Diversity and Universality*. National League for Nursing, New York.

Lewis, T., Synowiec, C., Lagomarsinoa, G. and Schweitzera, J. (2012) E-health in low- and middle-income countries: findings from the Centre for Health Market Innovations. *Bulletin of the World Health Organization* 90, 332–340.

Lievrouw, L. (2009) *Alternative and Activist New Media*. Polity Press, Oxford, UK.

Lin, P., Simoni, J.M. and Zemon, V. (2005) The health belief model, sexual behaviours and HIV risk among Taiwanese immigrants. *AIDS Education and Research* 17, 469–483.

Lin, Y., Osman, M. and Ashcroft, R. (2017) Nudge: concept, effectiveness, and ethics. *Basic and Applied Social Psychology* 39 (6), 293–306.

Linney, B. (1995) *Pictures, People and Power*. Macmillan Education Ltd, London.

Lister, C., West, J.H., Cannon, B., Sax, T. and Brodegard, D. (2014) Just a fad? Gamification in health and fitness apps. *Journal of Medical Internet Research* 2 (2), e9.

Lodge, M. and Wegrich, K. (2016) The rationality paradox of nudge: rational tools of government in a world of bounded rationality. *Law & Policy* 38 (3), 250–267.

Loibl, C., Sunstein, C.R., Rauber, J. and Reisch, L.A. (2018) Which Europeans like nudges? Approval and controversy in four European countries. *The Journal of Consumer Affairs*, 655–688.

Loss, J., Lindacher, V. and Curbach, J. (2014) Online social networking sites – a novel setting for health promotion? *Health and Place* 26, 161–170.

Luft, J. and Ingham, H. (1955) *The Johari Window: A Graphic Model for interpersonal relations*. University of California at Los Angeles, Extension Office, Western Training Laboratory in Group Development.

Lundahl, B.W., Kunz, C., Brownell, C., Tollefson, D. and Burke, B.L. (2010) Meta-analysis of motivational interviewing: twenty-five years of empirical students. *Research on Social Work Practice* 20, 137–160.

Lupton, D. (2012) M-health and health promotion: the digital cyborg and surveillance society. *Social Theory and Health* 10(3), 229–244.

Lupton, D. (2013) *Digitized Health Promotion: Personal Responsibility for Health in the Web 2.0 Era*. Sydney Health & Society Group Working Paper No. 5, Sydney, Australia.

Lupton, D. (2015a) Quantified sex: a critical analysis of sexual and reproductive self-tracking using apps. *Culture, Health and Sexuality* 17(4), 440–453.

Lupton, D. (2015b) Health promotion in the digital era: a critical commentary. *Health Promotion International* 30(1), 174–183.

Magill, M., Apodaca, T.R., Borsari, B., Gaume, J., Hoadley, A., Gordon, R.E.F., Tonigan, J.S. and Moyers, T. (2018) A meta-analysis of motivational interviewing process: technical, relational, and conditional process models of change. *Journal of Consulting and Clinical Psychology* 86(2), 140–157.

Maibach, E. and Parrott, R. (1995) *Designing Health Messages: Approaches from Communication Theory and Public Health Practice*. Sage, London.

Maio, G.R., Haddock, G.G. and Jarman, H.L. (2007) Social psychological factors in tackling obesity. *Obesity Reviews* 8 (Supplement 1), 123–125.

Mann, S. and Bailey, J.V. (2016) *Implementation of digital interventions for sexual health for young people*. Frontiers Public Health. Conference Abstract: 2nd Behaviour Change Conference: Digital Health and Wellbeing, London.

Manoff, R. (1985) *Social Marketing: New Imperative for Public Health*. Praeger, New York.

Marcano-Olivier, M.I., Horne, P.J., Viktor, S. and Erjavec, M. (2020) Using nudges to promote healthy food choices in the school dining room: a systematic review of previous investigations. *Journal of School Health* 90(2), 143–157.

Marks, D.F., Murray, M. and Estacio, E.V. (2018) *Health Psychology: Theory, Research & Practice*. 5th edition. Sage, London.

Marschang, S. (2014) *Health Inequalities and eHeatlh: Report of the eHealth Stakeholders Group*. European Public Health Alliance (EPHA), Brussels.

Marteau, T.M., Ogilvie, D., Roland, M. and Suhrcke, M. (2011) Judging nudging: can nudging improve population health? *British Medical Journal* 342, 263–265.

Martin, E., Blythe, R., Kularatna, S. and Carter, H. (2020) The economics of prevention. In: Fleming, M. and Baldwin, L. (eds) *Health Promotion in the 21st Century: New approaches to achieving health for all*. Allen & Unwin, London, pp. 15–36.

McGuire, W. (1989) Theoretical foundations of campaigns. In: Rice, R. and Atkin, C. (eds) *Public Communication Campaigns*. Sage, Newbury Park, California, pp. 43–65.

McLuhan, M. and Fiore, Q. (1967) *The Medium is the Message*. Penguin, Harmondsworth, UK.

Mda, Z. (1993) *When People Play People: Development Communication through Theatre*. Zed Books, London.

Mendelsohn, H. (1968) Which shall it be: mass education or mass persuasion for health? *American Journal of Public Health* 58, 131–137.

Meyer, J. and Land, R. (2005) Threshold concepts and troublesome knowledge (2): epistemological considerations and a conceptual framework for teaching and learning. *Higher Education* 49, 373–388.

Mezirow, J. (1981) A critical theory of adult learning and education. *Adult Education* 32, 3–24.

Mezirow, J. (2003) Transformative learning as discourse. *Journal of Transformative Education* 1, 58–63.

Michie, S., van Stralen, M.M. and West, R. (2011) The behaviour change wheel: a new method for characterising and designing behaviour change interventions. *Implementation Science* 6(42), doi.org/10.1186/1748-5908-6-42

Michie, S., Brown, J., Geraghty, A.W.A., Miller, S., Yardley, L., Gardner, B. et al. (2012) Development of StopAdvisor: a theory-based interactive internet-based smoking cessation intervention. *Translational Behavioral Medicine* 2, 263–75.

Michie, S., Atkins, L. and West, R. (2014) *The Behaviour Change Wheel: A Guide to Designing Interventions*. Silverback Publishing, London.

Mielewczyk, F. and Willig, C. (2007) Old clothes and an older look – the case for a radical makeover in health behaviour research. *Theory and Psychology* 17(6), 811–837.

Milburn, K. (1995) A critical review of peer education with young people with special reference to sexual education. *Health Education Research* 10, 407–420.

Miller, W.R. and Rollnick, S. (2002) *Motivational Interviewing: Preparing People for Change*, 2nd edition. Guildford Press, London.

Milligan, C., Roberts, C. and Mort, M. (2011) Telecare and older people: who cares where? *Social Science and Medicine* 72, 347–354.

Mittelstadt, B.D. and Floridi, L. (2016) The ethics of Big Data: current and foreseeable issues in biomedical contexts. *Science and Engineering Ethics* 22, 303–341.

Montreal Declaration (2018) *Montreal Declaration for a Responsible Development of Artificial Intelligence*. Available at: https://www.montrealdeclaration-responsibleai.com/the-declaration (accessed 7 April 2020).

Morrison, L., Moss-Morris, R., Michie, S. and Yardley, L. (2014) Optimizing engagement with Internet-based health behaviour change interventions: comparison of self-assessment with and without tailored feedback using a mixed methods approach. *British Journal of Health Psychology* 19, 839–855.

Nahmias, Y., Perez, O., Shlomo, Y. and Stremmer, U. (2019) Privacy preserving social norm nudges. *Michigan Technology Law Review* 26, 43–91.

Naidoo, J. and Wills, J. (2016) *Foundations for Health Promotion*. 4th edition. Elsevier, London.

National Health Service (NHS) (2017) *The Next Steps on the NHS Five Year Forward View in England*. HMSO, London.

Neter, E. and Brainin, E. (2019) Association between health literacy, eHealth literacy, and health outcomes among patients with long-term conditions. *European Psychologist* 24(1), 68–81.

Neuhauser, L., Kreps, G.L., Morrison, K., Athanasoulis, M., Kirienko, N. and Van Brunt, D. (2013) Using design science and artificial intelligence to improve health communication: chronology MD case example. *Patient Education and Counselling* 92, 211–217.

Norman, C. (2012) Social media and health promotion. *Global Health Promotion* 19(4), 3–6.

Norman, C. and Skinner, H. (2006) eHealth literacy: essential skills for consumer health in a networked world. *Journal of Medical Internet Research* 8(2), e9.

Nutbeam, D. (1998) Health promotion glossary. *Health Promotion International* 13, 349–364.

Nutbeam, D. (2000) Health literacy as a public health goal: a challenge for contemporary health education and communication strategies into the 21st century. *Health Promotion International* 15, 259–267.

Obrist, H.U. (2011) *Ai Weiwei speaks with Hans Ulrich Obrist*. Penguin, Harmondsworth, UK.

O'Neil, I. (2019) *Digital Health Promotion: A Critical Introduction*. Polity Press, Cambridge, UK.

Palmer, S., Tubbs, I. and Whybrow, A. (2003) Health coaching to facilitate the promotion of healthy behaviour and achievement of health-related goals. *International Journal of Health Promotion and Education* 41, 91–93.

Papacharissi, Z.A. (2010) *A Private Sphere: Democracy in a Digital Age*. Polity Press, Oxford, UK.

Peerson, A. and Saunders, M. (2009) Health literacy revisited: what do we mean and why does it matter? *Health Promotion International* 24, 285–296.

Pettigrew, S. (2015) Pleasure: an under-utilised 'P' in social marketing for health eating. *Appetite* 104, 60–69.

Pfeffer, I. and Strobach, T. (2017) Executive functions, trait self-control, and the Intention-Behavior Gap in physical activity behavior. *Journal of Sport & Exercise Psychology* 39, 277–292.

Piette, J.D., Lun, K.C., Moura, L.A., Fraser, H.S.F., Mechael, P.N., Powell, F.J., et al. (2012) Impacts of e-health on the outcomes of care in low- and middle-income countries: where do we go from here? *Bulletin of the World Health Organization* 90, 332–340.

Piwek, L., Ellis, D.A., Andrews, S. and Joinson, A. (2016) The rise of consumer health wearables: promises and barriers. *PLoS Medicine* 13(2), 1001953.

Pleasant, A. and Kuruvilla, S. (2008) A tale of two health literacies: public health and clinical approaches to health literacy. *Health Promotion International* 23, 152–159.

Pleasant, A., McKinney, J. and Rikard, R.V. (2011) Health literacy measurement: a proposed research agenda. *Journal of Health Communication* 16, 11–21.

Pratt, D.D. and Associates (2005) *Five Perspectives on Teaching in Adult and Higher Education.* Reprint of the 1998 edition with corrections. Krieger Publishing Company, Malabar, Florida.

Primack, B.A., Carroll, M.V., McNamara, M., Klem, M.L., King, B., Rich, M.O., et al. (2012) Role of video games in improving health-related outcomes: a systematic review. *American Journal of Preventive Medicine* 42(6), 630–638.

Prochaska, J.O. and DiClemente, C.C. (1983) Stages and processes of self-change of smoking: toward an integrative model of change. *Journal of Consulting and Clinical Psychology* 51, 390–395.

Purdy, M. (1997) Humanist ideology and nurse education – humanistic education theory. *Nurse Education Today* 17, 192–195.

Rajatonirina, S., Heraud, J., Randrianasolo, L., Orelle, A., Razanajatovo, N.H., Raoelina, Y.N., et al. (2012) Short message service sentinel surveillance of influenza in Madagascar, 2008–2012. *Bulletin of the World Health Organization* 90, 385–389.

Ramos, D. and Perkins, D. (2006) Goodness of fit assessment of an alcohol intervention program and underlying theories of change. *Journal of American College Health* 55, 57–64.

Rice, E., Haynes, E., Royce, P. and Thompson, S.C. (2016) Social media and digital technology use among Indigenous young people in Australia: a literature review. *International Journal for Equity in Health* 15, 81.

Rice, L. and Sara, R. (2019) Updating the determinants of health model in the Information Age. *Health Promotion International* 34, 1241–1249.

Roberts, R., Towell, T. and Golding, J.F. (2001) *Foundations of Health Psychology*. Palgrave, Basingstoke, UK.

Robinson, M. and Robertson, S. (2010) Young men's health promotion and new information communication technologies: illuminating the issues and research agendas. *Health Promotion International* 25, 363–370.

Rogers, C.R. (1969) *Freedom to Learn*. Merrill, New York.

Rogers, E.M. (1986) *Communication Technology: The New Media in Society*. The Free Press, New York.

Rogers, E.M. (1995) *The Diffusion of Innovations*, 4th edition. The Free Press, New York.

Rogers, E.M. (2003) *Diffusion of Innovations*, 5th edition. The Free Press, New York.

Rogers, E.M. and Shoemaker, F. (1971) *The Communication of Innovations*. The Free Press, New York.

Rogers, R.W. (1975) A protection motivation theory of fear appeals and attitude change. *Journal of Psychology* 91, 93–114.

Rogers, R.W. (1983) Cognitive and physiological processes in fear appeals and attitude change: a revised theory of protection motivation. In: Cacippo, J.R. and Petty, R.E. (eds) *Social Psychology: A Source Book*. Guilford Press, New York, pp. 153–176.

Rosenstock, I.M., Strecher, V.J. and Becker, M.H. (1988) Social learning theory and the health belief model. *Health Education Quarterly* 15, 175–183.

Roser, M. and Ortiz-Ospina, E. (2018) *Literacy*. Available at: http://www.ourworldindata.org (accessed 31 March 2020).

Rubak, S., Sandboek, A., Lauritzen, T. and Christensen, B. (2005) Motivational interviewing: a systematic review and meta-analysis. *British Journal of General Practice* 55, 305–312.

Rudd, R.E. (2015) The evolving concept of health literacy: new directions for health literacy studies. *Journal of Communication in Healthcare* 8(1), 7–9.

Sanders, C., Rogers, A., Bowen, R., Bower, P., Hirani, S., Cartwright, M., et al. (2012) Exploring barriers to participation and adoption of telehealth and telecare within the Whole System Demonstrator trial: a qualitative study. *BMC Health Services Research* 12, 220.

Saraceno, B., Van Ommeren, M., Batniji, R., Cohen, A., Gureje, O., Mahoney, J., et al. (2007) Barriers to improvement of mental health services in low-income and middle-income countries. *Lancet* 370, 1164–1174.

Sarafino, E. and Smith, T. (2016) *Health Psychology: Biopsychosocial Interactions*, 9th edition. John Wiley & Sons, Chichester, UK.

Seidenberg, P., Nicholson, S., Schaefer, M., Semrau, K., Bweupe, A., Masese, N., et al. (2012) Early infant diagnosis of HIV infection in Zambia through mobile phone texting of blood test results. *Bulletin of the World Health Organization* 90, 348–356.

Sfard, A. (1998) On two metaphors for learning and the dangers of choosing just one. *Educational Researcher* 27, 4–13.

Singh, B. (2011) The Power of New Media, The Youth Effect. Available at: http://www.youtheffect.org/bhavneetsingh/ (accessed 30 January 2012).

Shannon, C. and Weaver, W. (1949) *The Mathematical Theory of Communication*. University of Illinois Press, Urbana, Illinois. In: McQuail, D. and Windahl, S. (1993) *Communication Models for the Study of*

Mass Communication, 2nd edition. Longman, London.

Sheidaei, S., Jafarnejad, F., Mohammad Zadeh, F. and Taji Heravi, A. (2019) The effect of peer education on pregnant women's choosing mode of delivery. *Journal of Midwifery and Reproductive Health* 7(4), 1880–1887.

Shet, A., Arumugam, K., Rodrigues, R., Rajagopalan, N., Shubha, K., Raj, T., et al. (2010) Designing a mobile phone-based intervention to promote adherence to antiretroviral therapy in South India. *AIDS Behaviour* 14, 716–720.

Shove, E. (2010) Submission to the House of Lords Science and Technology Select Committee calling for evidence on behaviour change.

Sørensen, K., Pinheiro, P., Levin-Zamir, D., Bauer, U. and Orkan, O. (2019) *International Handbook of Health Literacy.* Policy Press (e-book).

South, J. (2005) Community Arts for Health: an evaluation of a district programme. *Health Education* 106, 155–168.

South, J., Bagnall, A. and Woodall, J. (2017) Developing a typology for peer education and peer support delivered by prisoners. *Journal of Correctional Health Care* 23 (2), 214–229.

Steinberg, S. (2006) *Introduction to Communication.* Juta and Co., Cape Town, South Africa.

Stephenson, A., McDonough, S., Murphy, M.H., Nugent, C.D. and Mair, J.L. (2017) Using computer, mobile and wearable technology enhanced interventions to reduce sedentary behaviour: a systematic review and meta-analysis. *International Journal of Behavioural Nutrition and Physical Activity* 14, 105.

Steptoe, A., Prekins-Porras, L., McKay, C., Rink, E., Hilton, S. and Cappuccio, F. (2003) Behavioural counselling to increase consumption of fruit and vegetables in low income adults: randomised trial. *British Medical Journal* 326, 855–858.

Stevely, A.K., Buykx, P., Brown, J., Beard, E., Michie, S., Meier, P.S. and Holmes, J. (2018) Exposure to revised drinking guidelines and 'COM-B' determinants of behaviour change: descriptive analysis of a monthly cross-sectional survey in England. *BMC Public Health* 18, 251, doi.org/10.1186/s12889-018-5129-y

Stevens, C. (2008) Social capital in its place: using social theory to understand social capital and inequalities in health. *Social Science & Medicine* 66, 1174–1184.

Sutton, S. (2005) Stage theories of health behaviour. In: Conner, M. and Norman, P. (eds.) *Predicting Health Behaviours*, 2nd edition. Open University Press, Buckingham, UK, pp. 223–275.

Sweeney, G.-M., Donovan, C.L., March, S. and Forbes, Y. (2016) Logging into therapy: adolescent perceptions of online therapies for mental health problems. *Internet Interventions*, 12.001.

Strategic Direction (2018) Influencing the influencers: using upstream social marketing to make changes at the top. *Strategic Direction* 34(12), 15–16.

Svenson, G. (1998) *European Guidelines for Youth AIDS Peer Education.* European Commission, Luxembourg.

Thaler, R.H. and Sunstein, C.R. (2008) *Nudge: Improving Decisions about Health, Wealth and Happiness*. Penguin, London.

Thirumurthy, H. and Lester, R. (2012) M-health for health behaviour change in resource-limited settings: applications to HIV care and beyond. *Bulletin of the World Health Organization* 90, 390–392.

Tones, K. (2002) Health literacy: old wine in new bottles? *Health Education Research* 17, 287–290.

UNAIDS (1999) *Peer Education and HIV/AIDS: Concepts, uses and challenges*. Joint United Nations Programme on HIV/AIDS (UNAIDS), Geneva.

Upton, D. and Thirlaway, K. (2014) *Promoting Healthy Behaviour: A Practical Guide. 2nd edition*. Routledge, Oxford, UK.

US Department of Commerce (2013) *Exploring the Digital Nation*. US Department of Commerce, Washington, DC.

Vannucci, A., Simpson, E.G., Gagnon, S. and McCauley Ohannessian, C. (2020) Social media use and risky behaviours in adolescents: a meta-analysis. *Journal of Adolescence* 79, 258–274.

Wachter, R.M. (2016) *Making IT Work: Harnessing the Power of Health Information Technology to Improve Care in England*. National Advisory Group on Health Information Technology in England, London.

Wakefield, M.A., Loken, B. and Hornik R.C. (2010) Use of mass media campaigns to change health behaviour. *The Lancet* 376, 1261–1271.

Warwick-Booth, L., Cross, R. and Lowcock, D. (2021) *Contemporary Health Studies: An Introduction.* 2nd edition Polity Press, Cambridge, UK.

Webb, T. L. Joseph, J., Yardley, L. and Michie, S. (2010) Using the Internet to promote health behaviour change: a systematic review and meta-analysis of the impact of theoretical basis, use of behaviour change techniques, and mode of delivery on efficacy. *Journal of Medical Internet Research* 12 (1), e4.

Werner, D. and Sanders, D. (1997) *Questioning the Solution: The Politics of Primary Health Care and Child Survival*. HealthWrights, Palo Alto, California

Weymann, N., Harter, M. and Dirmaier, J. (2014) Quality of online information on type 2 diabetes: a cross-sectional study. *Health Promotion International* 30(4), 821–831.

White, D.S. and Le Cornu, A. (2011) Visitors and residents: a new typology for online engagement [online]. *First Monday* 16(9). Available at: firstmonday.org/article/view/3171/3049 (accessed 22 April 2020).

Wills, J. and Earle, S. (2007) Theoretical perspectives on promoting public health. In: Earle, S., Lloyd, C.E.,

Sidell, M. and Spurr, S. (eds) *Theory and Research in Promoting Public Health*. Sage, London, pp. 129–162.

Windahl, S. and Signitzer, B. with Olson, J. (2009) *Using Communication Theory: An Introduction to Planned Communication*, 2nd edition. Sage, London.

Winter, S.J., Sheats, J.L. and King, A. (2016) The use of behaviour change technologies and theory in technologies for cardiovascular disease prevention and treatment in adults: a comprehensive review. *Progress in Cardiovascular Diseases* 58: 605–612.

WHO (World Health Organization) (1986) Ottawa Charter for health promotion. *Health Promotion* 1, *iii–v*.

WHO (World Health Organization) (2011) *mHealth: New Horizons for Health through Mobile Technologies. Global Observatory for eHealth series, no.3*. World Health Organization, Geneva.

WHO (World Health Organization) (2013) *Health Literacy*. World Health Organization, Copenhagen.

WHO (World Health Organization) (2016) The mandate for health literacy. Available at: www.who.int/health-promotion/conferences/9gchp/health-literacy/en/ (accessed 25 August 2020).

Yurt, S., Saglam Aksut, R. and Kadioglu, H. (2019) The effect of peer education on health beliefs about breast cancer screening. *International Nursing Review* 66, 498–505.

Zach, L., Dalrymple, P.W., Rogers, M.L. and Williver-Farr, H. (2011) Assessing internet access and use in a medically underserved population: implications for providing enhanced health information services. *Health Information and Libraries Journal* 29, 61–71.

Zarcadoolas, C., Pleasant, A. and Greer, D.S. (2005) Understanding health literacy: an expanded model. *Health Promotion International* 20, 195–203.

5 Professional Practice

JAMES WOODALL AND SIMON ROWLANDS[1]

This chapter aims to:
- explore the role of the settings approach to health promotion and the need for organizational change;
- discuss the importance of evidence-based practice and evaluation;
- describe some of the ethical issues in practising health promotion;
- suggest a means of overcoming the top-down/bottom-up tensions in practice;
- explore the need for developing partnerships between civil society, NGOs, and private and public sectors; and
- outline the skills and competencies of health promoters practising in the 21st century.

Introduction

It is clear from the preceding chapters that health promotion is not short on vision or strategy, and health promoters have developed practical ways of implementing those visions and ideas. This chapter does not have the 'answers', but does aim to make some suggestions about how steps can be taken to implement the vision.

It should be clear that we believe that top-down, programmatic approaches to change are not likely to be effective in tackling the complex, real-life problems that health promoters want to address. Such approaches also do not bring about sustainable development or sustainable, long-lasting solutions. There are no universal prescriptions or 'quick fixes' to the health problems facing the global community. What we do want is transformational change, in individuals, communities, organizations and governments – nothing short of transformational change will produce the desired redistribution of power required to bring about equity in health.

Later in this chapter, we suggest that the evolving, new relationships between the private sector, governments, the non-governmental or 'third sector', and civil society might be one way to move towards creating the kind of societies that people prefer to live in. There needs to be a move away from 'interventions' and a move towards working *with* people to implement change. If people are put at the centre of the change process, and if the way to transform communities and organizations is to develop networks based on cooperation, then there are clear implications for the professional–community relationship and for the skills required of health promoters. The skills and competencies of health promoters are discussed below, together with some ideas about what needs to happen in terms of taking on leadership roles for the health promotion agenda. The roles of professionals – 'experts' – are challenged by moving away from top-down approaches and this raises questions about the relationships between professionals and communities.

There needs to be practical ways of overcoming the top-down/bottom-up dichotomy, with new ways of working that properly reflect the 'messy' real life problems and the equally messy types of solutions required, which can be contextualized to the needs of specific situations and cultures. It cannot be the case that 'one size will fit all', and therefore ways of working need to be flexible, adaptable and adopt an action learning or action research approach.

To achieve a healthier society, we suggest that there must be: involvement of communities and citizens; healthy public policy building; and the development of organizations and organizational cultures towards health (Fig. 5.1).

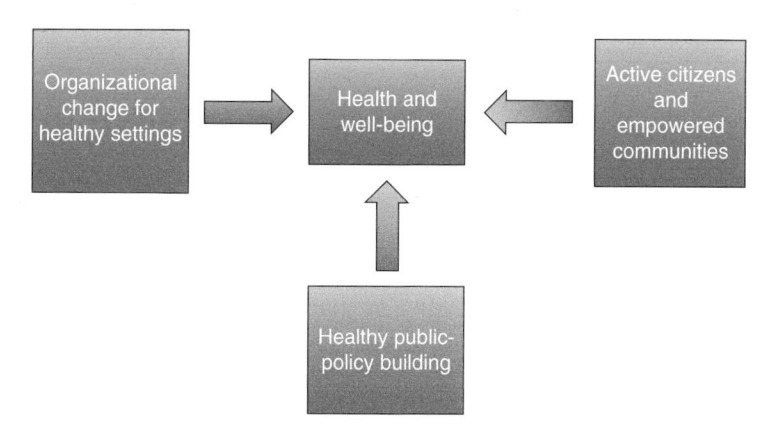

Fig. 5.1. Building blocks to create a healthier society.

The ways in which citizens and communities can be involved are described below in the examples of the People in Public Health Project, community health champions and the roles of community-based organizations in solid waste management. Some suggestions for ways in which organizations can contribute to producing healthier societies are also discussed.

Health promotion in its brief history has also not been short on rhetoric and idealism, and disagreements about the 'best' ways of working. We would assert that a hefty dose of pragmatism will help the implementation process; given that there are many routes to the same goal, what is important is that the journey begins. In this regard, we suggest that settings approaches offer one practical way to 'do' health promotion, and one section of this chapter therefore discusses in detail the strengths and weaknesses of this approach.

Evidence-based practice and the importance of evaluating health promotion work are also explored in this chapter as essential aspects of health promotion practice. Evidence-based practice and evaluation are linked in as much as the latter feeds into an understanding of what works and what does not, which then forms an evidence base. 'Research into practice' is another important activity, given that much health promotion research aims to 'make a difference'. Another section of this chapter considers ethics in health promotion work, although there is also a thread of ethics and exploration of the value base of health promotion work throughout the book. This chapter includes some examples of health promotion, which we consider show aspects of good practice and which might be of interest to illustrate 'good' health promotion on the ground.

This chapter therefore focuses on ways of working, and includes sections on: working in settings; working to change organizations; developing evidence-based practice and skills in evaluation; working ethically; working with active citizens and the third sector (or NGOs); working in ways that resolve the top-down/bottom-up conundrum; and the skills and competencies of health promoters. These sections are not in any particular order, except working in settings is logically followed by a section on organizational change, evidence-based practice and evaluation, which are linked, and the final section is in that position because it considers all of the rest in terms of what it means for the skills of health promoters. More simply, the chapter considers where health promotion can take place (in settings), and how we should work as effective and ethical promoters of health.

The Settings Approach to Health Promotion

The idea of promoting health through 'settings' has become a popular approach within health promotion practice, reflected through the diversity of global interventions now being implemented in traditional sites, such as schools, workplaces, universities and hospitals. There is, however, now a 'second wave' of environments in which settings-based activities are undertaken; this includes sports clubs and, of course, the virtual world. Health promotion can also operate in settings where there is a 'clash' of ideological and practical arrangements – prison is an example of this and this particular setting is used as an example in many sections of the chapter, given one of the authors' research focus. As an approach to 'doing' health promotion, the settings approach has provided practitioners with a tangible way to promote health, primarily because social systems have a huge bearing on people's lives and because they provide a distinct location for intervention. Some have said this suggests that the settings approach is one of the most successful and 'top rated' strategies to emerge from the Ottawa Charter (Torp et al., 2014).

However, despite the considerable strides made in practice, the theoretical framework underpinning the settings approach has not always been made explicit and a variety of words have been used, as shown in Box 5.1. Similarly, there have been difficulties in evidencing the outcomes of settings intervention and this has been suggested as one of the underpinning reasons why the approach has stalled and not had the impact that was originally anticipated (Woodall and Freeman, 2020). For example, it has now been some time since the establishment of the concept of the health-promoting prison and yet limited progress has taken place (Woodall, 2016). Moreover, health-promoting universities have been synonymous with the settings approach but the concept and practice, too, have been relatively slow to be adopted (Newton et al., 2016).

The underlying premise of the settings approach is that investments in health are made in social systems where health is not their primary remit. Fundamental to this is the belief that health is produced outside of illness (health) services and that effective health improvements require investment in social systems (Dooris, 2004). This was espoused in the Ottawa Charter, which argued that health was not primarily the outcome of medical intervention, but an ecological concept that embraced the interplay between social, political, economic and behavioural factors (Dooris et al., 1998): 'Health is created and lived by people within the settings of their everyday life; where they learn, work, play and love' (WHO, 1986a, p. v).

Consistent backing by the World Health Organization (WHO) through the late 1980s and 1990s (WHO, 1986b, 1991, 1997, 1998a, b) saw ecological views of health promotion, delivered through the settings approach, gain increasing momentum.

Proponents of the settings approach, like Green et al. (2000, p. 23), have suggested that settings can be conceptualized as both:

1. Physically bounded space-times in which people come together to perform specific tasks (usually oriented to goals other than health).
2. Arenas of sustained interaction, with pre-existing structures, policies, characteristics, institutional values and formal and informal social sanctions on behaviour.

This provides added scope to the WHO's (1998b, p. 19) definition of a setting for health:

> The place or social context in which people engage in daily activities in which environmental, organisational and personal factors interact to affect health and well-being…where people actively use and shape the environment and thus create or solve problems relating to health. Settings can normally be identified as having physical boundaries, a range of people with defined roles, and an organisational structure.

Arguably, this definition is now becoming more and more redundant with the rise in digital spaces and a virtual world that has expanded through the Covid-19 experience. Despite definitions and guidance being put forward within health promotion discourse, there remains some ambiguity as to what actually constitutes a 'setting'. The terms used for

---

Box 5.1. The settings approach: etymology.

A range of terminology has been used to denote settings-based approaches to health promotion. 'Health setting', 'health-promoting settings', 'settings for health', 'settings for health promotion', 'the settings approach' and 'the settings-based approach' are all terms commonly in use (Richmond, 2009). Whilst the semantic differences may seem trivial, the terms do carry different nuances (Richmond, 2009). Denman et al. (2002), for example, have drawn attention to the subtle semantic variations between organizations labelled as 'health-promoting settings' and those categorized as 'healthy settings'. Dooris (2006) notes the difference between a 'health-promoting setting' and a 'healthy setting', proposing that the former has a greater focus on people and a commitment to ensuring that the setting takes account of its external impacts.

health promotion in higher education, for example, have differed internationally. Europe and Latin America use the phrase 'health-promoting universities'; in the UK it is 'healthy universities' and in the USA a mixture of 'healthy campus' or 'healthy campus community' is used (Sarmiento, 2017). Galea *et al.* (2000), in their paper on healthy islands in the Western Pacific, attempt to provide some clarity by proposing a hierarchy of settings. They distinguish between contextual and elemental settings, explaining that:

> Elemental settings are contained within a broader contextual setting. Thus, a city may contain important elements, e.g. schools, hospitals and markets. Elemental settings directly affect the life of the people who live within them; they only affect others indirectly. (p. 170)

Similarly, Barić (1998) sees health-promoting settings made up of health-promoting units – operating somewhat like 'Russian dolls' (Dooris, 2006, p. 5).

Early commentators, like Hancock (1999), have argued that the settings approach has been one of the most successful strategies to emerge from the Ottawa Charter. However, others have been less supportive of the approach and have claimed that the settings approach has not fulfilled its true promise (Woodall and Freeman, 2020). Barić (1992, 1993, 1994, 1995) has consistently advocated the necessity to distinguish between 'health promotion in a setting' and a 'health-promoting setting'. Baric´ notes that 'health promotion in a setting' refers to any institution that has some kind of health promotion or education as part of its activities (Barić, 1992, 1993, 1994). In contrast, a 'health-promoting setting' reframes health promotion as an integral part of the organizational infrastructure (Barić, 1994) and includes:

- the creation of a healthy working and living environment;
- integration of health promotion into the daily activities of the setting; and
- creating conditions for the setting to reach out into the community (Barić, 1993, p. 19).

This thinking represents a shift in merely aiming various forms of health education at those who conveniently interact in a particular location (King, 1998; Paton *et al.*, 2005). Instead, a 'health-promoting setting' adopts an ecological approach in which the whole environment and culture is committed to promoting health in a coherent and integrated manner (Tones, 2001).

The Settings Approach and the Current Variability of Practice

In practice, variability of activity under the rubric of settings-based health promotion exists. Johnson and Baum (2001, p. 286), for example, highlighted a variety of interpretations in the meaning of a health-promoting hospital. They suggest that:

> Some hospitals do little more than move beyond providing health information and education to patients, while other initiatives achieve a significant re-orientation of their activities and institute significant organizational reform supported by strong policy and leadership.

This issue is not limited to hospitals, as variation of practice seems to exist across settings. However, variations in activities may arise from the extent to which organizations aspire to, or are able to achieve, the 'ideal' (Green *et al.*, 2019). High-security prisons, for example, tend to struggle in implementing the healthy prisons philosophy in contrast to lower-security establishments (Woodall, 2020). Often, practical limitations hinder the development of a settings approach including:

- translating the philosophy of the approach into tangible activities;
- competing forces acting against the health agenda;
- problems associated with health promoters being perceived as credible agents of change; and
- limitations in support structures, e.g. finance, time, training, expertise (Whitelaw *et al.*, 2001).

Whitelaw *et al.* (2001) have created a typology of settings activity. This consists of five types of settings-based activities and is presented in Table 5.1. The typology rests on the way health problems are framed and solutions are identified. For example, at one end, the solution and problem lie with the individual (passive model), whilst in contrast, the comprehensive/structural model views the solution and problem within the setting. In the passive model, for instance, the setting assumes a subordinate role within which traditional forms of education are employed. This clearly has some resonance with the medical and social concepts of health explored in Chapter 1.

Table 5.1. Overview of the 'types' of settings-based health promotion according to Whitelaw et al. (2001, p. 346).

Setting type	Description
'Passive' model	Both the problem and the solution lie with the behaviour and actions of the individual. Setting plays a passive role only providing access to population group. Traditional health education activities are at the heart of the work.
'Active' model	The problem lies within the behaviour of the individual; however, the solution is broadened to encompass features of the system in which the individual exists.
'Vehicle' model	The problem lies within the setting, the solution in learning from individually based projects. This is still focused on topic-based activities but does so with an expectation of moving beyond individual behaviour change to impacting on broader settings features.
'Organic' model	The problem lies within the setting, the solution in the action of the individuals. This approach focuses on strengthening collective participation, the focus is not on tangible health gains but reflects a desire for improved ethos or culture within the setting.
'Comprehensive/ structural' model	Both the problem and the solution lie within the setting. This approach sees that individuals are powerless to make any changes therefore enduring change can only come from within the system. The emphasis therefore targets broad settings policies and bringing structural change.

Joined-up Settings

Clearly, people connect with a range of settings throughout their lives and this can occur either in a concurrent or consecutive manner. Most people, for instance, spend time in a whole plethora of settings every day and week, whereas someone in prison may spend time solely in a prison and then move into the community.

A criticism of the settings approach is that it can only address individuals in certain organizations, not really adopting an ecological view to the way people live their lives. It is important to understand lay people's meanings of places and spaces (Gustafson, 2001) and to incorporate them into settings approaches. Settings having their own specific rules or culture (habitus), which can mean that one single behaviour or action might be allowed in one setting but sanctioned in another. For example, showing male emotion is generally frowned upon in the workplace, but allowed in a sport setting. This perhaps illustrates the power of settings themselves to determine behaviour. Equally, male cooking has historically been seen as women's work in the home and family setting, but viewed as a male activity in certain occupational settings (firemen, for instance) or as masculine demonstration of independence/survival in military settings.

People's lives are not as compartmentalized as the settings approach would suggest and often many problems experienced in one setting are often deep rooted in another (Poland et al., 2000; Dooris, 2005). Clearly, health does not acknowledge boundaries – it crosses a range of settings and situations. This has been exemplified particularly by the Covid-19 pandemic, which clearly showed no acknowledgment of borders, boundaries, organizations or contexts. By focusing on settings in isolation from the wider perspective, there is a danger that the approach fosters 'insularity and fragmentation' (Dooris, 2006, p. 5).

Settings work should not only focus on the organizations themselves, but also on the spaces (physical and metaphorical) that exist between them. People in prison moving from the prison back to the community is a prime example – so often people experience adverse consequences when their needs are not considered when shifting between these two settings. Mullen et al. (1995), similarly, point out the limitations in our understanding concerning the relationships 'between settings'. Resources and investment must be developed between work in different settings and the gaps between them bridged (Dooris, 2004). Dooris and Hunter (2007), for instance, note that settings initiatives should move away from operating on 'parallel tramlines' (p. 118) and should instead link with other settings, thereby moving beyond the physical boundaries towards a more 'orchestrated approach' (King, 1998, p. 129). Indeed, this links with the idea that settings must connect 'outwards', 'upwards' and 'beyond' health if the approach is to be successful (Dooris, 2013).

Challenges

The settings approach has offered health promotion a conceptual base that has allowed practice to be pursued across a far wider scope (Whitelaw et al., 2001). Whilst the settings approach is now recognized as an important means to tackle health inequalities, there remain some concerns about the effectiveness of settings initiatives.

The Potential Exclusion of Marginalized Sections of Society

Health promotion has been committed to reducing health inequalities since its inception and therefore any accusation that interventions or programmes should exacerbate inequalities is one to be taken seriously. Early settings-based approaches only managed to focus on 'legitimate sites of practice' (Green et al., 2000, p. 25) by focusing on large-scale, identifiable and easily accessible organizations. The danger was that, if this had continued, it may have potentially exacerbated health inequalities (Speller, 2006; Dooris and Hunter, 2007) by failing to consider groups who are found outside of these formal organizations (for example, the unemployed, illegal immigrants, children who truant from school and the homeless).

As the settings approach has developed, it has stimulated practice in 'non-traditional' arenas (Poland et al., 2000; Tones and Tilford, 2001). It has needed to become more expansive in order to reach diverse populations, but this has caused tensions in some places. The concept of health-promoting prisons has emerged despite the possible tensions between the core values of health promotion and imprisonment. Box 5.2 outlines the emergence of the health-promoting prison.

This continued shift towards focusing attention on 'non-traditional' settings will undoubtedly offer those once marginalized by a settings approach to have some contact with professionals to address key determinants of their health (Poland et al., 2000). The challenge ahead seems to be that those working within health promotion must continue to consider emerging settings to tackle health issues.

Not Keeping Pace with the Digital Age

A significant concern has been the inability of the settings approach to engage in the digital age and fully embrace the notion of 'virtual settings for health'. The exponential growth of the internet, and social media particularly, has created opportunities for health promotion to locate in 'virtual' settings, for example through the significant benefits to be gained from social networking (Moorhead et al., 2013), and yet the uptake and execution of this has not been forthcoming. The growth of the online 'setting' cannot be challenged – education, recreation and communication are now determined by the online space. As a brief example, a systematic review found several benefits of social media – including Facebook, Twitter, Wikipedia, YouTube, blogs, etc. – for health purposes (Moorhead et al., 2013). These benefits can be summarized as:

1. Providing access to a vast array of health issues.
2. Widening access to those who may not easily access health information.
3. Allowing delivery of information in a range of innovative and interesting ways.
4. Facilitating dialogue and collaboration.
5. Providing access to peer, social and emotional support.
6. Providing anonymity (or not).

It is highly debatable as to whether health promotion has engaged with virtual settings, but it is clear that this setting offers significant benefits to reach and engage. Of course, much caution is also needed because social media can increase the propensity for 'fake news'; harmful or erroneous information; and potentially political manipulation.

Evaluation

Accountability and demonstrating effectiveness are increasing requirements of health promotion practice. This is potentially where the settings approach falls. Indeed, one major drawback to settings-based health promotion has been the paucity of high-quality evaluation leading to 'an uneven and under-developed evidence base' (Dooris et al., 2007, p. 335). The 'Healthy Cities' project is a notable example. Regardless of the commitment and support from the academic community, very little research evidence has been generated for its success, with outcome evaluations proving particularly difficult (Baum, 2002; de Leeuw and Skovgaard, 2005). School settings are an exception, as the evidence base tends to be stronger and more robust in comparison with other organizations (Richmond, 2009). This has been facilitated, to some extent, by the standards and criteria developed for the 'health-promoting school' and other key texts (e.g. Barnekow et al., 2006), which have arguably made it easier to conduct evaluative studies.

Clearly, a settings approach provides researchers and academics with a number of unique challenges in regard to evaluation. The distinctiveness of many settings means that conducting randomized controlled trials and other experimental methods is very difficult (Green et al., 2000). These methods on their own would also tell us very little about the

Box 5.2. The emergence of health-promoting prisons.

Prisons are not necessarily in the primary business of promoting health (Smith, 2000), but do provide an opportunity to access marginalized groups. Those entering the criminal justice system have often been subjected to a lifetime of social exclusion, including poor educational backgrounds, low incomes, meagre employment opportunities, lack of engagement with normal societal structures, low self-esteem and impermanence in terms of accommodation (including bouts of homelessness) and relationships with family members (Social Exclusion Unit, 2002). Research has also consistently demonstrated that the prevalence of ill health in the prison population is higher than that reported in the wider community.

The notion of a health-promoting prison emerged in the mid-1990s under the guidance of the WHO. Commentators argue that the health-promoting prison should include all facets of prison life, from addressing individual health needs through to organizational factors and the physical environment (de Viggiani, 2009). The Ottawa Charter is a useful framework to envisage these facets of prison life and has been used by others to map health promotion work in prisons (Ramaswamy and Freudenberg, 2007; Woodall and South, 2011). Its application is demonstrated below.

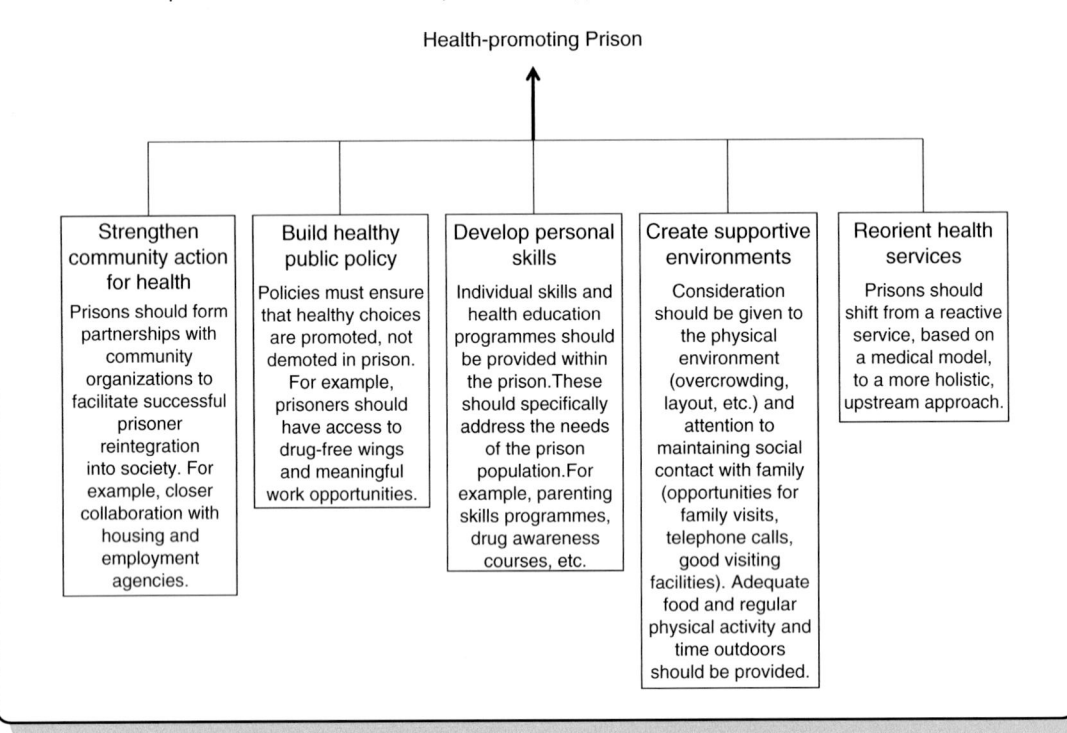

Health-promoting Prison

Strengthen community action for health	Build healthy public policy	Develop personal skills	Create supportive environments	Reorient health services
Prisons should form partnerships with community organizations to facilitate successful prisoner reintegration into society. For example, closer collaboration with housing and employment agencies.	Policies must ensure that healthy choices are promoted, not demoted in prison. For example, prisoners should have access to drug-free wings and meaningful work opportunities.	Individual skills and health education programmes should be provided within the prison. These should specifically address the needs of the prison population. For example, parenting skills programmes, drug awareness courses, etc.	Consideration should be given to the physical environment (overcrowding, layout, etc.) and attention to maintaining social contact with family (opportunities for family visits, telephone calls, good visiting facilities). Adequate food and regular physical activity and time outdoors should be provided.	Prisons should shift from a reactive service, based on a medical model, to a more holistic, upstream approach.

processes of the intervention (Poland *et al.*, 2000). This has also been noted by Downie *et al.* (1996, p. 90):

> The tendency to strait-jacket health promotion into models of biomedical evaluation focussing on outcomes ignores the creative, developmental components of health promotion and leads to a loss of opportunities to learn about approaches.

Reductivist methodologies may simply be inappropriate for measuring the success of settings initiatives, especially if researchers are asked to demonstrate positive health gains, which may be subjective and culturally contingent. Webb and Wright (2000) challenge researchers to view health promotion research with a postmodern lens, encouraging a re-consideration of the role of a single truth and embracing multiple narratives that reflect a range of perspectives. Furthermore, the problem of evaluation is not only a methodological and epistemological challenge but also a practical one. As an example, a prison setting can be a difficult environment to conduct research and may require intensive human resources especially when following-up prisoners to gain post-release data (Crundall and Deacon, 1997; Grinstead et al., 2001). This is partly due to offenders leaving prison lacking residential stability and not wanting any further contact with activities associated with the criminal justice system (Freudenberg, 2007). Time is also an important factor when evaluating settings-based projects, as sufficient time is needed to consider systems change and organizational development. Yet time is often a 'rare commodity' in health promotion programme evaluation (Kickbusch, 1995), where rapid, measurable success is frequently prioritized over determining longer-term achievements.

Dooris (2005, 2006) has outlined the main challenges that have inhibited the generation of a convincing evidence base. First, the funding structures for evaluative work are often focused on specific diseases and risk factor interventions. This would run counter to a comprehensive settings-based evaluation. Secondly, the heterogeneity between and across settings, coupled with the diversity and understanding of the approach, creates issues in transferability of research evidence. The 'conceptual variances', 'pragmatic influences' and differences in the 'size and type of setting' (Dooris, 2005) make building a substantive view of 'what works' challenging. Finally, there are problems with evaluating ecological and whole system approaches. Dooris, for instance, makes the valid point that if the settings approach is about integration within organizations, it can be argued that the greater the success, the more difficult the evaluation becomes. Therefore:

> Integrative approaches allow the language of 'health' to recede – and as the work becomes mainstreamed and the effectiveness of organization development becomes more apparent, 'health promotion' as an entity becomes more remote.
>
> (Dooris, 2005, p. 59)

Barić and Blinkhorn (2007) concur, as they see embedded health promotion and health education within organizations as a logical outcome of the settings approach. This leads to health promotion losing its professional identity as it develops into the core work of organizations. As a result, health promotion becomes difficult to assess or evaluate since it becomes integral to the function of a setting. Perhaps the ultimate evaluative indicator will be when health is so firmly embedded into the structure of organizations and settings the qualifying term 'healthy' or 'health promoting' is no longer required (Green et al., 2019).

Organizational Change

The settings approach throws into sharp relief the need for organizational change. The Bangkok Charter stated that all sectors and settings should advocate for health, invest in sustainable policies, actions and infrastructure to address the determinants of health, build capacity for policy development, develop leadership in health promotion and build strong partnerships with public, private, NGOs and international organizations and with civil society to create sustainable actions. If all sectors of government and all possible settings (schools, workplaces, sports stadia, clinics, cities, islands and so on) are to embrace the health promotion agenda, then radical change is required. There is a lot of literature on organizational change, but John Kotter's work is often the first cited (Kotter, 1996).

It would also be possible to adapt some of the individual behaviour change models to organizations – for example the stages of change model outlined in Chapter 4. Griffiths and Reynolds (2009) provide practical steps for organizational change in terms of embracing environmental issues, which include those that would help employees to be healthier, such as healthier transport plans. In terms of being change agents, Arneson and Ekberg (2005), in their study of empowerment in the workplace, found that when employees engaged in problem-based learning, with a non-directive facilitator, they developed an ability to reflect and be more self-aware, gained more self-direction and felt more empowered, such that they experienced greater psychological control over decision making.

If organizations are to change, we would argue that they need to become 'learning organizations'. Learning organizations are defined as those that facilitate the learning of all their members, continually transforming themselves (Pedler et al., 1991; Burgoyne, 1992). In short, a learning organization is one where 'people continually expand to create the results they truly desire, where new and expansive patterns of thinking are nurtured, where collective aspiration is set free, and where people are continuously learning how to learn together' (Senge, 1990, p. 3). This is in contrast to many organizations that rely on historical ways of doing things, are resistant to change, rely on hierarchies where most do not have to think about strategic direction and where people are not seen as intellectual capital to be harnessed for the development of the company or organizations. Pedler *et al.* (1991) outlined 11 dimensions of a learning organization, and this has been adopted in a number of different spheres with attempts to measure the extent to which an organization is a learning organization (de Villiers, 2008). A useful guide to learning organizations is provided by Serrat (2009), who highlights Kotter's steps to organizational change. This is an eight-step approach to embedding change in an organization. This includes:

1. Establish a sense of urgency.
2. Create a guiding coalition.
3. Develop a vision and strategy for the specific change.
4. Communicate the change vision and strategic plan.
5. Empower individuals for action.
6. Generate short-term wins.
7. Consolidate gains and produce more changes.
8. Anchor the new change in the culture.

In addition, as single organizations are not especially conducive to learning, they need to develop networks. In today's complex world, most organizations already have partners, or work with others in a supply chain analogy. The WHO (1998b), in its health promotion glossary, defines a network as 'a grouping of individuals, organizations and agencies organized on a non-hierarchical basis around common issues or concerns, which are pursued proactively and systematically, based on commitment and trust'. Networks function to exchange knowledge, to learn and to move agendas forward synergistically and in ways that would not be possible working alone. Increasingly, networks operate across the boundaries of private, public, voluntary or third sector, and with community involvement. The role of health promoters in facilitating organizational change and leading networks is discussed later in this chapter.

Changing does not necessarily need an infusion of cash, but thinking of new ways of working. Becoming a health-promoting school, a health-promoting workplace or a healthy market could have resource implications but could also achieve much simply by organizing and thinking in different ways. Organizing schoolchildren or workers to pick up litter, for example, does not need cash, but would considerably enhance the environment, reduce litter-based health problems and also provide exercise! The director of a major NGO in Tanzania realized that, on field trips, her driver did not have anything to do whilst she was in a community meeting; much of his time was, effectively, spent waiting around. He was encouraged to train as a peer educator, so that whilst she was engaged, he was too – talking to men in the community about health issues. He was keen on this development and was also learning IT skills (personal communication). This organization is therefore creating an environment where employees are stimulated and supported to learn (personal communication). Senge (1994) suggests that if organizations are to do things differently, and move from traditional, authoritarian organizations that control their workers, and are resistant to different ways of doing things, they need to develop in five areas:

1. Motivating individuals to learn, and to make the connections between their personal aspirations and the needs of the whole organization.
2. Challenging deeply rooted 'mental models' ('drivers are meant to drive, not talk to people').
3. Building long-term commitment in people by sharing the vision.
4. Developing dialogue so that people create genuine teams where they can think together.
5. Developing whole-systems thinking – which essentially integrates the previous four points.

Although Senge could be criticized as being optimistic about such sharing in a capitalist global economy and the fact that he ignores the power relations (and salary differentials!) between staff, there are important points that health promoters can take into their practice.

The role of health promoters in leading change is discussed below, but we now turn to a key dimension of working in health promotion, that of evidence-based practice.

Evidence-based Practice and Evaluation

Evidence and evaluation are of significant importance in underpinning the practice of health promotion, with an increasing emphasis on effectiveness, value for money and broader accountability. Increasing reference is made to the concept of evidence in the WHO health promotion declarations (Groot, 2011). Some commentators would argue that health promotion will be judged entirely on 'its ability to demonstrate in a scientific way that it is an effective field' (McQueen, 2001, p. 261). Evidence-based health promotion can be defined as the 'explicit application of research evidence when making decisions' (Wiggers and Sanson-Fisher, 1998, p. 126). If practitioners are *successfully* to effect change, then they should draw on existing evidence to enhance logical decision-making processes. Practitioners can use evidence in order to make decisions about a variety of key questions including: What are the *nature* and *determinants* of a health issue? What is the most appropriate approach that should be undertaken to address these determinants? What are the processes of *how* programmes should be implemented? How are programmes considered successful (Raphael, 2000)? In some contexts, the word 'evidence' conjures up notions of law courts and scientific forensic forms of evidence in order to support judgments about innocence or guilt – but we use evidence more casually, including in making decisions on what products to buy based on customer reviews and expert guidance. But the nature of what actually constitutes 'evidence' within health promotion is hotly contested and so raises questions about epistemological foundations underpinning different research methodologies (MacIntyre and Petticrew, 2000; Kelly *et al.*, 2002). Simplistically, the nature of evidence takes the form of qualitative and quantitative forms of data (Brownson *et al.*, 2009). The epistemological debates about the nature of evidence are outlined in the sections below. The same epistemological discourse underlies *how* to evaluate health promotion activity (Rootman *et al.*, 2001). Evaluation can be defined as 'the systematic examination and assessment of the features of an initiative and its effects, in order to produce information that can be used by those who have an interest in its improvement and effectiveness' (WHO, 1998b, p. 3).

Evaluating empowerment approaches to promoting health exemplifies the difficulties of effective evaluation and this has been widely discussed (Cross *et al.*, 2017). Although the term 'empowerment' is frequently used, the availability of high-quality research that demonstrates its success for improving individual health and wellbeing is fairly minimal (Woodall *et al.*, 2010). Hubley (2002), amongst others, comments on the disappointing number of evaluations demonstrating that empowerment has occurred. This is perhaps not surprising given that empowerment is a 'fuzzy' concept and problematic to measure (Green and South, 2006). Measuring the impact of empowerment on a community level is very difficult, not least because of methodological difficulties and the fact that the experience of being empowered may occur sometime after the 'intervention' (Baistow, 1994). A review by Woodall *et al.* (2010) found few published instances where empowerment approaches had made a difference to the actual health and wellbeing of communities. This is arguably because long-term health effects at a community-level are difficult to measure and because there is limited research on the benefits of community participation (South and Woodall, 2010). Despite the difficulties, it is essential that the pursuit of effective evaluation is prioritized.

Evidence-based practice and evaluation are explicitly linked through the health promotion planning cycle (Green and South, 2006, p. 5), in which evaluation of health promotion programmes feeds into the evidence base about what types of approaches are successful (or not) and under what conditions these effects happen. Knowing the answers to these types of evaluation questions ultimately strengthens the practical decision-making processes about what types of strategies should be implemented and whether successful projects can be translated into different settings and contexts. It has also proved useful when making decisions over which programmes or interventions to sustain, which to refine and which to discontinue.

In the following sections, the epistemological debates about the nature of evidence and the approaches used to evaluate health promotion practice are developed. Given that health promotion activities should address the wider social, environmental and economic determinants of health and be focused on 'upstream' rather than 'downstream' approaches, it then follows that of particular importance are programmes that feature action at community and policy level (Warwick-Booth *et al.*, 2012). Programmes at these levels of action are discussed to illustrate principles of both evidence-based practice and evaluation. Information about how practitioners can implement change by: (i) evaluating health promotion initiatives; (ii) using the existing evidence base within their own practice; and (iii) developing and enhancing the evidence base to support health promotion is discussed.

Epistemological and Methodological Issues Surrounding the Nature of Evidence and Evaluation

Epistemology is concerned with how knowledge is derived and what type of approaches we use to uncover knowledge. Evidence-based practice in health promotion originally borrowed epistemologies and frameworks developed for evidence-based *medicine* in the 1990s (Sackett *et al.*, 1996). Positivism, which underlies principles of evidence-based medicine, privileges objective factual knowledge by drawing on quantitative methodologies and design. Simply put, positivism defines reality only in terms of what is observed objectively and can be measured through our physical senses. Quantitative design such as experiments, cohort studies and case–control studies are used to answer questions about cause and effect. This question of cause and effect is central to both the evidence base of effectiveness of interventions and evaluation of health promotion initiatives. For example, we may wish to know if a health promotion intervention (cause) is effective in producing positive health outcomes (effects). One particular experimental design, the randomized control trial (RCT), has been heralded as the 'gold standard' and forms the basis of the type of evidence considered the most prized sitting at the top of a hierarchy (Box 5.3). The RCT forms the foundation of evidence-based medicine and clinical decision making and has been adopted by many Western countries. More latterly, hierarchical approaches to grading of evidence have been adopted by agencies such as the US Preventive Services Task Force and the National Institute for Clinical and Health Excellence in the UK.

The RCT is considered methodologically strong to assess cause and effect relationships and evidence of the effectiveness of interventions because of several features embedded in its design. The basic principles of an RCT design are that a sample is randomly allocated into either a comparison (control) group or an intervention group, but only the intervention group receives the intervention that is being assessed. This randomization attempts to ensure that both groups are similar in their characteristics, for example age and gender structures. This is important because if the characteristics of these two groups are different at the outset then any difference in effects (outcomes) between the groups at the end of the trial could be a result of the inherent differences between the groups at the outset of the trial. Any potential confounding factors that lead to changes in outcome will affect both the intervention and comparison groups equally and therefore any differences in outcomes can be attributed more confidently to the intervention.

The over-reliance and prioritization of RCTs as the strongest form of evidence has been heavily criticized especially within the context of health promotion as it applies principles, developed within the natural sciences and clinical settings, to social settings that cannot be easily controlled in an experimental fashion (Green and Tones, 1999; MacDonald and Davies, 1998). It is important to note that despite these criticisms, some commentators contend that experimental design and principles allied to positivism are useful frameworks within social sciences and naturalistic settings (MacIntyre and Petticrew, 2000). Epistemologically, social constructionism underpins criticism of positivist approaches to evidence. Social constructionism 'is the view that whatever any individual believes, is true for him or her' (Marks, 2002, p. 14). Within this school of thought, knowledge is subjective and constructed by the social world in which we live. Knowledge is derived from interpretation and meaning about events that exist in the social, cultural and political world. There is no single 'truth' as stated within positivist traditions, but different perspectives about truth are accepted and valued. Qualitative research methodologies and methods are strongly associated with evidence generated within social constructionist paradigms. Unlike positivists, the questions posed by social constructionists tend not to be ones of cause and effect, such as 'is an intervention effective?', but are concerned with how members of society (social actors) experience and give meaning to their world. Questions about *how* interventions lead to effects can be addressed by utilizing qualitative

---

Box 5.3. Example of hierarchical approach to grading evidence.

I. Strong evidence from at least one systematic review using meta-analyses of multiple well designed RCTs.
II. Strong evidence from at least one properly designed RCT of appropriate size.
III. Evidence from well designed trials without randomization.
IV. Evidence from cohort or case–control studies.
V. Evidence from expert committees, case reports, opinions and experience of respected authorities.

(Adapted from Marks, 2002; Petticrew and Roberts, 2003)

methodologies and methods. Pawson and Tilley (1997) refer to the black box of evaluation in which is contained the *processes* that lead to change. Health promotion places emphasis on valuing the perspectives of lay people who are the most important recipients of health promotion activity and therefore central to its practice. In addition, methods allied to action are empowerment and community development, which at the very least aim to place power and control of their health within the reach of lay people. Constructionist epistemologies, by acknowledging the valid multiple narratives of different perspectives, have the capacity to respect the accounts of lay people. Indeed, some would go as far as to say that lay people have expertise and only they can give valid data on their experiences and lives (Popay *et al.*, 1998; Prior, 2003). By drawing on qualitative forms of evidence, 'black boxes' can be illuminated bringing a richer picture of events and processes to practitioners and policy makers in their evidence-based decision making.

Using different forms of evidence to address different evidence-based questions is well received within health promotion circles. This *pragmatic* approach (Marks, 2002; Petticrew and Roberts, 2003) to utilization of differing forms of data in evidence-based practice and evaluation has led to the development of typologies of evidence (Table 5.2) rather than the hierarchical approach previously presented (Muir Gray, 1997; Petticrew and Roberts, 2003). There is a growing movement to synthesize different forms of evidence (Dixon-Woods *et al.*, 2004) and indeed several systematic reviews have been published that do not frame a review question of effectiveness but do frame questions about what is already known about an issue. For example, what is known about the facilitators and barriers to healthy eating? Shepherd *et al.* (2001) systematically reviewed and synthesized quantitative surveys, qualitative narratives and intervention studies in order to answer their initial review question rather than simply appraising RCTs.

Using pluralistic pragmatic approaches where 'the relative contributions that different kinds of [design] and methods can make to different kinds of research questions' (Petticrew and Roberts, 2003, p. 529) should be recognized and accepted in order to develop evaluation frameworks and research evidence to underpin decision making. Indeed, health promotion research is synonymous with having a broad and wide-ranging methodological toolkit. It is clear from the typology in Table 5.2 that the nature of evidence is contingent up on what research questions are posed. Many sources of evidence are often required to address complex initiatives. Rigorous evidence of outcomes may be evidenced using RCTs but evidence of how those outcomes were achieved and under what conditions and contexts they can be replicated is likely to come from qualitative data. Practitioners need to consider what they wish to find out and then draw on appropriate methodologies, designs and methods to address the issues.

Marks (2002) provides an excellent and much fuller discussion of the epistemological and methodological considerations of evidence used within public health.

Table 5.2. Example of typologies of evidence.

Research question	Type of research design					
	Qualitative	Survey	Case–control	Cohort study	RCTs	Systematic reviews
Effectiveness – does it work?				+	++	+++
Processes of delivery and implementation – how and why?	++	+				+++
Safety – good versus harm	++	++				+++
Cost effectiveness – it is worth buying for health gain produced?					++	+++
Appropriate – is it the right service?	++	++				++
Satisfaction with service or policy	++	++	+	+		+

Being an Evidence-based Practitioner

Governments in high-income countries and low and middle-income countries, as well as donor agencies, have had less resource in recent times and, therefore, budgetary allocations for public health and health promotion interventions need to be based on solid evidence (Owusu-Addo *et al.*, 2017). Two strategies exist for health promotion practitioners wishing to draw on research evidence to support their decision making. First, in some countries, national agencies have been commissioned to find, appraise, synthesize and produce evidence 'briefings' aiming to update practitioners in easy to digest bite-sized chunks largely focusing on what the most effective strategies to produce improved health outcomes are (Speller *et al.*, 2005). However, while this is a solid development to tackle the translation of evidence into practice, it is unlikely to address all the concerns of practitioners. In addition, within a developing countries context, culturally relevant evidence may not be published or widely disseminated – there continues to be discrepancies in the distribution of 'where' evidence is produced with a continued predominance of literature from the UK, Australia, Canada and USA. Systematic reviews tend to be undertaken on issues specific to Western health priorities and where relevant systematic reviews do exist it may not be possible to implement interventions because of limited resources and infrastructures available to practitioners (McMichael *et al.*, 2005). The second strategy necessitates building capacity for practitioners to find and appraise evidence themselves and apply it to their own practice. Muir Gray (1997) and Brownson *et al.* (2003) outline the steps and skills in the process of evidence-based decision making (Box 5.4).

Framing Evidence-based Questions

The overwhelming majority of existing evidence pertains to questions of effectiveness of interventions but as we have suggested in the typology of evidence, not all questions of interest to practitioners relate to whether an intervention works. Practitioners implementing initiatives are concerned with what are the best ways of working with different partners, sectors and clients. Commissioners of health promotion interventions may be interested in framing questions about which interventions are most equitable, acceptable and accessible to clients and therefore more likely to be effective (Rada *et al.*, 1999).

Searching for Evidence

Evidence can be in the form of practical experience and may not be published. However, these forms of evidence are not thought to be reliable or robust enough to be used for rational decision making (Box 5.3). Typically, a body of evidence is needed to make sound judgements. If half the existing evidence is not found, then it is not possible to make balanced decisions about evidence. Evidence that underpins decision making is likely to be obtained via academic databases such as Social Science Citation Indices and the Science Citation Indices or PubMed. Specialist evidence databases such as the Campbell Library of Systematic Reviews give full details of completed and ongoing systematic reviews in education, crime and justice, and social welfare; Evidence for Policy and Practice Information (EPPI) Centre and Cochrane Database Systematic Reviews contains the full text of regularly updated systematic reviews of the effects of health interventions carried out by the Cochrane Collaboration. The rise in open-access publications, offering free, unrestricted online access to research evidence, has helped researchers and practitioners in locating evidence. Some examples of journals that frequently feature health promotion studies using open-access platforms include: *BMJ Open*; *BMC Public Health*; and *Global Health (PLoS ONE)*.

Box 5.4. Steps and skills in the process of evidence-based decision making.

1. Ability to *frame* evidence-based questions.
2. Ability to *find* evidence that addresses the stated questions.
3. Ability to *assess the quality* of the evidence.
4. Ability to *determine* whether the results of the research can be *transferred* to the practitioners' local context and client group.
5. Ability to communicate and disseminate evidence to other practitioners.

Grey literature such as paper-based reports that are not available electronically are also potentially useful sources of evidence. An excellent guide about how to search for evidence can be found in Craig and Smyth (2002).

Appraising Evidence

This step in the process is important as practitioners should be able go beyond what the descriptive findings of the research state to a more critical understanding of the *methodological* rigour about how the research was designed and conducted. If research is poorly designed and implemented the findings themselves are untrustworthy, whatever findings are presented. Criteria and checklists to assess different types of evidence have been developed in order to allow systematic and consistent judgements to be made about the methodological quality of the research undergoing assessment. Rychetnik (2002) provides a useful discussion in this area.

Transferability of Evidence into Local Context

To assess whether existing evidence can be transferred to other settings and situations, detailed descriptions of the design, development, delivery and context of an initiative should be available. It may be that interventions that are effective and acceptable in one setting or context may fail in another. Context refers to the social and cultural environment and the particular political and organizational system in which the research takes place. Wang *et al.* (2005) have developed a useful set of questions (e.g. are the characteristics of the target population comparable between the study setting and the local setting?) to aid judgements to be made about transferability of initiatives.

Dissemination of Evidence into Practice

Crucial to the processes of evidence-based decision making is communication of existing evidence to practitioners who can rationally make judgements about what strategies should be used to undertake health improvement and how they should be implemented. Research indicates that resources designed to disseminate evidence-based information are unlikely to facilitate change in decision making unless they are linked to a knowledge management process that includes practitioner engagement (Armstrong *et al.*, 2007). Innovative work has involved practitioners and service users being actively involved in the development of evidence-based guidelines to promote and support breastfeeding. This approach 'allowed a transparent, accountable process for formulating recommendations based on scientific, theoretical, practical and expert evidence, with the added potential to enhance implementation' because of the strong engagement with practitioners and service users (Renfrew *et al.*, 2008, p. 3). This type of approach involving relevant stakeholders is considered a principle of good practice.

Evidence-based Policy Making

As suggested in the introduction, existing evidence clearly informs us that in order to address health inequities and increase life expectancy for those countries that have poorer health outcomes, we need to tackle the social, environmental, economic and political determinants of health. This necessitates acting at policy and community level. Unpicking processes about *how* a policy is implemented and whether it can give rise to evidence of effectiveness is complex (see Chapter 3). It has been suggested that policy and community action cannot be evaluated to produce an evidence base because the causal chain leading from the policy (cause) to health outcomes (effects) is not straightforward and many other policy interventions are also acting on populations. Teasing out single attributable effects is problematic. Asthana and Halliday (2006) analysed 125 systematic reviews and concluded that the current evidence base favours those interventions based on individual lifestyle factors and educational approaches. However, the evidence base for interventions addressing the wider determinants of health via policy making is much weaker. Nevertheless, systematic reviews do exist about policy and community action. For example, the health effects of volunteering (Casiday *et al.*, 2008), interventions that aim to increase employee participation or control (Egan *et al.*, 2007) and the effects on health and health inequalities of partnership working (Smith *et al.*, 2009) have all been assessed using systematic review approaches. Bambra *et al.* (2010) also provide a systematic review of evidence where social determinants have been the focus of action. Within the context of developing countries, some optimistic commentators contend that the evidence-based global health policy movement has taken many important strides with the development of organizations such as the Evidence to Policy initiative (E2Pi), which aims to help narrow the gap between evidence synthesis and practical policy making in global health (Yamey and Feachem, 2011). An interesting study highlighted that policy makers were persuaded by surprising forms of evidence such as *timely stories*, especially if they were combined with scientific evidence. Where academics and researchers were able to produce stronger evidence for health improvement and financial reductions in governmental departmental budgets, the evidence was more likely to be persuasive and actioned (Petticrew *et al.*, 2004). It is this type of research that will enable a stronger interplay between academics, policy makers, communities and practitioners.

Evaluative and Research Culture in Health Promotion Practice

Wimbush and Watson (2000) reiterate that differing stakeholders will have different evaluation questions and that these will be addressed by drawing on appropriate epistemologies, methodologies and methods.

Given the previously stated link between evaluation and evidence, it is important that health promotion develops a stronger evaluative and research culture in which practitioners embed process, impact and outcome evaluation at the outset of their programmes. The epistemological and methodological debates about how to evaluate have already been discussed earlier.

Nutbeam (1998) provides one framework for defining the outcomes associated with health promotion activity such as education, social mobilization and advocacy. These activities are linked to: the immediate health promotion outcomes (programme impact measures); the intermediate health outcomes (modifiable determinants of health); and the desired long-term health and social outcomes (reductions in morbidity, avoidable mortality and disability, improved quality of life, functional independence and equity). Green and South (2006) also provide practical frameworks for the practitioner wishing to embark on rigorous evaluations of initiatives including more complex community-based programmes. Dissemination of evaluation evidence is crucial: (i) if good practice is to be translated across settings, sectors and clients; (ii) if approaches that are ineffective are not to be repeated; and (iii) if evaluation can feed into developing a stronger evidence base within health promotion.

In summary, all forms of high-quality, robust data can be used as evidence and form the spine of developing stronger evaluative culture. There are methodological strengths of each design and method if they are applied correctly to stated evidence and research questions. There are challenges facing practitioners when undertaking evidence-based decision making, but progress has been made addressing many of these. It is important to state that generating and implementing evidence is not a perfect process. A realistic goal is stated by Muir Gray (1997, p. 48): 'The absence of excellent evidence does not make evidence-based decision making impossible: what is required is the best evidence available, not the best evidence possible.' The developing evidence base for Covid-19 and how this has changed over time, and as new data come in, and how it has been translated into practitioner action (or not) is a recent example of working with the best evidence at the time.

Health promotion is developing a unique research culture and indeed some have argued that there are a number of key characteristics that makes health promotion distinct (Woodall *et al.*, 2018). These are:

1. Application to real-world contexts – health promotion research has direct applications to solving 'real world' issues and tends to avoid 'blue sky' research, which focuses more on theoretical rather than applied issues. Indeed, Whitehead *et al.* (2003) have suggested how the tenets of action research, i.e. research designed explicitly to feed into and inform practice, resonate strongly with health promotion research.
2. Research values – health promotion's value-base, derived from the Ottawa Charter (WHO, 1986a), is clear in espousing ways of working that are enabling and empowering and that support individuals and communities to gain control over their own health. Some claim that health promotion research should reflect this and have an emphasis on control-enhancing action with 'values related to inclusion and participation' explicitly woven into the research design (Lahtinen *et al.*, 2005).
3. Relinquishing professional control – the process of health promotion researchers as 'co-researchers with the participants in the co-production of knowledge' (Cross and Warwick-Booth, 2016, p. 9) is a distinctive feature of health promotion research. Such participatory approaches in health promotion

research, and the evidence that they derive, asks people to adopt different attitudes to knowledge production and to reject traditional models of evidence or evidence hierarchy that may inadvertently favour experimental approaches or positivist ideas (Whitehead et al., 2003).

4. Expansive methodological toolkit – the fourth area of distinctiveness is the expansive methodological toolkit that health promotion researchers can and should draw upon in their practice. Inherently interdisciplinary and not dogmatically tied to research paradigms, views or perspectives, health promotion research should be flexible and diverse to address the issue being explored or investigated.

The additional abilities and competencies of health promotion practitioners are addressed later in this chapter, but first we turn to thinking about practising ethically.

Working Ethically

This is not the only place in the book where 'ethics' are considered, as clearly we have a strand throughout the book of considering the values base, moral issues and ethics of what we do. Here, however, we present some of the detailed issues facing practitioners. Sindall (2002) has argued that 'health promotion can no longer take its own moral credentials for granted'. He calls for debate about whether health promotion needs its own set of ethics in the same way that public health or medicine has, and for the development of a coherent ethical framework upon which to base health promotion practice. Clearly, with macro-level issues such as privacy, the right to interfere in people's lives, 'social engineering', the use of persuasion or coercion, 'nudging' and a whole raft of other ethical dilemmas, health promotion needs to engage with such a debate, in the interests of developing the profession.

Discussion of ethics in public health work often takes as its point of departure the tenets of health care ethics, and it is worth looking at these first. Indeed, many workers enter health promotion by first having worked in health care. Health care is usually concerned with patients or clients and thus the power differentials between them and the professionals who are caring for them raise ethical issues. Abuses of power are an obvious hazard, and a system of ethics has developed, which aims to protect the relatively vulnerable. Thus, the principles of autonomy (not doing anything that goes against a person's wishes), non-maleficence (not doing harm), beneficence (doing good) and justice (treating people equally and with respect) provide a foundation for the doctor–patient relationship. These key principles apply to health promotion work, too, but there are key differences between health promotion and health care work, and additional issues to consider. As we are dealing with healthy populations, and not necessarily with those who have identified themselves as in need of help, different kinds of 'contracts' between professionals and the community apply.

As health promotion is tacitly concerned with creating a 'good' global society, with positive ramifications for health, it is inevitably bound up with ethical and moral questions. We are making judgments about what kind of society we want to live in. Cribb and Duncan (2002) make a distinction between customary ethics and reflective ethics. The former refers to those aspects of everyday life that we hold to be part of custom or normative practice and are expected patterns of good behaviour; an example they give is that everyone 'knows' it is wrong to steal from a host, or to turn up very late for an event. However, 'Nothing can be accepted simply on the basis that it is customary. We have to be able to critically reflect on, and challenge, customary ethics' (Cribb and Duncan, 2002, p. 155). Otherwise, societies would be static with no room for change. Clearly, certain 'customary practices' that *have* been challenged as unethical – forced sex within marriage, female genital mutilation and beating of children, to name a few – had been seen as 'normal' aspects of life until challenged. Each of these issues has been taken up by health promoters and other social reformers, and many have been made illegal. The relationship between legality and morality is a complex one, and one that changes over time. Aspects of sexuality, for example, have variously been seen as legal and illegal, moral and immoral, in different historical times and in different cultures. Whereas we view being gay, lesbian, bisexual or transgendered as needing to be legal and being moral, this would not be the case in those countries where gay people are persecuted with impunity, or where homosexuality is illegal. Some countries such as Uganda have recently not only discussed making homosexuality illegal, but making it a criminal offence not to report to the authorities if someone knows someone who is gay. The murder of the gay rights activist David Kato shows how much a matter of life and death this is. If health promoters are to work with sensitive areas such as sexuality, HIV/AIDS and reproductive health, then they must sort out their own ideas and understand their own moral codes!

Not Doing Harm

Arguably, the most important ethical principle is to do no harm. Some examples will be provided here from the area of weight and obesity. O'Hara and Gregg (2006) provide an interesting example of a discussion about the harm that programmes focusing on obesity can cause. Arguing that the weight-centred paradigm has stigmatized overweight and obese people, and that interventions to promote weight loss are not particularly effective and can produce psychological distress, they espouse instead a 'Health at every size' model as an alternative. There *has* been an increase in the stigma faced by obese children (Latner and Stunkard, 2003). However, whilst we would agree that the obsession with weight in Western countries is unhealthy, it is also the case that obesity *does* have health consequences, and many children and adults are unhappy when obese or overweight (Dixey, 1998a; McElhone *et al.*, 2005). Not to act in the face of expressed health needs would also be unethical. At least, obesity prevention programmes need to make sure that they build in measures to ensure that they do not cause harm, such as measures of self-esteem, over the life of the project.

Dixey (1998a, b) has speculated on whether the focus on not being too fat has resulted in disordered eating, and also whether tackling one issue (child pedestrian accidents) has led to another – that of children becoming overweight due to lack of exercise and a rise in sedentary activities within the home, and to increased parental distress.

Voluntarism, Autonomy and Informed Choice

It goes without saying that it is unethical to coerce people. Rohinton Mistry's novel *A Fine Balance* (1996) graphically describes the rounding up of poor men, street dwellers and those with no power to resist during India's forced sterilization campaigns. This shameful period in the mid-1970s saw a policy of population control targeting men who already had two or more children, for compulsory vasectomies, but in the process and to meet quotas, other powerless men were also forced to have the operation. The other example that is often raised when discussing voluntarism is China's one-child policy. These examples are extreme, and are likely to occur in only a small number of countries. However, other issues do affect very large numbers of people, and another obvious example is of female genital mutilation and other traditional practices harmful to women. Where female genital mutilation is performed on girls, there is clearly no consent, and where it is performed on young women, there cannot be said to be consent given the strength of the cultural norms sanctioning the practice. Health promoters have made huge efforts to work on this issue, but it is very persistent.

Health promotion works with the whole community, not only those 'at risk' or identified as in need. People thus do not necessarily ask for, or want, health communications or public service type broadcasts. They might not be able to avoid them, even if they wanted to, in the same way that commercial advertising is hard to escape. They do not sign consent forms, as patients are expected to. 'Voluntarism' is thus difficult to estimate, especially when health educators and promoters are trained in how to develop 'persuasive messages'. Commercial advertisers, too, are adept at the art of persuasion, using emotional appeals with impunity. Is there really any such thing as 'free choice'? Or are we fooling ourselves that our actions are not influenced by significant others, by our socialization and by persuasive arguments?

Where there are democratic systems of decision making in place, decisions are easier to assess in terms of ethics. Adding fluoride or chlorine to water supplies usually raises its head in such cases; it is not possible to provide each person in a region with the means to consent. If a whole region makes the democratic decisions to add fluoride, then the consequences are easier to take than if a despot made that decision. Likewise, if decisions are made in democratic fora, they are easier to 'swallow', even if some people feel that their autonomy is compromised. Also, if actions compromise autonomy but save lives, it could be argued that those people saved have increased their ability to live autonomous lives in the future (as otherwise they would have been dead).

Surprisingly often in the health promotion literature, reference is made to 'captive audiences', and whilst most writers mean nothing sinister by this, it runs contrary to the ethos of voluntarism, and does need to be deconstructed!

Imposing Health Values

Downie *et al.* (1990) seem to overcome the moral dilemma of health promoters imposing their own values by taking a fundamentalist position, asserting that health is to be valued above all other values; health promotion 'endeavours to persuade people to adopt certain lifestyles, and is committed to furthering certain values'. This view is perhaps the honest one – health promoters often *do* believe that a healthy life is one where people prioritize health rather than hedonism or seeming recklessness. They would rather that people make the 'right' choices after hearing the evidence, rather than deciding to carry on with their 'unhealthy' behaviours. Ewles and Simnett (1985), in a 'whose life is it anyway?' fashion, question the 'ethical justification' for the imposition of these 'healthist' values, and seem to say that one set of values is just as good as another – for example, if some people prefer to live a sedentary life of enjoyment involving alcohol and tobacco, who are we to say that this is 'wrong'? Dixey (1999) has raised similar concerns regarding beliefs in settings where religious ideas may be more culturally important than 'scientific' worldviews; in seeing it as important to wear a helmet on a motorcycle, a whole range of cultural issues were uncovered in Nigeria:

> The dominant discourse of contemporary health promotion tends to see fatalism as atavistic and unhelpful. However, 'fatalism' may be a rational perspective in the social and economic circumstances, and who can judge whether there are gods or a God who predetermine people's fate? Health promotion needs to recognise its secular, modernist, individualist biases, and its preoccupation with control and empowerment.
>
> (Dixey, 1999, p. 206)

The Right to Intervene

We have agreed that states have a moral obligation to create the conditions in which people can be healthy. It also has a role in those cases where people are particularly vulnerable, such as with children, frail elderly, those with learning disabilities or those who are otherwise compromised. States, in short, have a stewardship role (Calman, 2009). Most citizens accept that the state has a right to curtail certain freedoms in the public interest – most recently exemplified during Covid-19 with many countries forcing people to stay indoors – but the whole issue of the relationship between the authority of the state and the individual is a complex one, and varies between societies. To a European, for example, the importance of the right for individuals to 'bear arms' (carry guns), so much a part of American culture, is baffling. This libertarian approach, which privileges the rights of individuals over the collective, runs counter to the 'social contract' assumed in many parts of the world. Those societies find it easier to accept John Stuart Mill's principle, that the state has the right to intervene when one person's actions harm other people.

Rationing – Deciding Who to Work With

Canada's Saskatchewan province's (Saskatchewan Health, 2002) guide to health promotion suggests that in deciding how best to use resources, decisions have to be made as follows:

Using the best available data and evidence on population health issues and effectiveness of interventions, weigh each possible issue in terms of:

- the degree of impact on population health status (as measured by mortality, morbidity, quality of life);
- the availability and effectiveness of interventions to address the issue;
- the cost to the community of pertinent health or social conditions and their treatment and prevention; and
- the potential to reduce health inequities.

(Saskatchewan Health, 2002, p. 20)

Not Acting – Doing Nothing

When we do nothing, we are supporting the status quo, which is itself a political act. Further, as Edmund Burke is reputed to have said, 'the only thing necessary for the triumph of evil is for good people to do nothing'. Doing nothing is one of the options available in the Nuffield 'intervention ladder' (Box 5.5). Each of the options presents ethical challenges.

Whilst it would be unethical to act not knowing whether a course of action was going to be effective, if we waited until all the evidence was watertight, no action might take place at all. The importance of evidence-based practice has been addressed earlier in this chapter, but here we want to stress this as an ethical issue. When to invoke the precautionary principle was mentioned in Chapter 3 of the previous edition (Warwick-Booth *et al.*, 2013), and there are many examples where thousands of lives would have been saved if that principle had been invoked. That asbestos could be a potential hazard to health was noted in the last years of the

> **Box 5.5. The intervention ladder.**
>
> The ladder of possible government actions is as follows:
>
> - **Do nothing** or simply monitor the current situation.
> - **Provide information.** Inform and educate the public, for example as part of campaigns to encourage people to walk more or eat five portions of fruit and vegetables per day.
> - **Enable choice.** Enable individuals to change their behaviours, for example by offering participation in an NHS 'stop smoking' programme, building cycle lanes, or providing free fruit in schools.
> - **Guide choices through changing the default policy.** For example, in a restaurant, instead of providing chips as a standard side dish (with healthier options available), menus could be changed to provide a healthier option as standard (with chips as an option available).
> - **Guide choices through incentives.** Regulations can be offered that guide choices by fiscal and other incentives, for example offering tax-breaks for the purchase of bicycles that are used as a means of travelling to work.
> - **Guide choice through disincentives.** Fiscal and other disincentives can be put in place to influence people not to pursue certain activities, for example through taxes on cigarettes, or by discouraging the use of cars in inner cities through charging schemes or limitation of parking spaces.
> - **Restrict choice.** Regulate in such a way as to restrict the options available to people with the aim of protecting them, for example removing unhealthy ingredients from foods, or unhealthy foods from shops or restaurants.
>
> (adapted from Griffiths and West, 2015)

19th century, but it was not banned until 100 years later, by which time it had caused thousands of deaths in Europe (European Environment Agency, 2002). As their report states,

> Preventive and precautionary public action … requires a minimum measure of agreement between governments and stakeholders about the approach to causality under conditions of uncertainty, ignorance, disputed values and the high stakes of 'being wrong' in both directions, i.e. failing to reduce harmful exposures; or taking precautionary measures that turn out to be unnecessary.
>
> (European Environment Agency, 2002, p. 3)

Manipulating Behaviour

Health promoters potentially tread a thin line between educating, persuading and manipulating behaviour. 'Behaviour change' paradigms do not seem to see any problems with persuading or with 'persuasive interventions'. 'Nudging', for instance, was mentioned in Chapter 4. There has been much debate in the health promotion literature about the use of shock tactics as a means to change behaviour. The idea is to use the fear of consequences in order to shock people into doing something about their health. Ethical questions aside, evidence on the effectiveness of shock tactics is inconclusive. A very early study by Janis and Fresbach (1953) on persuading people to brush their teeth regularly found that approaches using high levels of fear resulted in them being less likely to brush their teeth. It seems that when fear increases, compliance in following the solution decreases or resistance to the message becomes manifest. However, other studies have showed that fear appeals can have positive effects (Boster and Mongeau, 1984), but often their sustainability and longevity are questionable. Protection Motivation Theory (Rogers, 1983) helps to explain how using shock tactics might work: the motivation to take action is based on the individual's appraisal of the health threat and its solution, and the ability of the individual to take a particular action in dealing with the threat is important. Witte and Allen (2000) believe that fear can motivate an individual to take action as long as s/he believes they are able to protect themselves. An example of a fear approach is given by Hale and Dillard (1995, p. 65), who describe a 'well known fear appeal' campaign to reduce illegal drug use: 'The commercial shows an egg, a frying pan and then the egg frying. The voice-over says: "This is your brain. This is your brain on drugs. Any questions?" The intent of the message is to demonstrate that drug use kills brain cells.'

Curtis *et al.*'s (2011) work on the role of disgust in people's aversion to dirt and disease suggests that one of the most effective ways to get people to wash their hands after using public toilets is to put up a sign saying 'Is the person next to you washing their hands?', shaming them into washing their own hands. The Community-Led Total Sanitation movement in Nepal and Sierra Leone goes one step further and makes no apologies for using name and shame approaches.

The example of naming and shaming raises the question of whether the means justify the ends – if serious causes of mortality such as childhood diarrhoea in poor countries are caused by some community members' poor hygiene, why should they not be called to account? This consequentialist or utilitarian argument would assert that if the greatest happiness of the greatest number is served by a certain course of action, then that course is justified. In our Community-Led Total Sanitation example, if a few people feel humiliated, then that is the price a few must pay for the greater good. The utilitarian standpoint is usually contrasted with the deontological or rules-based approach, where it is argued that if a rule exists (e.g. that people should never be deliberately humiliated) then this should hold, whatever the consequences.

Hale and Dillard (1995, p. 78) end their chapter on fear appeal by saying that

> Fear appeals have enormous persuasive potential and can promote better health. The effectiveness depends in large part on the structure of the message. At the least, an effective fear appeal must include a severe threat, evidence suggesting the target is especially vulnerable to the threat, and solutions that are both easy to perform and effective.

We would say that severe threats are unethical; interestingly, Hale and Dillard do not discuss ethical dilemmas. This area remains contentious, as often people only do recognize the need to change actions and practices when their concerns are raised, and when they experience a degree of cognitive dissonance (which health promoters deliberately try to raise). Perhaps at least Hale and Dillard's subtitle – 'Too much, too little or just right?' – is helpful when considering what degree of concern, interest and attention (but not fear!) to raise with people and communities.

We cannot do justice here to the very large number of ethical issues facing the practice of health promotion and readers will need to follow this up elsewhere. We now turn to thinking about new ways of working with people in the 21st century, and specifically we consider new citizenship roles.

Active Citizenship – a New Role for Empowered People?

An implicit theme in this book concerns the relative roles of government, the private or commercial sector, the non-governmental sector and the community. Community participation was discussed in Chapter 2. In this chapter, we expand on what we could call civil society. We have stressed the importance of empowered people being able to take control of the factors that determine their health, and thus to take control of their own lives. Citizenship is a progression from being a 'community member' as it implies an active, engaged and fully participating citizenship in order to bring about the 'good society'. How should health promoters work alongside these empowered citizens? The idea of people taking a more active citizenship role has been adopted by both left and right politicians. Indeed, the idea of a 'whole of society' approach to achieving maximum heath gains is becoming increasing recognized (Public Health England, 2015).

We have also argued that it is the role of governments to ensure the health and safety of their populations. The commercial or business sector is often seen as developing products and ways of operating that harm health – either through employment practices that do not prioritize worker health, such as in poor factory conditions, or sweat shops, or by selling products that are clearly harmful, such as tobacco or 'junk' food. Private medicine and the pharmaceutical industry, too, have been accused of distorting health care, in promoting those areas that can be profitable and turning health into a commodity. This is obviously a simplified picture, and the private sector can obviously play a positive and constructive role in society, not least because it provides jobs and creates incomes. What is of interest here, however, is first how the political and policy landscapes have shifted such that the boundaries between these sectors have become blurred (Walt, 1994); secondly, how the non-governmental sector (NGOs) has emerged as a key players; and thirdly, how empowered, active citizens can play a role in counteracting the agenda of the other sectors. Laverack (2013) has described the various forms of protest and demonstration used by citizens in what he calls 'community activism'. Some of these include: protest marches; demonstrations and involving individuals using their bodies to stop machinery; and sit-ins. We have witnessed the

'Occupy' movements, where across major cities in Europe and the USA people have occupied spaces near the financial centres of those cities in order to question the relationship between governments and the major financial institutions, and to question what is seen as the systemic failure of the international financial system to bring about economic stability and prosperity for ordinary people.

The 21st century tacitly questions what it means to be a citizen – an active, engaged citizen:

> Upon what is citizenship based? In discussions about rights and responsibilities, obligations and entitlements, belonging and participation, a set of questions keeps insisting: how does one imagine oneself in connection with a community, a culture or a nation?
>
> (Frosh, 2001, p. 62)

There is also an implicit assumption that the

> ... citizen in the information age requires a different range of skills and taken-for-granted knowledge to his/her predecessor and those skills and assumptions are constantly shifting. Without these skills individuals cannot properly perform their citizenship role. They lack the knowledge which would allow them to choose and argue on public-political issues and are therefore excluded from full citizenship.
>
> (Crossley, 2001, p. 40)

According to Kubow et al. (2000, p. 134), 'effective citizenship first requires the internalisation of a set of civic ethics or values'; a good person and a good citizen can be distinguished by the latter's engagement with civic society, contributing in some way to the public good. It is virtuous to be involved in community action, and it transcends self-interest. This participative citizenship, according to Kymlicka and Norman (1995, p. 293), holds the 'intrinsic value of political participation for the participants themselves'.

This implies that people participate in civil society for intrinsic rewards. It contrasts with the 'instrumental' motivation in theories of participation, where it is assumed that people are motivated by extrinsic rewards, such as gaining work experience, gaining new social contacts and so on. Parry et al. (1992) propose three other categories of motivation: the communitarian, educative and expressive. In practice, the boundaries between these motivations are blurred for people, and people may be motivated by a wish to express themselves, be educated and to identify with their communities, plus getting something out of the experience, which furthers their career or simply makes their life more meaningful and enjoyable. A communitarian model, however, suggests that where people strongly identify with their community, they are more likely to increase their participation, and, in turn, increased participation leads to greater identification with the community. By being more involved, people enhance their sense of belonging, are able to express themselves and somehow earn a sense of validation. Archer (2007, p. 7) suggests that we act as citizens 'to promote our concerns ... to advance or protect what we care about most'. But why are some people more willing (and able) to cooperate with others (Karsten et al., 2000)? Clearly, those with some power already, and with skills and confidence, will be more likely to 'get involved'. Thus community assemblies, local councillors and lay involvement generally tend to over-represent the middle classes, the better educated and those with time and other resources to spare. However, as South et al. (2011) show, there are ways in which professionals can support people in civic engagement, such as in contributing to public health. In the UK, for example, a framework for mapping and understanding the myriad strategies purporting to take a community-centred approach to health has been developed. A conceptual map, described as a 'family' of approaches, categorized community-centred approaches under four areas: (i) strengthening communities; (ii) volunteer and peer roles; (iii) collaborations and partnerships; and (iv) access to community resources (South et al., 2017).

The changing relationships between the private, governmental and community levels can also be illustrated by taking a look at solid waste management. Management of waste produced by everyday life is a major problem to be solved by all societies. In countries such as England, there have been attempts to create more upstream solutions – to use less packaging, to recycle and to reduce waste – rather than expect a local council to collect waste from households and take it to landfill sites. This has resulted in a changed relationship between municipal authorities and citizens – the 'good' citizen sorts waste for recycling at the household level, takes climate change seriously and, in short, takes responsibility for some of his/her actions around waste creation. In poorer countries, where there are less well-developed systems of local government and a low tax base to pay for services, different solutions have been found. In Kenya, Uganda, Tanzania and Zambia, the municipal authorities have franchised the collection of waste to community-based organizations, community-based enterprises and small and medium enterprises, so that they generate income for themselves and also provide a valuable public service (Tukahirwa, 2011). At Leeds Beckett University, we were involved for more than a decade in providing support for aspects of these initiatives in Tanzania and Zambia, and have seen how they can empower women by providing income and social support (especially in the women-only or women-run organizations; Foster et al., 2012).

Arguably, adults and young people gain experiences earlier in life, which lead to civic responsibility – or not. Clearly, children do have agency, and it is important to foster this in terms of them becoming active citizens as young people and also later in life. Where children are asked, they are 'very interested in their communities and, if given the opportunity, are willing to become involved in changing community conditions to promote their own well-being' (Kalnins et al., 2002, p. 231). The Child-to-Child initiative (Pridmore, 1999) was successful in encouraging children's involvement, and fostering the development of social responsibility, partially through its apprenticeship approach (Rogoff, 1993). It asserted that children could be partners with adults to improve health, though at times it has had to challenge the allegation that it 'uses' children as health educators. It has been shown to develop children's full participation and potential, and to make significant positive differences in adulthood (Serpell et al., 2011). The Child-to-Child initiative has been evaluated latterly and shown to have had a role in developing civic responsibility in Zambia. An empowerment approach was developed in a rural primary school, using Child-to-Child approaches. It fostered cooperative learning, democracy in the classroom and social responsibility. In following up pupils, now adults, the evaluation showed that they had a sense of personal

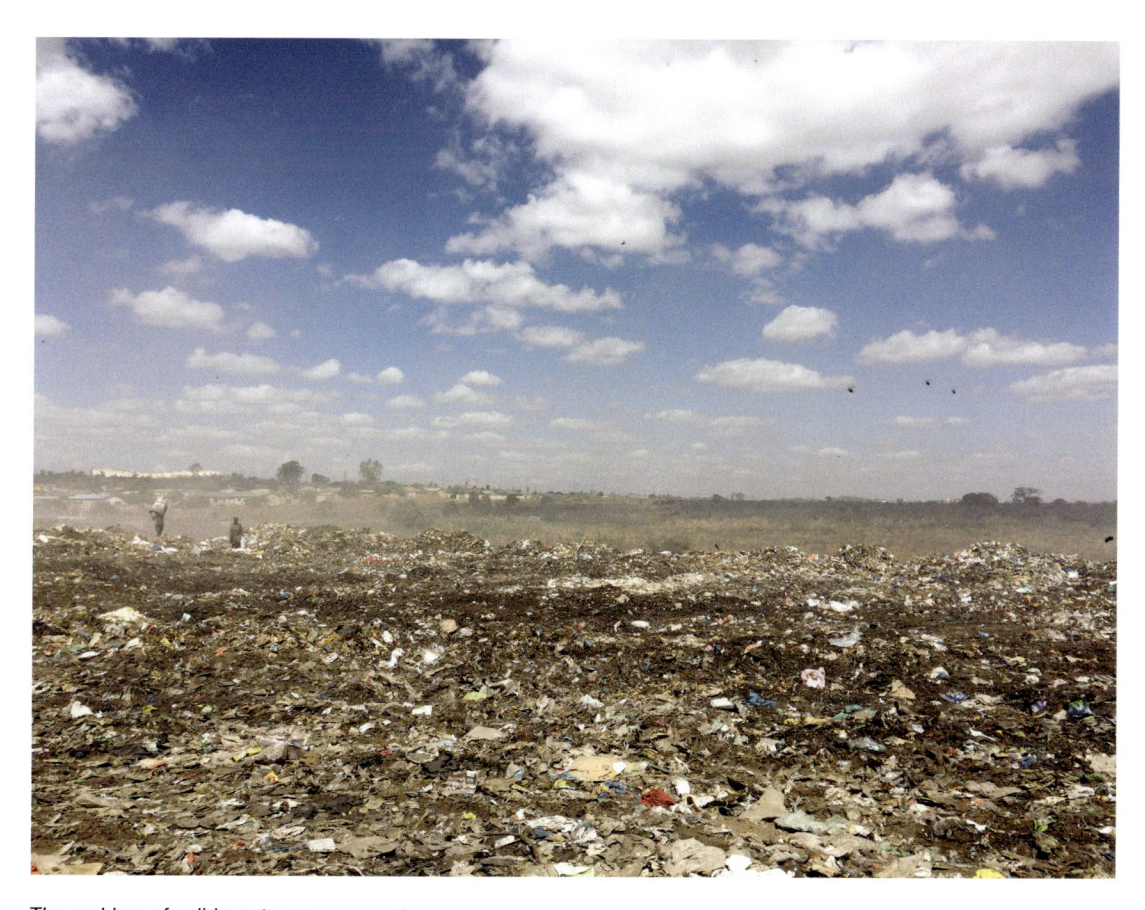

The problem of solid waste management.

agency conducive to being active citizens in their current lives (Serpell *et al.*, 2011).

The Non-governmental or 'Third Sector'

The discussion so far has suggested that new forms of relationships are being created between the state, its citizenry, the private sector and what is increasingly being called the third sector. Pearce (2006) provides an overview of the key debates in the development discourse, as one of a collection of useful chapters in the book edited by Eade (2006). During the 1990s in particular, there was something of an 'explosion' of NGOs (Fisher, 1997). Salamon (1993, p. 1) has gone so far as to suggest that this explosion, at least in the 'third world', may 'prove to be as significant to the latter twentieth century as the rise of the nation-state was to the latter nineteenth century'. NGOs cover a range of types and scales of organizations, from large bodies with resources at their disposal to those run by one or two individuals from their own homes. The term 'NGO' covers community-based organizations, grass-roots organizations and people's organizations as well as the more familiar international NGOs such as Oxfam. These groups are creating new opportunities for citizen engagement through coming together to form organizations. Some have become very powerful players, especially where they deliver services traditionally offered by government. The development of the third sector further blurs the boundaries between the four sectors, whilst Fisher (1997, p. 440) comments that 'political scientists are re-evaluating the role of voluntary associations in building vibrant civil societies and their impact on the relationship between society and the state'. What is interesting is the process by which activists have found ways of challenging established structures, changing the rules of engagement; NGOs represent new forms of associations, can manoeuvre themselves into political spaces and can tackle issues not high on government agendas. The emphasis on processes has led one commentator to suggest: 'NGOs are not things, but processes, and instead of asking what an NGO is, the more appropriate question then becomes how "NGO-ing" is *done*' (Hilhorst, 2003, p. 5).

This sector is seen optimistically by some, who see it as an expansion of civil society and as a means for people to bring about the kind of society they want to live in – as many NGOs are fuelled by moral concerns, faith or politics. The sector asserts that there is more to it than 'being not for profit'; the values of the third sector are distinctive, have meaning to the sector and have been encapsulated as:

- empowering people;
- pursuing equality;
- making voices heard;
- transforming lives;
- being responsible;
- finding fulfilment;
- doing a good job; and
- generating public wealth (Blake *et al.*, 2006).

There are thousands of NGOs doing health promotion work. Recent scandals have questioned the lack of regulation and oversight within international NGOs. It can be an unregulated business that often operates in places and contexts where the law does not reach fully. Moreover, the duplication of efforts has been criticized – there are many hundreds of NGOs working in the HIV/AIDS field, for example – but Fisher suggests that whereas the impermanence and fluidity of these organizations and associations could be a weakness, 'the space created in their passing may contribute to new activism that builds up after them' (Fisher, 1997, p. 459). In other words, the political landscape has been permanently changed and there are now four sectors, with permeable boundaries, as suggested in Box 5.6.

Here we have called the citizen sector the fourth sector. It is not clear where a major, wealthy philanthropic foundation might sit, with more money to

---

Box 5.6. The four sectors of communal life.

Public sector	Government, local authorities, public bodies, public sector workers
Private sector	Businesses, industry
Third sector	NGOs, charities, foundations, formal civil society groups, associations
Fourth sector	Citizens, people, communities, volunteers, user groups, self-help groups

spend on health than many governments, and run by a businessman; or which sector might accommodate one of the women's community-based organizations mentioned above, which is a members' organization but run for profit, delivering a service that in another country might be run by a local council. The injunction to participate, get involved, be active, *will* lead to new groupings.

Osaghae (1995, p. 194) warns of using Western models to analyse civil society, as they fail to appreciate the role of rural, kinship and ethnic-based associations – 'there is a clear misrepresentation of the Western connotation of civil society to the African situation'. He chastises the Western preoccupation with the role of civil society organizations in challenging the power of the state and argues that there is a need to focus more on the 'traditional' self-preservationist functions of civil society in Africa (Osaghae, 1995, p. 195). He argues that these associations have functioned more as 'shadow states', providing social welfare for groups and individuals when these have not been provided by the state. Box 5.7 provides a case study of a seemingly successful association in India.

These forms of voluntary associations and ways of people coming together to take action raise what in health promotion circles is called the bottom-up/top-down dilemma.

Box 5.7. Case study of the Voluntary Health Association of India (from http://www.vhai.org/)

The Voluntary Health Association of India (VHAI) is a non-profit, registered society formed in 1970. It is a federation of 27 State Voluntary Health Associations, linking together more than 4500 health and development institutions across the country. We are one of the largest health and development networks in the world. VHAI advocates people-centered policies for dynamic health planning and programme management in India. We initiate and support innovative health and development programmes at the grassroots with the active participation of the people.

VHAI strives to build up a strong health movement in the country for a cost-effective, preventive, promotive and rehabilitative health care system. We work towards a responsive public health sector and responsible private sector with accountability and quality service. VHAI promotes health issues of human rights and development. The beneficiaries of VHAI's programme include health professionals, researchers, social activists, government functionaries and media personnel.

Objective

VHAI's primary objective is to make health a reality for the people of India by promoting community health, social justice and human rights related to the provision and distribution of health services in India. VHAI tries to achieve these goals through campaigns, policy research, advocacy, need based training, media and parliament interventions, publications and audio visuals, dissemination of information and running of health and development projects in difficult areas. VHAI works for people-centered policies and their effective implementation. It sensitizes the general public on important health and development issues for evolving a sustainable health movement in the country with due emphasis on its rich health and cultural heritage.

Our Goal

- To ensure social justice, equity and Human Rights in the provision and distribution of health services to all, with emphasis on the less privileged millions.
- To promote and strengthen a medically rational, culturally acceptable and economically sustainable Health Care System in the country.
- To develop sustainable and innovative strategies to ensure health and overall community development in remote and vulnerable areas through various grassroot level initiatives.
- To provide relief and rehabilitation in areas affected by disasters and calamities and help the affected rebuild a better life for themselves.

Our Path

- Health Policy Research and Policy interventions for a cost-effective promotive and preventive Health Care System.
- Advocacy and lobbying with policy makers.
- Supporting voluntary efforts through formation and strengthening of similar developmental initiatives.
- Initiating sustainable Health and Development programmes at the grassroots.
- Developing communication strategies aimed at promoting campaigns and Health education.
- Dissemination of information to wide range of audience.
- Effective Networking with Government, UN and voluntary organizations.
- Responding to disasters and calamities.

Resolving the Top-down/Bottom-up Conundrum

A central tension exists in health promotion as to how to resolve the problem of connecting bottom-up problem solving with top-down policy making and top-down programmatic interventions. In certain instances, anti-social behaviour clearly needs to be restrained, and also we would argue that in *every* area of discrimination, legislation is needed to change institutional culture and behaviour. In relation to people with disabilities, for example, Barrett *et al.* (2003, p. 229) suggest that:

> It is agreed that policies which focus on awareness raising may alter attitudes to some extent, but will not change structural, institutional behaviour and this will not reduce inequality. Legislation is required to change institutional behavior rather than relying on persuasion.

Legislation is conventionally thought of as the singular example of top-down activity but what matters is the *process* of policy making, and that it is inclusive, participatory and ultimately democratic. The predominant discourse of the Ottawa Charter and subsequent iterations of health promotion methods is of community development; in practice, however, many health promotion textbooks espouse planning models and typical programme cycles where a scoping study or needs assessment is carried out, an intervention is designed, appraised, approved, implemented, managed to fruition and evaluated – all with varying degrees of community 'consultation' or 'participation' but the control stays with the funders and professionals. The latter's priorities may be accountability to funders, cost effectiveness and reaching targets for coverage, number of people included and so on. The well-known North Karelia Project on coronary heart disease was an early example of a massive intervention, which does appear to have had some success (Tones and Tilford, 2001). In the present century, the mood seems to have swung against these large-scale projects and towards 'local solutions for local problems', which keys into not only the zeitgeist but also the funding landscape.

Beattie's model (Beattie, 1991) has become a mainstay of health promotion textbooks, offering a way of seeing relationships between more negotiated ways of taking action in relation to more authoritative or top-down methods, and at both individual and collective levels. The model, made up of a vertical and horizontal axis, is useful in terms of helping individual workers to see where they fit in the spectrum, and in making the point that on many issues, a full range of actions (i.e. actions in each quadrant of Beattie's diagram) is required. Table 5.3 takes this discussion further by outlining the characteristics of top-down and bottom-up approaches.

Table 5.3. The different characteristics of top-down and bottom-up approaches (adapted from Laverack and Labonté, 2000).

Characteristic	Top-down approaches	Bottom-up approaches
Role of agents	Outside agents define the issue, develop strategies to resolve the issue, involve the community to assist with solving the issue.	Outside agents act to support the community in the identification of issues which are important and relevant to their lives and enable them to develop strategies to resolve these issues.
Power relationships	Power-over by the outside agent.	Power with and power from within. Outside agent surrenders some of their control.
Design	Defined short- to medium-term time frame, fixed budget and large scale.	Long-term without a fixed time frame or design. Uses participatory approach and small scale.
Objectives	Objectives are determined by outside agent and are usually concerned with changing specific behaviours to reduce disease and improve health.	Community identifies objectives, which are negotiated with outside agent. These may be concerned with disease and behaviours, but also with community empowerment outcomes and political and social changes.
Implementation	Decisions over budget, strategy, administration, etc. essentially rests with outside agent.	Decisions are constantly being negotiated between the outside agent and the community.
Evaluation	Evaluation concerned with targets and outcomes often determined by the outside agents.	Evaluation concerned with process and outcomes, and inclusion of the participants.

For some issues, a top-down, authoritative approach is needed because it is a matter of public safety – for example, many countries have laws protecting the public in terms of regulations surrounding food handling by retailers (to avoid food poisoning), or laws on speeding, driving after consuming alcohol and car maintenance. There are areas of public safety that are so important that they cannot be left to personal choice. The limits to top-down approaches and the use of law were discussed above in the section on ethics.

What we wish to discuss here is not so much these areas where the law or tough regulation is necessary, but rather approaches to health promotion when working with communities or in health education, and, more broadly, in developing healthy public policy or organizational change. Many health initiatives adopt a 'public address system' approach where messages are simply transmitted by an outside agent in a diffusionist model. That 'agent' is seen as having superior insight into the needs of the 'recipient' community and has produced an idea that it is believed will benefit that community. Paolo Freire describes in a stark way how well-meaning professionals actually commit acts of 'cultural invasion' in their belief that they have the answers to other people's problems (Freire, 1972). Central to health promotion thinking and values is that change occurs from below – impositions from the top and without clear and supportive frameworks for implementation are unlikely to produce change. As far back as 1976, Rogers (1976) was calling for a new paradigm arguing that this approach doesn't work. Community-led approaches with full ownership of stakeholders and strong partnerships are more likely to bring about sustainable change. Moreover, Walker (quoted in Attwood et al., 2003, p. 4) suggests, 'Bright ideas dreamt up at the centre sink time and time again ... [due to] ... the absence of a grassroots delivery system that is both accountable and effective'. Attwood et al. (2003, p. 5) write about 'Mad Management Virus', which believes that 'Programmatic top-down approaches always work', and 'The more inspection and control, the better the outcome'. The Mad Management Virus sets targets and believes that these will produce specified results; it also believes that these methods have no harmful effects on people's morale, levels of trust or engagement. In contrast,

> Positive and successful paradigms of change put users and communities at the centre, taking the view that effective lateral cooperation around action and learning can transform communities of place, interest, practice or influence.
>
> (Attwood et al., 2003, p. 7)

The aid sector, development and health promotion abound with examples where programmatic, top-down initiatives were ineffective and resulted in both rejection by the community and unsustainable interventions. As an example from the sphere of schooling, Wrigley (2000) argues that to bring about school improvement, top-down initiatives fail and only an empowerment approach will work. Attwood et al. (2003, p. 11) suggest a whole systems approach: 'Innovators employing whole systems methodologies seek to work in the uncomfortable spaces where the top-down collides with the horizontal and networked world of implementation. Restraining the top-down impulse in order to create virtuous cycles of hope, collective innovation and pride of purpose is what this book is all about.' The book is recommended as very useful further reading.

That people have to come up with their own solutions was recognized by the seminal work of Everett Rogers on the diffusion of innovations, whilst both Carl Rogers and Paolo Freire believed that all people have within them the ability to come up with their own solutions, as we discussed in Chapter 4. E. Rogers was interested in why some farmers adopted innovations (such as new types of seed) more readily than others. In summarizing a large body of evidence on effective adoption of new ideas by communities (Rogers and Shoemaker, 1971), they developed a matrix, which showed that where people identified both the need for change, and came up with their own solutions, change was more likely to be implemented and long-lasting than where these were identified by outsiders. It could be hypothesized that the greater the level of outside 'intervention', as in a 'public address system' approach, the less participation there will be and the less conscientization will occur.

These questions raise important dilemmas for health promotion professionals in terms of how to work with communities and organizations. Laverack and Labonté (2000) have proposed a 'middle-out' way of working, which provides a role for workers to liaise with those above (the policy makers and so on), and the communities on the ground or 'below' – not that we like this sense of a hierarchy, but the terminology is what has become custom and practice. They also show how a 'parallel track' approach could keep a programme on track whilst also meeting empowerment objectives and methods (Fig. 5.2).

Stage 1. Programme design phase	Empowerment characteristics
How has the programme design taken into consideration the empowerment characteristics? Identification Appraisal Approval	Programme time frame Programme size Attention to marginalized groups Conflict management

'Programme Track'   'Empowerment Track'

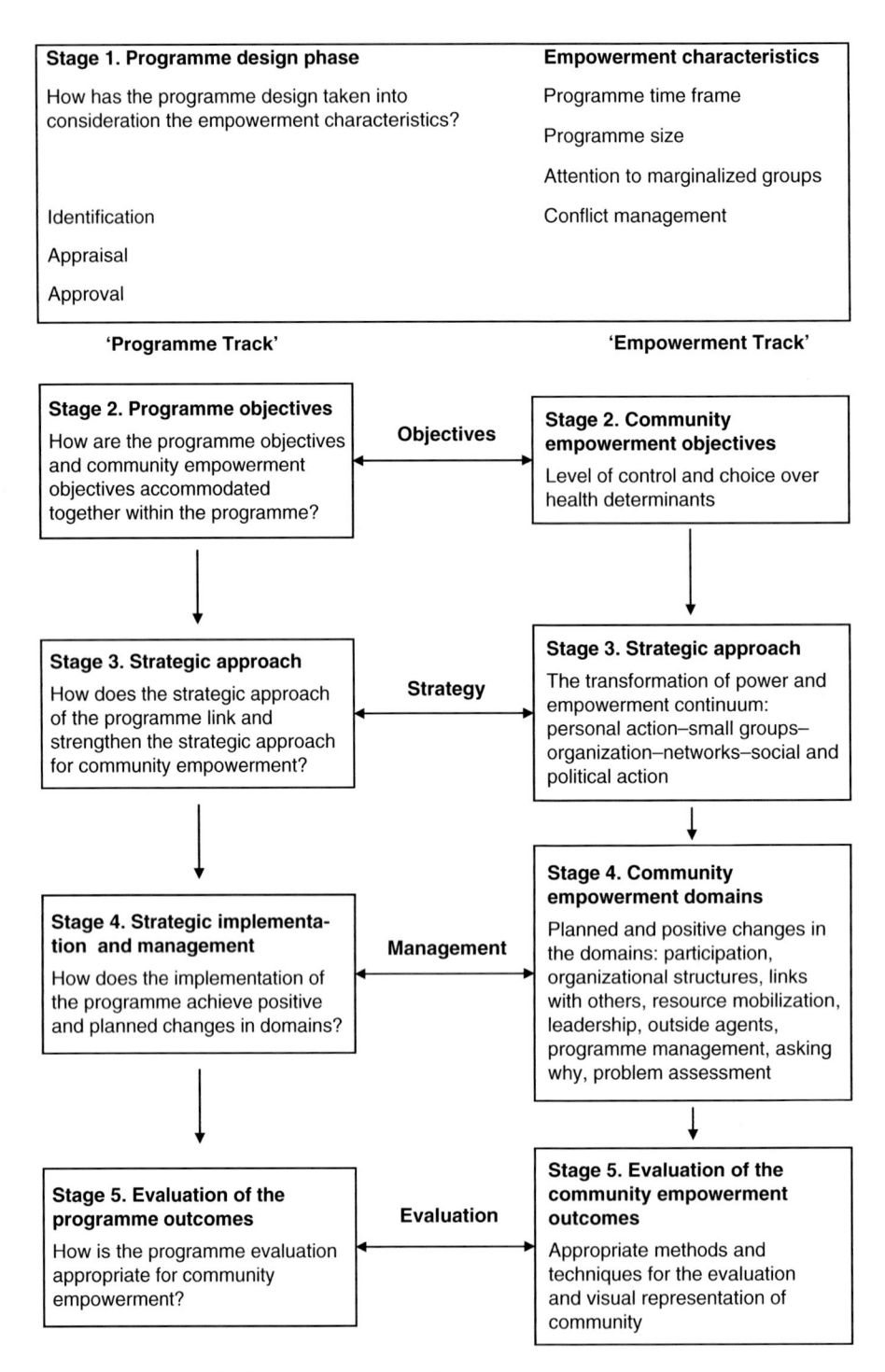

Stage 2. Programme objectives	Objectives	Stage 2. Community empowerment objectives
How are the programme objectives and community empowerment objectives accommodated together within the programme?	↔	Level of control and choice over health determinants

Stage 3. Strategic approach	Strategy	Stage 3. Strategic approach
How does the strategic approach of the programme link and strengthen the strategic approach for community empowerment?	↔	The transformation of power and empowerment continuum: personal action–small groups–organization–networks–social and political action

Stage 4. Strategic implementation and management	Management	Stage 4. Community empowerment domains
How does the implementation of the programme achieve positive and planned changes in domains?	↔	Planned and positive changes in the domains: participation, organizational structures, links with others, resource mobilization, leadership, outside agents, programme management, asking why, problem assessment

Stage 5. Evaluation of the programme outcomes	Evaluation	Stage 5. Evaluation of the community empowerment outcomes
How is the programme evaluation appropriate for community empowerment?	↔	Appropriate methods and techniques for the evaluation and visual representation of community

Fig. 5.2. The accommodation of bottom-up approaches into top-down programmes.

This still raises issues for the ways in which those with expertise can work with communities. Many people have skills that they have taken years to acquire, are motivated to work with communities in need and sometimes themselves come from backgrounds that are not that dissimilar from the communities in question. How can this expertise be harnessed and used appropriately, avoiding 'cultural invasion', insensitive top-down programme planning and taking into account the skills and knowledge of the community members? An example might be that a dietician with a commitment to working with parents in a poor housing area in Leeds would see it as obvious to offer nutrition and 'healthy eating on a budget' classes in local Children's Centres. The class would be advertised and take-up, typically, would be low. Those parents might not see this as a priority, or might want to tackle a more pressing issue such as the poor quality of the local green spaces and children's play areas. If a health promoter worked with these parents, who gained knowledge and confidence in tackling the local council about their issues, they might in the future identify other issues on which they wanted some input. One of these could be thinking about how to grow more of their own food, to develop a food cooperative, and also to learn about cooking … in which case they might approach the dieticians and invite them to work alongside them.

One initiative in which we were involved was a project with ten primary schools in Leeds to consider how they could promote more exercise and healthier eating with the longer-term goal of preventing obesity. The medically trained on the team assumed that we go into the schools with a prescription for what they needed to do in order to achieve reductions in children's body mass indexes (BMIs). The health promoters on the team were seeing the process very differently – that we would approach the school staff and ask them if they wanted to develop their own action plan for setting about the objectives. In this way, each school had a different plan, but they were all geared towards making the school a healthier place in terms of eating and exercise. The staff 'owned' the ideas and thus had an investment in bringing them to fruition. The process evaluation showed that the schools had changed in terms of their thinking and organizational cultures, but the measures such as BMI did not show any changes. If the latter was the yardstick for success, it would have been said that the project was a failure; in fact, significant differences had occurred in the schools. The point of relating this experience here is that organizational change needs to put the people in that organization at the heart of the initiative.

Skills of Health Promoters

What does all this indicate for the development of health promoters as professionals? A compounding factor is that it appears from some of the discussion above and from a number of studies (Carter et al., 2009; South et al., 2011) that training lay people to perform health promotion work can be as effective, if not more so, than when professionals do that work (Bagnall et al., 2015). Carter et al. (2009) have shown how lay people are more effective at taking accurate blood pressures (and people do not get as stressed) than physicians. Peer support in prisons has been shown to be as effective and more acceptable as interventions delivered by professionals (Bagnall et al., 2015). Moreover, village health workers, working on a voluntary basis have a long history in many countries (Campbell and Scott, 2011). Labonté and Laverack (2010) provide a critical commentary on the whole debate about developing community capacity for health promotion. All this has implications for the notion of professionalism, professionalization and how professionals work alongside both communities and lay workers. Evans (2008, p. 23) has attempted to define 'professional' – it is an 'articulated perception of what lies within the parameters of a profession's collective remit and responsibilities', but as Holroyd (2000, p. 39) points out, 'Professionalism is not some social-scientific absolute, but a historically changing and socially constructed concept in-use'. There is agreement that professional work incorporates a body of knowledge, a set of ethics, often a professional body, which regulates its members, and also a commitment to learning, professional updating and continuous professional development. It is not at all clear what the 'profession' of health promotion is, or what the health promotion professional would look like. One attempt to clarify this has been the discussions that led to the Galway Consensus, which, as the name signifies, is a global consensus on the competencies for the specialist health promoter.

The Galway Consensus

A team of academics and practitioners, including John Allegrante, Collins Airhihenbuwa, Maurice

Mittelmark and Margaret Barry, has been instrumental in developing the Galway consensus, arguing (Allegrante et al., 2009; Barry et al., 2009) the critical need to consider what skills and competencies are required by health promoters in addressing current health challenges, such as tackling health inequities and social determinants of health, and promoting healthy ageing and positive mental health. The Sustainable Development Goals (SDGs) and the report of the WHO Commission on Social Determinants of Health call for actions that require a complex mix of technical skills, expertise and leadership. Once identified, these need to inform the basis of education and training development of health promoters, so there are important implications for colleges and universities.

The eight domains identified are:

1. **Catalysing change** – Enabling change and empowering individuals and communities to improve their health.
2. **Leadership** – Providing strategic direction and opportunities for participation in developing healthy public policy, mobilizing and managing resources for health promotion, and building capacity.
3. **Assessment** – Conducting assessment of needs and assets in communities and systems that leads to the identification and analysis of the behavioural, cultural, social, environmental and organizational determinants that promote or compromise health.
4. **Planning** – Developing measurable goals and objectives in response to assessment of needs and assets, and identifying strategies that are based on knowledge derived from theory, evidence and practice.
5. **Implementation** – Carrying out effective and efficient, culturally sensitive and ethical strategies to ensure the greatest possible improvements in health, including management of human and material resources.
6. **Evaluation** – Determining the reach, effectiveness, and impact of health promotion programmes and policies. This includes utilizing appropriate evaluation and research methods to support programme improvements, sustainability and dissemination.
7. **Advocacy** – Advocating with and on behalf of individuals and communities to improve their health and wellbeing and building their capacity for undertaking actions that can both improve health and strengthen community assets.
8. **Partnerships** – Working collaboratively across disciplines, sectors and partners to enhance the impact and sustainability of health promotion programmes and policies.

The Galway meetings have had representation from all parts of the globe and it is felt that the skills outlined apply to people practising anywhere in the world. Prior to the Consensus, a number of attempts had been made by the professional associations representing health promotion to outline the core skills, and to differentiate these from public health skills. There has, however, been a continual absence of consensus on what these competencies should look like in different parts of the world.

The competency approach has been criticized by some; Eraut (2004, p. 264), for example, notes that 'from a learning viewpoint, competence is a moving target'. Professional learning is an ongoing process through practice (Eraut, 2001), and it is difficult to measure professional competence and professional learning (Daley, 2001) and to provide assurance of competence, particularly relating to informal learning such as in reflective practice (Friedman and Philips, 2004). Often competencies are measured against professional and occupational standards, but their rigidity can lead to a mechanical assessment of professional competence, which is not suited to the dynamism and complexity of the current public health environment (Cole, 2000). In relation to health promotion, Naidoo and Wills (2005, p. 10) have argued:

> The concept of competence has aroused much controversy. It can be seen as narrow and mechanistic, focusing on tasks and not enabling practitioners to acquire the value base essential for critical practice. All practitioners need to be not just technicians but reflective practitioners with a professional literacy. Competencies cannot cover all types of activities nor the personal processes entailed in health improvement. In specifying a range of activities in which the practitioner must perform, the role of theory and understanding is diminished. 'Knowing' becomes merely preparation for 'doing' with no requirement to reflect on theoretical bases or make sense of working practice.

The debate about a competence-based approach notwithstanding, recent decades have seen a twin track of developing the competencies for health promotion specialists and of encouraging those who could who do some health promotion as part of their main role, to develop health promotion (or at least health education) skills. The latter has usually been linked with the Ottawa Charter's call to reorient health services. We can perhaps identify *three* levels:

1. **Specialist health promoters**: those who have health promotion (or an equivalent) in their job

title and who work for all of their time in health promotion activity; these might be health trainers, health improvement officers, etc.

2. A range of workers who have a health promotion function as part of their role, such as housing officers, social workers, community workers, nurses, doctors, clinical officers, midwives, teachers, youth workers, play workers, dieticians, pharmacists, counsellors; these workers need to have skills to enable them to do health promotion.

3. Workers who need to have a health promotion awareness, such as transport planners, architects, leisure and hospitality management workers, education officers, politicians, policy makers, etc.; these workers need to be aware of how their actions impact on health and to be aware of how they can contribute to health-promoting settings.

The Galway Consensus perhaps relates most to the first of these groups. For the second and third groups, if more preventive and upstream ways of working are to be adopted, there are implications for the kinds of skills required by *all* those who can contribute to public health – whether currently working within the health (care) service, such as nurses, physiotherapists, occupational therapists, dentists, pharmacists, or outside of it, as planners, community workers, environmental health officers, housing officers, teachers … and many more. In the UK, there has been a plethora of discussion papers about the development of the public health workforce to make sure it is 'fit for purpose'. As noted, there is much variation on how this may look, but it is unsurprising that consensus has not been fully realized given that within England all public health activity operates within local government where it could be expected consensus may be easier to reach. Much of this discussion has historically been restricted to those working within the National Health Service (NHS) and there have been similar discussions in other countries about how health workers can contribute to broader public health goals. This picks up on the relatively neglected aspect of the Ottawa Charter, of reorientating health services.

A lot is known about the roles of various cadres of health workers in effective health communication, and behaviour change in terms of source credibility. Health visitors, for example, are seen as respected and credible educators by new mothers (Weeks *et al.*, 2005). Dieticians have a mixed response in terms of perceptions of their effectiveness in giving health messages (Hancock *et al.*, 2011). Much could be gained by training health workers in health promotion skills and recent years have seen interest in the role of pharmacists, and also in the role of other workers who have contact with the public, including barbers and hairdressers (Linnan and Ferguson, 2007). One of the areas of development has been in helping people to make appropriate and timely use of health care services, which is an important aspect of health education. Late presentation (for example of cancers) tends to be associated with lower socio-economic status in the UK and other developed countries. Health workers can also play a large role in encouraging parents to present children for the full range of vaccinations and in encouraging women to present early for antenatal care. Research shows that poor attitudes of health care workers is one determinant of under-utilization of services in India (Navaneetham and Dharmalingam, 2002), Jordan (Obermeyer and Potter, 1991), Pakistan (Stephenson and Hennink, 2004), Mali (Gage, 2007) and Ethiopia (Mekonnen and Mekonnen, 2003), and improvements in perceived quality of service have led to greater utilization in Bangladesh (Koenig *et al.*, 1997). These 'poor attitudes' are perhaps not surprising given the conditions many workers find themselves in. Health workers in Asia and Africa are often underpaid, lack opportunities for professional development, have high workloads and poor morale, and work in health services with poor infrastructure. Insufficient supply of health workers due to low numbers being trained in the first place is also a major factor, related to the low level of capacity of higher education institutions, particularly in many African countries (Dovlo, 2005; Dixey and Green, 2009). (This issue is explored further in Chapter 6.)

Many working in health promotion take on a training role, especially training others in health promotion skills. This is not mentioned in the eight domains of the Galway Consensus, but it is an important aspect, and some health promotion workers have an exclusive training role. There is a surprising lack of literature on the qualities that are held by highly skilled and effective trainers and how to measure these. Another relatively neglected area of work in the literature on skills is that of handling information, running public resource centres and the sorts of skills held by librarians, IT specialists, journalists and media personnel.

The Public Health Skills and Career Framework was published in 2008 (Public Health Resource Unit, 2008) as a tool for describing the kinds of skills needed across the entire public health workforce, and was intended to recognize everyone's contribution to improving health, even if not in posts traditionally seen as 'health work' and those for whom 'health work' is a part of their job alongside other responsibilities. The framework provides an outline of which skills are required, which can then be used to commission a range of education and training opportunities that might provide those skills. A range of providers have responded, and offer education and training across the various levels of the framework; the concept of a skills escalator has also developed, whereby staff, once on the 'escalator', can progress. The framework has given impetus to the discussion about what kinds of skills are needed by any workers who come into contact with the public and who thus might have opportunities to carry out opportunistic or more structured health promotion activities. Naidoo *et al.* (2003) have discussed the framework's role in developing the public health workforce and described how it might work in relation to working with asylum seekers in England. Latterly, 'health trainers' have emerged as the newest addition to the public health workforce as an innovative means of tackling inequalities and helping individuals to think about their health and lifestyle.

Leadership

Arguably the chief task of specialist health promoters is to play a leadership role, and other competencies fall under this. As change agents and advocates, partnership builders and planners, such workers are expected to *lead* health promotion into the 21st century. St Leger (2001) has commented on the need for the next generation of health promotion leaders who are not only technically competent, but who are also able to lead theoretical developments, to reflect on the purpose of health promotion and to relate health promotion to broader social issues. As specialist health promoters are involved in working with communities and, increasingly, with organized, active citizens, in developing healthy public policy, and working with governments, civil servants, with the complex NGO scene, developing health communication strategies, working with media organizations and negotiating the complex world of PR and public messaging, leading on organizational change to create healthy settings and raise positive health awareness across all sectors, there is a need to develop clear leadership skills. There is not the scope in this book to elaborate on leadership, and whole books are available on this. What we would say is important is that leadership remains true to health promotion principles. This requires the adoption of the new thinking about leadership, as Attwood *et al.* (2003, p. 17) comment: 'The new leadership "game" is engagement and involvement, not hierarchical domination, and effective leadership involves the many rather than the few.' They quote Drath and Palus (1994, in Attwood, 2003, p. 17), who liken ideas of 'the powerful individual taking charge' to the 'whitecaps on the sea – prominent and captivating', but with no recognition of the 'far vaster and more profound phenomenon out of which such waves arise'. In opposition to this 'heroic form of leadership', Attwood *et al.* (2003) argue that leaders should provide coherent frameworks within which others have space to think, to decide things for themselves, and to decide what needs changing and what does not. Thus, effective leaders develop 'holding frameworks':

> ... the job of leadership is both to set in motion the processes by which the container or framework is established, and to ensure that it operates like a membrane so that those involved (stakeholders in the issues concerned) are affected by the uncertainties of the external environment in ways that support rather than stultify their sense-making and learning.
> (Attwood, 2003, pp. 61–62)

The notion of holding frameworks derives from psychotherapy, where, as it can be imagined, the therapist provides a space in which to facilitate a client to work out solutions. If there is real belief that people have within them the capability of producing solutions to their own problems, and are not powerless (which we have said is central to health promotion values), then in one way the task of leadership is straightforward – it is simply to get everyone in the same space, and to have the facilitation skills to manage the engagement, resolve potential conflict and move to resolutions. (In practice, it is more complicated!) The framework can provide a set of values, purpose and strategic direction; the leader also needs to understand the 'big picture' and keep this in focus. In bringing about significant change, for example developing a Healthy City initiative, there would be considerable complexity, multiple stakeholders and a very long-term vision. Thus, leaders in health promotion often find themselves managing networks, or even networks of networks. Networking is a skill in its own right and although linked to partnership building, it is distinct from that. The importance of networks in organizational learning and knowledge transfer and management was discussed above.

If health promoters are to get health promotion onto agendas, and mobilize organizations and communities, they need to be able to play leadership roles in networks. Part of this role involves 'knowledge renewal' (Ballantyne, 2000) or knowledge exchange. The leadership roles include: energizing and encouraging people to share experiences; 'code breaking' or helping people break into each other's worlds and language; diffusing knowledge, letting it circulate, be tested, tried out and incorporated into new practices (Senge, 1994; Horsman, 2004). Working with networks throws up a number of issues, as identified by Attwood *et al.* (2003, p. 154):

- How are the effectiveness, quality and success of networks to be defined and evaluated, and how would these be agreed?
- How can networks be effectively led?
- How are they to be governed – who is eligible to join, how should behaviour be regulated and conflicts resolved?
- Where does accountability rest – in the participating organizations or within the network, or somewhere else?
- How can the network be supported in terms of overheads, infrastructure and so on, and how are these to be managed?

Summary

This chapter has attempted to discuss some challenges in the practice of health promotion, ending on the challenges in terms of the skills required to do health promotion work. Some of these challenges reoccur in the next chapter, particularly when discussing capacity building for health promotion at a societal level rather than the individual level, as we have done here. Working ethically, developing evaluation skills and evidence-based practice are contentious areas and we do not pretend to have produced all the answers here. It remains to be seen whether settings approaches will really 'deliver'. Many factors run counter to organizations wishing to become healthier settings, not least the imperative in some sectors to be profitable or show 'value for money'. However, as we suggest in the next chapter, health promotion is an optimistic profession, and the future development of health promotion will be explored next.

Note

[1] The previous version of this chapter entitled 'Practising Health Promotion' was written by Rachael Dixey, James Woodall and Diane Lowcock.

Further Reading

Green, J. and South, J. (2006) *Evaluation*. Open University Press, Maidenhead, UK.

Green, J., Cross, R., Woodall, J. and Tones, K. (2019) *Health Promotion: Planning and Strategies*, 4th edition. Sage, London.

Scriven, A. and Hodgins, M. (2012) *Health Promotion Settings: Principles and Practice*. Sage, London.

References

Allegrante, J.P., Barry, M., Airhihenbuwa, C.O., Auld, E., Collins, J.L., Lamarre, M-C., Magnusson, G., McQueen, D.V., Maurice, B. and Mittelmark, M. on behalf of the Galway Consensus Conference (2009) Domains of core competency, standards, and quality assurance for building global capacity in health promotion: the Galway Consensus Conference Statement. *Health Education & Behavior* 36, 476–482.

Archer, M. (2007) *Making Our Way Through the World. Human Reflexivity and Social Mobility*. Cambridge University Press, Cambridge, UK.

Armstrong, R., Waters, E., Crockett, B. and Keleher, H. (2007) The nature of evidence resources and knowledge translation for health promotion practitioners. *Health Promotion International* 21, 76–83.

Arneson, H. and Ekberg, K. (2005) Evaluation of empowerment processes in a workplace health promotion intervention based on learning in Sweden. *Health Promotion International* 20, 351–359.

Asthana, S. and Halliday, J. (2006) *What Works in Tackling Health Inequalities? Pathways, Policies and Practice through the Lifecourse*. The Policy Press, Bristol, UK.

Attwood, M., Pedler, M., Pritchard, S. and Wilkinson, D. (2003) *Leading Change. A Guide to Whole Systems Working*. The Policy Press, Bristol, UK.

Bagnall, A.-M., South, J., Hulme, C., Woodall, J., Vinall-Collier, K., Raine, G., Kinsella, K., Dixey, R., Harris, L. and Wright, N.M. (2015) A systematic review of the effectiveness and cost-effectiveness of peer education and peer support in prisons. *BMC Public Health* 15, 1–30.

Baistow, K. (1994) Liberation and regulation? Some paradoxes of empowerment. *Critical Social Policy* 14, 34–46.

Ballantyne, D. (2000) Internal relationship marketing: a strategy for knowledge renewal. *International Journal of Bank Marketing* 18, 274–286.

Bambra, C., Gibson, M., Sowden, A., Wright, K., Whitehead, M. and Petticrew, M. (2010) Tackling the wider social determinants of health and health inequalities: evidence from systematic reviews. *Journal of Epidemiology & Community Health* 64, 284–291.

Barić, L. (1992) Health promoting hospitals. *Journal of the Institute of Health Education* 30, 141–148.

Barić, L. (1993) The settings approach – implications for policy and strategy. *Journal of the Institute of Health Education* 31, 17–24.

Barić, L. (1994) *Health Promotion and Health Education in Practice: Module 2 – the Organisational Model*. Barns Publications, Altrincham, UK.

Barić, L. (1995) Implications for policy and strategy. In: Theaker, T. and Thompson, J. (eds) *The Settings Based Approach to Health Promotion: Conference Report*. Hertfordshire Health Promotion, Welwyn Garden City, UK.

Barić, L. (1998) *People in Settings*. Barns Publications, Altrincham, UK.

Barić, L. and Blinkhorn, A. (2007) Consumer-driven embedded health promotion and health education. *International Journal of Health Promotion and Education* 45, 87–92.

Barnekow, V., Buijs, G., Clift, S., Bruun Jensen, B., Paulus, P., Rivett, D. and Young, I. (2006) *Health-promoting Schools: A Resource for Developing Indicators*. European Network of Health Promoting Schools, Copenhagen.

Barrett, E., Heycock, M., Hick, D. and Judge, E. (2003) Issues in access for disabled people: the case of the Leeds transport strategy. *Policy Studies* 4, 227–242.

Barry, M., Allegrante, J., Lamarre, M-C., Auld, E. and Taub, A. (2009) The Galway Consensus Conference: international collaboration on the development of core competencies for health promotion and health education. *Global Health Promotion* 16, 5–11.

Baum, F. (2002) Health and greening the city. Setting for health promotion: the importance for an evidence base. *Journal of Epidemiology and Community Health* 56, 897–898.

Beattie, A. (1991) Knowledge and control in health promotion: a test case for social policy and social theory. In: Gabe, J., Calnan, M. and Bury, M. (eds) *The Sociology of the Health Service*. Routledge and Kegan Paul, London.

Blake, G., Robinson, D. and Smerdon, M. (2006) *Living Values: A Report Encouraging Boldness in Third Sector Organisations*. Common Links, London.

Boster, F.J. and Mongeau, P.A. (1984) Fear arousing persuasive messages. In: Bostrom, R. (ed.) *Communication Year Book*, Volume 8. Sage, Newbury Park, California, pp. 330–375.

Brownson, R.C., Baker, E.A., Leet, T.L. and Gillespie, K.N. (2003) *Evidence Based Public Health*. Oxford University Press, Oxford, UK.

Brownson, R.C., Fielding, J.E. and Maylahn, C.M. (2009) Evidence-based public health: a fundamental concept for public health practice. *Annual Review of Public Health* 30, 175–201.

Burgoyne, J. (1992) *Creating a Learning Organization*. Royal Society of the Arts Paper, London.

Calman, K. (2009) Beyond the 'nanny state': stewardship and public health. *Public Health* 123, 6–10.

Campbell, C. and Scott, K. (2011) Retreat from Alma Ata?: the WHO's report on task shifting to community health workers for AIDS care in poor countries. *Global Public Health* 6, 125–138.

Carter, M., Karwalajtys, T., Chambers, L., Kaczorowski, J., Dolovich, L., Gierman, T., Cross, D. and Laryea, S. (2009) Implementing a standardised community-based cardiovascular risk assessment program in 20 Ontario communities. *Health Promotion International* 24, 325–333.

Casiday, R., Kinsman, E., Fisher, C. and Bambra, C. (2008) *Volunteering and Health: What Impact Does it Really Have?* Volunteering England, London.

Cole, M. (2000) Learning through reflective practice: a professional approach to effective continuing professional development among healthcare professionals. *Research in Post-Compulsory Education* 5, 23–38.

Craig, J.V. and Smyth, R.L. (2002) *The Evidence Based Practice Manual for Nurses*. Churchill Livingstone, London.

Cribb, A. and Duncan, P. (2002) *Health Promotion and Professional Ethics*. Blackwell, Oxford, UK.

Cross, R. and Warwick-Booth, L. (2016) Using storyboards in participatory research. *Nurse Researcher* 23, 8–12.

Cross, R., Woodall, J. and Warwick-Booth, L. (2017) Empowerment: challenges in measurement. *Global Health Promotion* 26, 93–96.

Crossley, N. (2001) Citizenship, intersubjectivity and the lifeworld. In: Stevenson, N. (ed.) *Culture and Citizenship*. Sage, London, pp. 33–46.

Crundall, I. and Deacon, K. (1997) A prison-based alcohol use education program: evaluation of a pilot study. *Substance Use & Misuse* 32, 767–777.

Curtis, V., de Barra, M. and Aunger, R. (2011) Disgust as an adaptive system for disease avoidance behaviour. *Philosophical Transactions of the Royal Society B: Biological Sciences* 366, 389–401.

Daley, B.J. (2001) Learning and professional practice: a study of four professions. *Adult Education Quarterly* 52, 39–54.

De Leeuw, E. and Skovgaard, T. (2005) Utility-driven evidence for healthy cities: problems with evidence generation and application. *Social Science & Medicine* 61, 1331–1341.

de Viggiani, N. (2009) *A Healthy Prison Strategy for HMP Bristol*. Project report. University of the West of England, Bristol, UK.

De Villiers, W.A. (2008) The learning organisation: validating a measuring instrument. *The Journal of Applied Business Research* 24, 11–20.

Denman, S., Moon, A., Parsons, C. and Stears, D. (2002) *The Health Promoting School: Policy, Research and Practice*. Routledge, London.

Dixey, R.A. (1998a) Healthy eating in schools, overweight and 'eating disorders': are they connected? *Educational Review* 50, 29–35.

Dixey, R.A. (1998b) Improvements in child pedestrian safety: have they been gained at the expense of other health goals? *Health Education Journal* 57, 60–69.

Dixey, R.A. (1999) Fatalism, accident causation and prevention: issues for health promotion from an exploratory study in a Yoruba town, Nigeria. *Health Education Research* 14, 197–208.

Dixey, R.A. and Green, M. (2009) Sustainability of the health care workforce in Africa: a way forward in Zambia. *The International Journal of Environmental, Cultural, Economic and Social Sustainability* 5, 301–310.

Dixon-Woods, M., Agarwal, S., Young, B., Jones, D. and Sutton, A. (2004) *Integrative Approaches to Qualitative and Quantitative Evidence*. Health Development Agency, London.

Dooris, M. (2004) Joining up settings for health: a valuable investment for strategic partnerships? *Critical Public Health* 14, 37–49.

Dooris, M. (2005) Healthy settings: challenges to generating evidence of effectiveness. *Health Promotion International* 21, 55–65.

Dooris, M. (2006) Health promoting settings: future directions. *Promotion & Education* 13, 4–6.

Dooris, M. (2013) Expert voices for change: bridging the silos: towards healthy and sustainable settings for the 21st century. *Health and Place* 20, 39–50.

Dooris, M. and Hunter, D.J. (2007) Organisations and settings for promoting public health. In: Lloyd, C.E., Handsley, S., Douglas, J., Earle, S. and Spurr, S. (eds) *Policy and Practice in Promoting Public Health*. Sage, London.

Dooris, M., Dowding, G., Thompson, J. and Wynne, C. (1998) The settings-based approach to health promotion. In: Tsouros, A., Dowding, G., Thompson, J. and Dooris, M. (eds) *Health Promoting Universities: Concept, Experience and Framework for Action*. WHO, Copenhagen.

Dooris, M., Poland, B., Kolbe, L., Leeuw, E.D., McCall, D. and Wharf-Higgins, J. (2007) Healthy settings. Building evidence for the effectiveness of whole system health promotion – challenges and future directions. In: McQueen, D.V. and Jones, C.M. (eds) *Global Perspectives on Health Promotion Effectiveness*. Springer, New York.

Dovlo, D. (2005) Wastage in the health force: some perspectives from African countries. *Human Resources for Health* 3(6).

Downie, R.S., Fyfe, C. and Tannahill, A. (1990) *Health Promotion: Models and Values* Oxford University Press, Oxford, UK.

Downie, R.S., Tannahill, C. and Tannahill, A. (1996) *Health Promotion. Models and Values*. Oxford University Press, Oxford, UK.

Eade, D. (ed.) (2006) *Development, NGOs and Civil Society*. Oxfam, Oxford, UK.

Egan, M., Bambra, C. and Thomas, S. (2007) The psychosocial and health effects of workplace reorganisation: a systematic review of interventions that aim to increase employee participation or control. *Journal of Epidemiology & Community Health* 61, 945–954.

Eraut, M. (2001) Do continuing professional development models promote one-dimensional learning? *Medical Education* 35, 8–11.

Eraut, M. (2004) Informal learning in the workplace. *Studies in Continuing Education* 26, 247–273.

European Environment Agency (2002) *Late Lessons from Early Warnings: The Precautionary Principle 1896–2000*. Environmental issue report No. 22, European Environment Agency.

Evans, L. (2008) Professionalism, professionality and the development of education professionals. *British Journal of Educational Studies* 56, 20–38.

Ewles, L. and Simnett, I. (1985) *Promoting Health: A Practical Guide to Health Education*. John Wiley & Sons, Chichester, UK.

Fisher, W.F. (1997) DOING GOOD? The politics and antipolitics of NGO practices. *Annual Review of Anthropology* 26, 439–464.

Foster, S., Dixey, R., Oberlin, A. and Nkhama, E. (2012) 'Sweeping is women's work': employment and empowerment opportunities for women through engagement in solid waste management in Tanzania and Zambia. *International Journal of Health Promotion and Education* 50, 203–217.

Freire P (1972) *Pedagogy of the Oppressed*. Penguin, London.

Freudenberg, N. (2007) Health research behind bars: a brief guide to research in jails and prisons. In: Greifinger, R.B., Bick, J. and Goldenson, J. (eds) *Public Health Behind Bars. From Prisons to Communities*. Springer, New York.

Friedman, A. and Philips, M. (2004) Continuing professional development: developing a vision. *Journal of Education Work* 17, 361–376.

Frosh, S. (2001) Psychoanalysis, identity and citizenship. In: Stevenson, N. (ed.) *Culture and Citizenship*. Sage, London, pp. 62–73.

Gage, A.J. (2007) Barriers to the utilisation of maternal health care in rural Mali. *Social Science & Medicine* 65, 1666–1682.

Galea, G., Powis, B. and Tamplin, S.A. (2000) Healthy islands in the Western Pacific: international settings development. *Health Promotion International* 15, 169–178.

Green, J. and South, J. (2006) *Evaluation*. Open University Press, Maidenhead, UK.

Green, J. and Tones, K. (1999) Towards a secure evidence base for health promotion. *Journal of Public Health Medicine* 21, 133–139.

Green, J., Cross, R., Woodall, J. and Tones, K. (2019) *Health Promotion. Planning and Strategies*. Sage, London.

Green, L.W., Poland, B.D. and Rootman, I. (2000) The settings approach to health promotion. In: Poland, B.D., Green, L.W. and Rootman, I. (eds) *Settings for Health Promotion. Linking Theory and Practice*. Sage, Thousand Oaks, California.

Griffiths, J. and Reynolds, A. (2009) How to help organisations to take action. In: Griffiths, J., Rao, M., Adshead, F. and Thorpe, A. (2009) *The Health Practitioner's Guide to Climate Change, Diagnosis and Cure*. Earthscan, London.

Griffiths, P.E. and West, C. (2015) A balanced intervention ladder: promoting autonomy through public health action. *Public Health* 129, 1092–1098.

Grinstead, O., Zack, B. and Faigeles, B. (2001) Reducing postrelease risk behavior among HIV seropositive prison inmates: the health promotion program. *AIDS Education and Prevention* 13, 109–119.

Groot, E. (2011) Use of evidence in WHO health promotion declarations: overview, critical analysis, and personal reflection. *Reflective Practice* 12, 507–513.

Gustafson, P. (2001) Meanings of place: everyday experience and theoretical conceptualisations. *Journal of Environmental Psychology* 21, 5–16.

Hale, J. and Dillard, J.P. (1995) Fear appeals in health promotion campaigns: too much, too little or just right? In: Maibach, E. and Parrott, R. (eds) *Designing Health Messages*. Sage, Thousand Oaks, California.

Hancock, R.E.E., Bonner, G. and Madden, A.M. (2011) A qualitative examination of patient experiences of dietetic consultations. *Journal of Human Nutrition and Dietetics* 24, 284–285.

Hancock, T. (1999) Creating health and health promoting hospitals: a worthy challenge for the twenty-first century. *International Journal of Health Care Quality Assurance* 12, 8–19.

Hilhorst, D. (2003) *The Real World of NGOs: Discourses, Diversity and Development*. Zed Books, London.

Holroyd, C. (2000) Are assessors professional? *Active Learning in Higher Education* 1, 28–44.

Horsely, K. (2007) Storytelling, conflict and diversity. *Community Development Journal* 10, 109.

Horsman, D. (2004) An investigation of the extent to which the University of Bradford compares to other higher education institutions (HEIs) in the UK in developing a learning and knowledge management climate. MEd Thesis, University of Bradford, UK.

Hubley, J. (2002) Health empowerment, health literacy and health promotion: putting it all together. Available at: http://www.hubley.co.uk/ (accessed 23 August 2010).

Janis, I.L. and Fresbach, S. (1953) Effects of fear arousing communications. *Journal of Abnormal and Social Psychology* 48, 78–92.

Johnson, A. and Baum, F. (2001) Health promoting hospitals: a typology of different organizational approaches to health promotion. *Health Promotion International* 16, 281–287.

Kalnins, I., Hart, C., Ballantyne, P., Quartaro, G., Love, R., Sturis, G. and Pollack, P. (2002) Children's perceptions of strategies for resolving community health problems. *Health Promotion International* 17, 223–232.

Karsten, S., Kubow, P., Matrai, Z. and Pitiyanuwat, S. (2000) Challenges facing the twenty-first century citizen: views of policy makers. In: Cogan, J.J. and Derricott, R. (eds) *Citizenship for the 21st Century: An International Perspective in Education*. Kogan Page, London, pp. 109–130.

Kelly, M., Swann, C., Killoran, A., Naidoo, B., Barnett-Paige, E. and Morgan, A. (2002) *Methodological Problems in Constructing the Evidence Base in Public Health*. Health Development Agency, London.

Kickbusch, I. (1995) An overview to the settings based approach to health promotion. In: Theaker, T. and Thompson, J. (eds) *The Settings Based Approach to Health Promotion: Conference Report*. Hertfordshire Health Promotion, Welwyn Garden City, UK.

King, L. (1998) The settings approach to achieving better health for children. *New South Wales Public Health Bulletin* 9, 128–129.

Koenig, M., Hossain, M.B. and Whittaker, M. (1997) The influence of quality of care upon contraceptive use in rural Bangladesh. *Studies in Family Planning* 28, 278–289.

Kotter, J.P. (1996) *Leading Change*. Harvard Business School Press, Boston, Massachusetts.

Kubow, P., Grossman, D. and Ninomiya, S. (2000) Multidimensional citizenship: educational policy for the 21st century. In: Cogan, J. and Derricot, R. (eds) *Citizenship for the 21st Century: An International Perspective on Education*. Kogan Page, London, pp. 131–150.

Kymlicka, W. and Norman, W. (1995) Return of the citizen: a survey of recent work on citizenship theory. In: Beiner, R. (ed.) *Theorizing Citizenship*. State University of New York Press, Albany, New York, pp. 283–322.

Labonté, R. and Laverack, G. (2010) Capacity building in health promotion, Part 1: For whom? And for what purpose? *Critical Public Health* 11, 111–127.

Lahtinen, E., Koskinen-Ollonqvist, P., Rouvinen-Wilenius, P., Tuominen, P. and Mittelmark, M.B. (2005) The development of quality criteria for research: a Finnish approach. *Health Promotion International* 20, 306–315.

Latner, J.D. and Stunkard, A.J. (2003) Getting worse: the stigmatization of obese children. *Obesity Research* 11, 452–456.

Laverack, G. (2013) *Health Activism. Foundations and strategies*. Sage, London.

Laverack, G. and Labonté, R. (2000) A planning framework for accommodation of empowerment goals within health promotion planning. *Health Policy and Planning* 15, 255–262.

Linnan, L. and Ferguson, Y.O. (2007) Beauty salons: a promising health promotion setting for reaching and promoting health among African American women. *Health Education and Behavior* 34, 517–530.

Macdonald, G. and Davies, J.K. (1998) Reflection and vision: proving and improving the promotion of health. In: Davies, J.K. and Macdonald, G. (eds) *Quality, Evidence and Effectiveness in Health Promotion: Striving for Certainties*. Routledge, London.

Marks, D.F. (2002) *Perspectives on Evidence-based Practice*. Health Development Agency, London.

Macintyre, S. and Petticrew, M. (2000) Good intentions and received wisdom are not enough. *Journal of Epidemiology & Community Health* 54, 802–803.

McElhone, S., Walker, J., Christie, D., Sahota, P., Dixey, R. and Rudolf, M.C.J. (2005) What sort of quality of life do obese children and adolescents in the UK have? *Obesity Reviews* 6 (Supplement 1), 133.

McMichael, C., Waters, E. and Volmink, J. (2005) Evidence-based public health: what does it offer developing countries? *Journal of Public Health* 27, 215–221.

McQueen, D.V. (2001) Strengthening the evidence base for health promotion. *Health Promotion International* 16, 261–268.

Mekonnen, Y. and Mekonnen, A. (2003) Factors influencing the use of maternal healthcare services in Ethiopia. *Journal of Health, Population and Nutrition* 21, 374–382.

Moorhead, S.A., Hazlett, D.E., Harrison, L., Carroll, J.K., Irwin, A. and Hoving, C. (2013) A new dimension of health care: systematic review of the uses, benefits, and limitations of social media for health communication. *Journal of Medical Internet Research* 15, e85.

Muir Gray, J.M. (1997) *Evidence Based Healthcare*. Churchill Livingstone, London.

Mullen, P.D., Evans, D., Forster, J., Gottlieb, N.H., Kreuter, M., Moon, R., O'Rourke, T. and Strecher, V.J. (1995) Settings as an important dimension in health education/promotion policy, programs, and research. *Health Education Quarterly* 22, 329–345.

Naidoo, J. and Wills, J. (2005) *Public Health and Health Promotion: Developing Practice*, 2nd edition. Bailliere Tindall, London.

Naidoo, J., Orme, J. and Barrett, G. (2003) Capacity and capability in public health. In: Orme, J., Powell, J., Taylor, P., Harrison, T. and Grey, M. (2003) *Public Health for the 21st Century: New Perspectives on Policy, Participation and Practice*. Open University Press, Maidenhead, UK.

Navaneetham, K. and Dharmalingam, A. (2002) Utilisation of maternal health care services in Southern India. *Social Science & Medicine* 55, 1849–1869.

Newton, J., Dooris, M. and Wills, J. (2016) Healthy universities: an example of a whole-system health-promoting setting. *Global Health Promotion* 23, 57–65.

Nutbeam, D. (1998) Evaluating health promotion: progress, problems and solutions. *Health Promotion International* 13, 27–44.

O'Hara, L. and Gregg, J. (2006) The war on obesity: a social determinant of health. *Health Journal of Australia* 17, 260–263.

Obermeyer, C.M. and Potter, J.E. (1991) Maternal health care utilisation in Jordan: a study of patterns and determinants. *Studies in Family Planning* 22, 177–187.

Osaghae, E.E. (1995) The study of political transitions in Africa. *Review of African Political Economy* 64, 183–197.

Owusu-Addo, E., Cross, R. and Sarfo-Mensah, P. (2017) Evidence-based practice in local public health service in Ghana. *Critical Public Health* 27, 125–138.

Parry, G., Moyser, G. and Day, N. (1992) *Political Participation and Democracy in Britain*. Cambridge University Press, Cambridge, UK.

Paton, K., Sengupta, S. and Hassan, L. (2005) Settings, systems and organization development: the healthy living and working model. *Health Promotion International* 20, 81–89.

Pawson, R. and Tilley, N. (1997) *Realistic Evaluation*. Sage, London.

Pearce, J. (2006) Development, NGOs, and civil society: the debate and its future. In: Eade, D. (ed.) *Development, NGOs and Civil Society*. Oxfam, Oxford, UK.

Pedler, M., Burgoyne, J. and Boydell, T. (1991) *The Learning Company: A Strategy for Sustainable Development*. McGraw-Hill, Maidenhead, UK.

Petticrew, M. and Roberts, H. (2003) Evidence, hierarchies, and typologies: horses for courses. *Journal of Epidemiology Community Health* 57, 527–529.

Petticrew, M., Whitehead, M., Macintyre, S., Graham, H. and Egan, M. (2004) Evidence for public health policy on inequalities: 1: the reality according to policymakers. *Journal of Epidemiology Community Health* 58, 811–816.

Poland, B.D., Green, L.W. and Rootman, I. (2000) Reflections on settings for health promotion. In: Poland, B.D., Green, L.W. and Rootman, I. (eds) *Settings for Health Promotion. Linking Theory and Practice*. Sage, Thousand Oaks, California.

Popay, J., Williams, G., Thomas, C. and Gatrell, A. (1998) Theorising inequalities in health: the place of lay knowledge. *Sociology of Health and Illness* 20, 619–644.

Pridmore, P. (1999) *Participatory Approaches to Promoting Health in Schools: A Child to Child Training Manual*. Institute of Education/CTC, London.

Prior, L. (2003) Belief, knowledge and expertise: the emergence of the lay expert in medical sociology. *Sociology of Health and Illness* 25, 41–57.

Public Health England (2015) *A Guide to Community-centred Approaches for Health and Wellbeing*. Crown, London.

Public Health Resource Unit (2008) Public Health Skills and Career Framework. PHRU, London. Available at: http://www.sph.nhs.uk/sph-files/PHSkills-Career Framework_Launchdoc_April08.pdf (accessed 10 February 2012).

Rada, J., Ratima, M. and Howden-Chapman, P. (1999) Evidence based purchasing of health promotion: methodology for reviewing evidence. *Health Promotion International* 14, 177–187.

Ramaswamy, M. and Freudenberg, N. (2007) Health promotion in jails and prisons: an alternative paradigm for correctional health services. In: Greifinger, R.B., Bick, J. and Goldenson, J. (eds) *Public Health Behind Bars: From Prisons to Communities*. Springer, New York.

Raphael, D. (2000) The question of evidence in health promotion. *Health Promotion International* 15, 355–367.

Renfrew, M.J., Dyson, L., Herbert, J., McFadden, A., McCormick, F., Thomas, J. and Spiby, H. (2008) Developing evidence-based recommendations in public health – incorporating the views of practitioners, service users and user representatives. *Health Expectations* 11, 3–15.

Richmond, K.M. (2009) Factories with fences: the effect of prison industries on female inmates. Unpublished PhD thesis, University of Maryland, Maryland.

Rogers, E.M. (1976) Communication and development: the passing of a paradigm. *Communication Research* 3, 213–240.

Rogers, E.M. and Shoemaker, F. (1971) *The Communication of Innovations*. The Free Press, New York.

Rogers, R.W. (1983) Cognitive and physiological processes in fear appeals and attitude change: a revised theory of protection motivation. In: Cacippo, J.R. and Petty, R.E. (eds) *Social Psychology: A Source Book*. Guilford Press, New York, pp. 153–176.

Rogoff, B. (1993) Observing sociocultural activity on three planes. In: Wertsch, J.V., del Rio, P. and Alvarez, A. (eds) *Sociocultural Studies of Mind*. Cambridge University Press, New York, pp. 139–163.

Rootman, I., Goodstadt, M., Hyndman, B., McQueen, D.V., Potvin, L., Springett, J. and Ziglio, E. (eds) (2001) *Evaluation in Health Promotion. Principles and Perspectives*. WHO, Geneva.

Rychetnik, L. (2002) Criteria for evaluating evidence on public health interventions. *Journal of Epidemiology & Community Health*. 56, 119

Sackett, D.L., Rosenberg, W.M.C., Gray, J.A.M., Haynes, R.B. and Richardson, W.S. (1996) Evidence-based medicine: what it is and what it isn't. *British Medical Journal* 312, 71–72.

Salamon, L.M. (1993) *The Global Associational Revolution: The Rise of the Third Sector on the World Scene*. Occasional paper 15, Institute of Policy Studies, Johns Hopkins University, Baltimore, Maryland.

Sarmiento, J.P. (2017) Healthy universities: mapping health-promotion interventions. *Health Education* 117, 162–175.

Saskatchewan Health (2002) A population health promotion framework for Saskatchewan regional health authorities. Regina, Canada.

Senge, P.M. (1990) *The Fifth Discipline: The Art and Practice of the Learning Organization*. Doubleday Currency, New York.

Senge, P.M. (1994) *The Fifth Discipline Field Book: Strategies and Tools for Building a Learning Organization*. Nicholas Brealey Publishing, London.

Serpell, R., Mumba, P. and Chansa-Kabali, T. (2011) Early educational foundations for the development of civic responsibility: an African experience. In: Flanagan, C.A. and Christens, B.D. (eds) *Youth Civic Development: Work at the Cutting Edge: New Directions for Child and Adolescent Development* 134, 77–93.

Serrat, O. (2009) A primer on organisational learning, knowledge solutions. *Asian Development Bank* 6, 1–6.

Shepherd, J., Garcia, J., Oliver, S., Harden, A., Rees, R., Brunton, G. and Oakley, A. (2001) *Young People and Healthy Eating: A Systematic Review of Barriers and Facilitators*. EPPI-Centre, Social Science Research Unit, London.

Sindall, C. (2002) Does health promotion need a code of ethics? *Health Promotion International* 17, 201–203.

Smith, C. (2000) Healthy prisons: a contradiction in terms? *The Howard Journal of Criminal Justice* 39, 339–353.

Smith, K.E, Bambra, C. and Joyce, K.E. (2009) Partners in health? A systematic review of the effects on health and health inequalities of partnership working. *Journal of Public Health* 31, 210–221.

Social Exclusion Unit (2002) *Reducing Re-offending by Ex-prisoners*. Crown, London.

South, J. and Woodall, J. (2010) *Empowerment and Health & Well-being: Evidence Summary*. Centre for Health Promotion Research, Leeds Metropolitan University, Leeds, UK.

South, J., Meah, A. and Branney, P. (2011) 'Think differently and be prepared to demonstrate trust': findings from public hearings, England on supporting lay people in public health roles. *Health Promotion International* doi:10.1093/heapro/dar022

South, J., Bagnall, A.-M., Stansfield, J.A., Southby, K.J. and Mehta, P. (2017) An evidence-based framework on community-centred approaches for health: England, UK. *Health Promotion International* 1–11.

Speller, V. (2006) Developing healthy settings. In: Macdowall, W., Bonell, C. and Davis, M. (eds) *Health Promotion Practice*. Open University Press, Maidenhead, UK.

Speller, V., Wimbush, E. and Morgan, A. (2005) Evidence-based health promotion practice: how to make it work, *Promotion & Education* 12, 15–20.

Spicker, P. (2006) *Policy Analysis for Practice. Applying Social Policy*. The Policy Press, Bristol, UK.

St Leger, L. (2001) Building and finding the new leaders in health promotion: where is the next wave of health promotion leaders and thinkers? Are they emerging from particular regions, and are they less than 40 years old? *Health Promotion International* 16, 301–303.

Stephenson, R. and Hennink, M. (2004) Barriers to family planning service use among the urban poor in Pakistan. *Asia-Pacific Population Journal* 19, 5–26.

Tones, K. (2001) Health promotion: the empowerment imperative. In: Scriven, A. and Orme, J. (eds) *Health Promotion: Professional Perspectives*, 2nd edition. Palgrave, London.

Tones, K. and Tilford, S. (2001) *Health Promotion, Effectiveness, Efficiency and Equity*. Nelson Thornes, Cheltenham, UK.

Torp, S., Kokko, S. and Ringsberg, K.C. (2014) *Promoting Health in Everyday Settings: Opportunities and Challenges*. Sage, London.

Tukahirwa, J.T. (2011) Civil society in urban sanitation and solid waste management: the role of NGOs and CBOs in metropolises of East Africa. PhD thesis, University of Wageningen, Netherlands.

Walt, G. (1994) *Health Policy. An Introduction to Process and Power*. Zed Books, London.

Wang, S., Ross, J.R. and Hiller, J.E. (2005) Applicability and transferability of interventions in evidence-based public health. *Health Promotion International* 21, 76–83.

Warwick-Booth, L., Cross, R. and Lowcock, D. (2012) *Health Studies: An Overview of Contemporary Perspectives*. Polity Press, Cambridge, UK.

Warwick-Booth, L., Dixey, R. and South, J. (2013) Healthy Public Policy. In: Dixey, R. *et al.* (eds) *Health Promotion: Global Priciples and Practices*. CAB International, Wallingford, UK.

Webb, D. and Wright, D. (2000) Postmodernism and health promotion: implications for the debate on effectiveness. In: Watson, J. and Platt, S. (eds) *Researching Health Promotion*. Routledge, London.

Weeks, J., Scriven, A. and Sayer, L. (2005) The health promoting role of health visitors: adjunct or synergy. In: Scriven, A. (ed.) (2005) *Health Promoting Practice: The Contribution of Nurses and Allied Health Professionals*. Palgrave Macmillan, Basingstoke, UK, pp. 31–44.

Whitehead, D., Taket, A. and Smith, P. (2003) Action research in health promotion. *Health Education Journal* 62, 5–22.

Whitelaw, S., Baxendale, A., Bryce, C., Machardy, L., Young, I. and Witney, E. (2001) 'Settings' based health promotion: a review. *Health Promotion International* 16, 339–352.

WHO (1986a) Ottawa Charter for health promotion. *Health Promotion* 1, iii–v.

WHO (1986b) *Ottawa Charter for Health Promotion. First International Conference on Health Promotion, Ottawa*, 17–21 November. WHO Regional Office for Europe, Copenhagen.

WHO (1991) *Third International Conference on Health Promotion*. Sundsvall, Sweden. WHO, Geneva.

WHO (1997) *Jakarta Declaration on Leading Health Promotion into the 21st Century*. WHO, Geneva. Available at: http://www.who.int/healthpromotion/conferences/previous/jakarta/declaration/en/index1.html (accessed 12 October 2012).

WHO (1998a) *Health 21 – The Health for All Policy for the WHO European Region – 21 Targets for the 21st Century*. WHO, Copenhagen.

WHO (1998b) *Health Promotion Glossary*. WHO, Geneva.

Wiggers, J. and Sanson-Fisher, R. (1998) Evidence-based health promotion. In: Scott, R. and Weston, R. (eds) *Evaluating Health Promotion*. Stanley Thornes, Cheltenham, UK.

Wimbush, E. and Watson, J. (2000) An evaluation framework for health promotion: theory, quality and effectiveness. *Evaluation* 6, 301–321.

Witte, K. and Allen, M. (2000) A meta analysis of fear appeals: implications for effective public health campaigns. *Health Education and Behavior* 27, 591–615.

Woodall, J. (2016) A critical examination of the health promoting prison two decades on. *Critical Public Health* 26, 615–621.

Woodall, J. (2020) Health promotion co-existing in a high-security prison context: a documentary analysis. *International Journal of Prisoner Health,* doi: 10.1108/IJPH-09-2019-0047

Woodall, J. and Freeman, C. (2020) Where have we been and where are we going? The state of contemporary health promotion. *Health Education Journal*. Available at: https://doi.org/10.1177/0017896919899970

Woodall, J. and South, J. (2011) Health promoting prisons: dilemmas and challenges. In: Scriven, A. and Hodgins, M. (eds) *Health Promotion Settings: Principles and Practice*. Sage, London, pp. 170–186.

Woodall, J., Raine, G., South, J. and Warwick-Booth, L. (2010) *Empowerment & Health and Well-being: Evidence Review*. Centre for Health Promotion Research, Leeds Metropolitan University, Leeds, UK.

Woodall, J., Warwick-Booth, L., South, J. and Cross, R. (2018) What makes health promotion distinct? *Scandinavian Journal of Public Health* 46, 118–122.

Wrigley, T. (2000) Misunderstanding school improvement. *Improving Schools* 3, 23–29.

Yamey, G. and Feachem, R. (2011) Evidence-based policymaking in global health – the payoffs and pitfalls. *Evidence-Based Medicine* 16, 97–99.

6 Towards the Future of Health Promotion

RUTH CROSS, LOUISE WARWICK-BOOTH AND SALLY FOSTER[1]

This chapter aims to:
- explore the role of the epistemic and academic community of health promoters;
- suggest that there are new and emerging public health problems to take into account;
- reinforce the need to defend the radical intent of the Ottawa Charter and to develop further anti-oppressive practice;
- describe how the health promotion discourse is changing, and moving into new realms of wellbeing;
- reinforce the importance of hearing lay voices and understanding 'healthworlds'; and
- present some ideas for moving forward the value base of health promotion.

Introduction

This chapter has the task of reflecting on the state of health promotion in the 21st century. It would perhaps require another book to consider fully where health promotion is going, its potential as a social movement to bring about a fairer, more just world in which everyone has good health and can achieve their potential, and whether contemporary health promotion has the answers to the issues of the 21st century and its concomitant threats to health. This begs the question of what characterizes the 21st century; we suggest that globalization and climate change are two of the defining features, amongst others. What this chapter does is start to address some of these questions and suggest what the academic community can offer.

We have noted several implementation gaps throughout this book, in terms of, for example, the rhetoric and reality of closing inequalities in health and the potential gap between the ideology of empowerment and health promotion practice. This includes the failure to close the gap between intentions (such as in the original aims of the Ottawa Charter) and progress on the ground. This chapter considers the slow, uneven progress towards developing health promotion globally by considering its tardy implementation in the continent of Africa. The politically fraught nature of developing health promotion will be exemplified by charting its fortunes in England, where currently health promotion is in a major decline. The chapter illustrates how language reflects power, and that the discourse around public health in England has quietly dropped 'health promotion'. This reminds us that discourse not only reflects reality, but it helps to construct it, and as that construction can shut off other ways of seeing, it is very powerful.

The epistemic health promotion community has drawn attention to the ways in which the radical intent of the initial key documents and conferences, which brought paradigm shifts in thinking and which are essential milestones in our history, has been diluted by the political forces that have no interest in prioritizing social justice in health. Hall and Taylor (2003) suggest that as soon as the Alma-Ata conference was over, primary health care came under attack and papers abound with the notion of a retreat from Alma-Ata, such as Campbell and Scott (2011). The health promotion community has been vocal in defending the legacy of Ottawa and Alma-Ata but as *health promotion* remains a contested concept, there has been disagreement amongst that community too. Our view is that the original radicalism *has* indeed been diluted, though the high-level activities on social determinants have restored some of this.

Leadership in health promotion for the 21st century has never been more essential. What has been already won needs to be guarded and energy is required to stay involved in the politics of implementing the vision. Health promotion is an intellectual activity applied practically. Academic health promotion plays an essential role in developing the theory behind practice; it also plays a crucial role in defending health promotion, developing the evidence base to show whether and how it works. By academic, we do not merely mean those who work in universities or other higher education institutions (HEIs), but all those who contribute to the literature on health promotion, to theory-building, evaluation studies and so on. They could be working in para-statal bodies, NGOs, government or as freelancers, as well as in HEIs.

The academic community, in our view, has a fivefold role:

1. To maintain a watch on the implementation of the vision, to ensure that health promotion ideas remain radical and do not become distorted and diluted, and thus to carry out analysis, such as discourse analysis, to ensure this.
2. To continually refresh the theoretical base, move across disciplinary boundaries, and draw on relevant ideas which can enrich understanding and thus inform practice.
3. To challenge health inequities and oppressive practice and to present critiques of systems of stratification or divisions which mean that people cannot reach their full potential.
4. To suggest ways of theorizing and understanding key challenges of the 21st century – among them, globalization, climate change, engaging with communities and the 'search for meaning'.
5. To take seriously the need to develop the evidence base for health promotion, publishing both what works and what doesn't, whilst also defending the value base, and bearing in mind that 'what really counts can't always be counted'.

These five dimensions are not in any particular order – they are all important.

It goes without saying, too, that the academic community needs to publish, but more than that, needs to dialogue and engage with policy makers and others in power. In addition, we would argue that HEIs, including universities such as our own, have a fourfold role:

1. To carry out high-quality research that makes a difference on the ground.
2. To develop capacity in health promotion, thus developing the health promotion workforce and adding to human resources for health.
3. To engage with communities.
4. To model a settings approach by becoming health-promoting universities.

Implementing the Vision of Health Promotion

The changing discourse of health promotion

Academics and practitioners have questioned whether health promotion has strayed from its radical roots based in the Alma-Ata Declaration and the Ottawa Charter, and also whether progress has been made on primary health care or on Ottawa's five action areas (Baum and Sanders, 1995; Hall and Taylor, 2003). Whilst challenges remain, Potvin and Jones (2011, p. 247) suggest that 'the significance of the Ottawa Charter lies in its longevity as a mouthpiece for the field of health promotion. It continues to confirm a vision, orient action, and underpin the values that comprise health promotion today.' Much progress has been made in creating health in all policies, though Sparks (2011) warns against the 'misdirection' generated by opponents of such approaches. Developing health in all policies has been key to the modern health promotion movement but has come under attack by those who wish to 'roll back the state' in the current neo-liberal climate. Despite evidence (Baum and Fischer, 2014), those on the political right use arguments about individual freedom and the 'nanny state' to dispense with the idea of regulation and legislation to promote health. Petterson (2011) argues that the need for health promoters to become involved in policy making remains present.

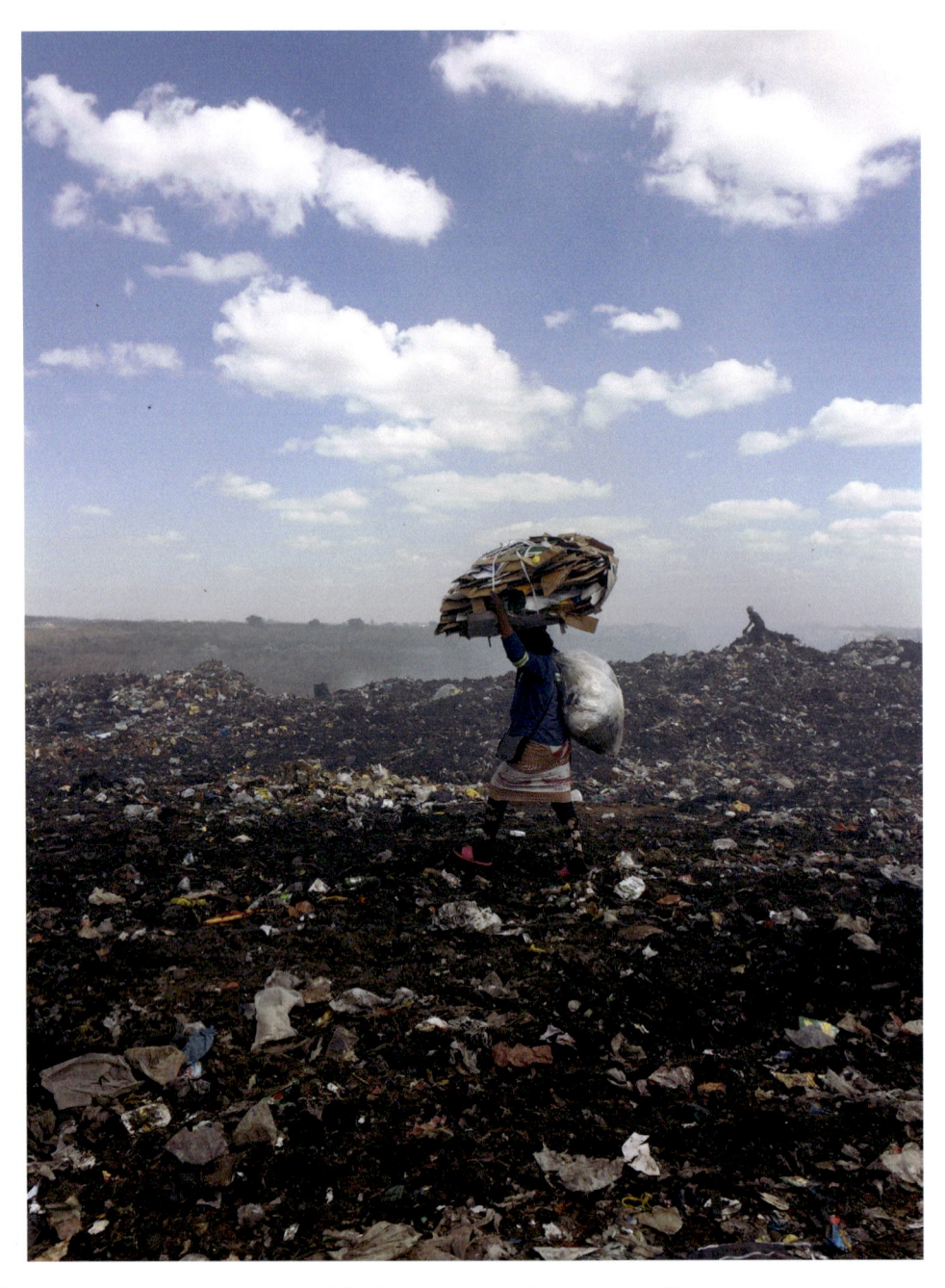

The dump site in Lusaka, Zambia – highlighting the importance of environmental issues.

The environmental movement has given attention to the emphasis on supportive environments, and the application of newer concepts such as social capital has led impetus to the creation of strong communities, and there has been some development of personal skills. The newer cadres of health workers such as health trainers are increasingly contributing to the development of personal skills, confidence and health literacy, and the development of skills frameworks (such as the UK Public Health

Skills and Knowledge Framework; UKPHSKF) can be seen as positive. Viens and Vass (2020) report that whilst such frameworks can support public health practice, those working in health promotion need to be aware of them. Their survey of UK practitioners found low levels of awareness with only 38.4% of respondents saying that they had accessed the framework.

The final area of action, reorienting health services has perhaps been the most disappointing and most difficult to see progress in. Not only has the radical vision of Alma-Ata failed to materialize in bringing full primary care to developing countries, but in those 'industrialized countries' represented in Ottawa, there has been a corresponding lack of a shift in emphasis towards prevention, primary (rather than tertiary) care, or increased funding for health promotion within health care. The importance of health care services, whilst recognized in higher income countries, is underplayed in countries where good quality health care, and access to it, is taken for granted (except in countries such as the USA where millions do not have free health care). Yet Petterson (2011, p. ii173) states that:

> health promotion is as relevant for the twenty-first century as ever. The challenges and opportunities are evident; the increasing global burden of non-communicable diseases, ageing populations, harmful use of alcohol, social determinants and fair societies improved governance and more.

Secondly, however, there is a lack of incorporation of what is known about people's help-seeking behaviours into service planning. There are many studies about people's behaviours in relation to health and illness, from uptake of services such as immunization and screening to illness behaviours and seeking medical help. For instance Chen *et al.*'s (2006) work on lay beliefs about hepatitis among North American Chinese shows why they do not seek health care in the form of vaccinations – because they saw hepatitis as caused by harmful food, alcohol, stress and lack of adequate rest, as much as infection, and strategies to prevent it were more likely to involve tackling stress and getting rest. Similarly, Carruth (2014) explored ideas about health and illness in the Somali Region of Ethiopia, and found that complex ideas that included the importance of 'balance between bodily fluids or humours and divine causality ("Allah is the cause of all disease")' (p. 407) then led to people engaging in 'medical pluralism' – that is not only using biomedical help but also ethnomedical and faith healing systems (in this case therapeutic camel milk, Qur'anic spiritual healing and herbal remedies). In relation to this choice of health systems, Pescosolido *et al.* (2019) discuss the complexity of contemporary utilization behaviour in their global view of population use of allopathic and alternative medical systems. Therefore, recognising that people move between medical systems is crucial for any interventions.

The role of gender in help seeking behaviours has also been much studied, demonstrating that men's actions are very much linked to hegemonic concepts of masculinity (see, for example, Seidler *et al.*, 2016, on how traditional masculine gender norms may deter men from seeking help for depression). The challenge here is to effectively reorient interventions and services, and this is the focus of the strategy on the health and wellbeing of men of the WHO European Region (2018). Men's sheds have been one type of initiative and Misan *et al.* (2017) explore the scope for health promotion in such sheds for older men in Australia. And, also in Australia, Gwyther *et al.* (2019) evaluate community and school-based health promotion programmes relevant to young males aged 12–25 years. Finally, in the UK, Robertson *et al.* (2015; 2018) look at what works in terms of promoting mental health and wellbeing among boys and men. Thus, the evidence base for a reorientation of services is growing.

Discourse analysis has also been used to dissect the texts enshrining the basic principles and goals of the modern health promotion movement. Discourse analysis of this kind helps to illustrate how 'social movement frames gain wide appeal but over time lose the progressive formulation that incited their production or, more are used to counter progressive goals' (Naples, 2003, p. 89). In other words, the radical nature behind the original movement becomes diluted and subverted by the 'powers that be'. Discourse analysis starts with the premise that language is central to the creation of discourse/s and therefore that language is central in reflecting and perpetuating power structures (Lupton, 1992). Discourses thus create 'regimes of truth' (Lessa, 2006, p. 285), which come to be 'hegemonic', i.e. those regimes of truth come to be accepted as the norm, keeping in place the status quo in terms of power structures. Scott-Samuel and Springett (2007) put this clearly when they write:

> Gramsci, Foucault and Bourdieu have all pointed to the relationship between discourse (that is, knowledge associated with a particular theme – such as public

health) and power. Their mutual nature ensures that as a particular discourse becomes more prominent, the power of the groups whose interests it represents increases. Just as discourse shapes relations of power, the latter in turn shape how and by whom discourse is influenced over time.

They argue that health promotion discourse has changed in England, resulting in a dramatic decline in its fortunes. Porter (2006) compared the Ottawa Charter and the Bangkok Charter using critical discourse theory to analyse how the health promotion discourse significantly changed from 1986 to 2005. She argues that the language of the Bangkok Charter has become far more timid; whereas the Ottawa Charter *directed* and said, 'we must', Bangkok merely makes suggestions and calls for certain actions to take place. Whilst Ottawa was framed in terms of a 'new social movement' discourse (emphasizing empowerment, action on social determinants, community participation), Bangkok replaces this with a 'new capitalism' discourse, where adjustments to health status are made by changes to the economy. Whereas sociology and ecology framed Ottawa, resulting in a stress on a 'socio-ecological' approach, Bangkok privileges economics – 'Discursively, this proposes cleaning up messes of new capitalism, but not questioning their sources' (p. 77). Porter (2006) describes a move from 'participatory democracy' to 'global technocracy'. The social justice equity agenda of Ottawa is described as being replaced by a concern to improve health opportunities. She argues that discourse analysis suggests that the holistic view of health within Ottawa has been lost, people have become consumers, and there is a shift from workers and their needs to employers' roles. Duncan (2013) offers a historical analysis of the fortunes of specialist health promotion noting its failure in England, and the wider political environment in which health promotion is being practised in the UK remains challenging (Warwick-Booth *et al.*, 2018b).

Raphael (2003) also noted how health promotion discourse in Canada shifted through the adoption of the term 'population health', which has served to depoliticize health promotion; moreover, despite being a world leader (Pederson *et al.*, 2005) in the development of health promotion, Raphael argues that the approach in reality in Canada is still very downstream and medically oriented. More recently his discourse analysis (Raphael, 2011) of the social determinants of health (SDH) shows varying responses to this agenda. He identifies seven discourses, ranging from conservative to radical; at one end, SDH is seen merely as being concerned with identifying those in need of health and social services, a problem that will be solved by extending service provision to those groups. At the other extreme are discourses that see SDH resulting from economic and political structures and their justifying ideologies, and as centring on identifying those classes and interests that benefit from social and health inequalities. The more conservative discourse is capable of derailing the original intent of the Marmot review and its later follow-up assessment. Furthermore, particular groups, through their ability to influence and sponsor the dominant discourse, are able to promote their own interests; they have a 'voice'. Kickbusch *et al.* (2016) argue that neoliberal values need wider study because of the global corporate interests at play which serve to propagate non-communicable diseases.

This next section considers the challenges facing health promotion in sub-Saharan Africa and later discusses how 'health promotion' has lost its place in England. Across European countries, health promotion is achieved via a range of different approaches. In comparing health promotion for older adults in Germany, Italy, the Netherlands and Poland, Arsenijevic and Groot (2020) found different models of implementation, but no documents to specifically address health promotion policies for older adults, thus reporting concerns that this was gradually disappearing from the national agenda in all four countries. Health promotion remains alive and well, however, in the Scandinavian countries, for example. Whereas the Ottawa Charter was principally concerned with the health of 'industrialized nations', and the Lalonde report with developing new approaches to the ill health of an affluent society, the Alma-Ata Declaration in 1978 was a more relevant cornerstone on which to reorient health and health care in resource-poor countries, and it was only really the Jakarta Declaration that made prominent the needs of the 'developing' world. After Jakarta, subsequent international conferences, particularly Mexico, addressed the glaring equity gaps between the richest and poorest countries. This is not to say that the Ottawa Charter is inappropriate for resource-poor countries, but that such countries have a range of health issues not faced by wealthy, industrialized nations. Jones (2019) argues that health promotion needs decolonizing to better enable it to deal with contemporary challenges such as the likely health impacts of climate change upon Indigenous communities.

More positively, Mercer (2020) reports that at the 164th Meeting of the Executive Committee of the Pan American Health Organization/World Health Organization (held in Washington, DC, during June 2019), it was recommended a series of changes be made to the conceptual map of health policies in the Americas, which situates health promotion as a central strategy and possible action plan in achieving equity and social justice.

Bringing health promotion about in sub-Saharan Africa

Africa is a huge continent and generalizations about it are usually not a good idea, though it is essential to counter the negative view and misperceptions of Africa held by some in the global North (Dixey, 2013). For example, whereas Africa is seen as famine-ridden, only one of the 20 largest famines (in terms of lives lost) during the 20th century occurred in Africa (Keneally, 2011). The use of the word Africa can work as a pseudonym for poverty, corruption, conflict and marginalization so such usage should be resisted. However, that is not to say that health and development challenges do not exist. Veary *et al.* (2019) note the increasing population growth across the continent and the associated challenges that this brings for public health with increased numbers of younger people living in urban areas. The loss of trained health care personnel in sub-Saharan Africa, due to migration, death and other factors, is a continuous threat to the sustainability of health systems in many states. The 'health worker crisis' refers to the severe shortage of trained health staff – doctors, nurses, allied health professionals – that characterizes most African health care systems (WHO, 2006). Labonté *et al.* (2015) use the term 'brain drain' to describe the high proportions of health professionals including doctors and nurses who, once trained and educated in their own countries, leave to work in higher-income locations with better pay and conditions (Labonté *et al.*, 2015). The emphasis on expensive, curative care in poorer countries was challenged by the Declaration of Alma-Ata (WHO, 1978), which attempted to divert more funding into primary care, accessible to the majority, rather than into tertiary care in the urban centres. Ironically, the lack of trained health (read 'medical') staff *has* resulted in the need to rethink how health care is provided, resulting in cadres of village health workers, public health officers and clinical officers, all of which can be provided more cheaply than expensively trained doctors.

The crisis of health care staff has been cited as one reason why sub-Saharan Africa would not meet the Millennium Development Goals (MDGs) (Economic Commission for Africa, 2005). Easterly (2009) notes, however, that the MDG campaign frequently and unfairly referred to the failure of sub-Saharan Africa, which was disadvantaged from the outset because of the way the goals were organized and measured.

The state of health promotion in Africa has also been the subject of critical analysis (Sanders *et al.*, 2008; Amunyunzu-Nyamongo and Nyamwaya, 2009). The Nairobi Conference was the first international health promotion conference organized in Africa, enabling more Africans to participate. Catford's (2010, p. 3) conference reflections describe Africa's opportunity 'to light the way' forward for health promotion, thus closing the obvious 'implementation gap' between the rhetoric and the reality. He commended the 'vitality, level-headedness and commitment' of African participants, despite the 'lack of resources and infrastructure' available for health promotion in their countries. Dixey (2013) argues that whilst health promotion has increased in presence across Africa after Nairobi, problematic infrastructure limits capacity for it to be further implemented, and Eurocentrism in the field of health promotion still serves as a barrier. There are, of course, health challenges that need attention across Africa, but in some instances health promotion is working well to address these. Sampson *et al.* (2013, p. 353) report the use of community based interventions in Ghana, Nigeria and South Africa as well as school-based programmes in Swaziland, Namibia and Kenya that are examples of efforts to advance health promotion and disease prevention for cardiovascular diseases, though they call for more developed intersectoral partnership approaches to tackle the 'unfinished agenda' in this area.

Anugwom (2020, p. 11) argues that there is a need to give attention to health promotion in Africa, because it still has a tendency to be focused upon the medical model, and, furthermore, specific disciplinary challenges remain such as:

- Poor definition and rudimentary elaboration of expected health outcomes;
- Ambiguous elaboration of factors and conditions to be targeted in health promotions;
- Ambiguity of health promotion policies and guidelines;

- Lack of capacity (or inadequate capacity) to develop, implement and evaluate health promotion programmes;
- A general context of inadequate investment in health promotion; underdeveloped sectoral collaboration;
- Low political will and commitment to health promotion programmes as well as institutional corruption and resource mismanagement.

Anugwom (2020, p. 11)

Therefore, despite substantial 'health promotion' or health education type activity in Africa, it is not 'big picture health promotion', occurring at a policy level and true to the Ottawa Charter – addressing the SDH or concerned with tackling inequalities, empowerment and with people taking control of their health. On the other hand, there *is* 'small picture' health promotion, which can be seen as an adjunct to the medical enterprise, concerned with health education, encouraging people to make better use of preventative health services and so on. Moving into more radical 'big picture' health promotion remains challenging. The 'implementation gap' continues.

If African colleagues are to take forward the health promotion agenda in Africa, the academic infrastructure also needs strengthening. Outside South Africa, the academic infrastructure for health promotion is under-developed, and where health promotion *is* offered, it tends to be as part of a medically dominated university public health department. Before 1960, only 18 of the 48 sub-Saharan countries had a university (Sawyerr, 2002), despite which African universities are acknowledged to have performed well in terms of producing human resources to replace colonial officials (Ajayi *et al.*, 1996). However, in the interconnected global knowledge economy of the 21st century, and the marketization trajectory that universities in the global North have been on for some time, African universities continue to face challenges (Warwick-Booth *et al.*, 2018b). Yet, the importance of learning remains central to tackling the many challenges that remain in Africa, as it underpins workforce development (Welter *et al.*, 2017).

Understanding the Demise of 'Health Promotion' in England

The history of health promotion in England demonstrates the way in which the dominant ideology and the views of the government in power affect policy towards health and its determinants. For a number of years there has been a great deal of pessimism among the health promotion community in England about the political direction of change (Scott-Samuel and Wills, 2007). Scott-Samuel and Springett (2007, p. 211) show how 'the words health promotion have been steadily disappearing from the public health discourse in England'. During the 1970s, the Labour government continued to emphasize health education and narrow lifestyle approaches; it did not appear to recognize the shifts being fostered by the Lalonde report. The arrival of the Thatcher government in 1979, and its suppression of the Black report into inequalities in health, did not presage a new dawn, but, surprisingly, health promotion did 'develop and even flourish in the context of local government and the non-statutory sector' (Scott-Samuel and Springett, 2007, p. 212). Despite a government 'diametrically opposed to [a] social justice agenda' (Scott-Samuel and Wills, 2007, p. 116), the 1980s saw a period of health promotion activism, where the settings approach, strong Healthy Cities networks, the Health For All movement and fora provided by journals such as *Radical Community Medicine* and the pressure group Public Health Alliance, 'temporarily liberated health promotion from the distortions of biomedicine and placed it firmly in the hands of the local state' (Scott-Samuel and Springett, 2007, p. 213). Later, when the National Health Service (NHS) was reorganized, public health came under the newly formed Primary Care Trusts, and health promoters were thus embedded within the health (sickness) service, which many felt was a step back in that placing health promotion services within local government is more helpful than placing them within the NHS, where officers have to exempt themselves from political activities. However, this move was reversed following The Health and Social Care Act of 2012, which led to the implementation of large-scale structural reforms to health and care systems in England (Secretary of State for Health, 2012; Department of Health, 2012a, b; Local Government Information Unit, 2012). From April 2013, local government councils once again became responsible for key public health staff, functions and services. In addition, a national public health agency, Public Health England (PHE), was established to provide nationwide leadership and co-ordination (Department of Health, 2011). Milne (2018) argues that these changes have weakened relationships between public health and the

NHS, but more positively have led to improvements in the quality of commissioning, in part driven by significant public health budget cuts. Peckham *et al.* (2017) argue that whilst this structural change offered potential for health promotion and associated health improvements, in reality it has been a significant challenge because of both reorganization and resource constraints threatening the future of locally based public health systems.

The broader political environment of austerity has led to local authorities having to make difficult decisions about service provision related specifically to health (Milne, 2018), and to cut back on wider services that support both health and quality of life (Alston, 2018). Previous governments (New Labour 1997–2010) received criticism for their attempts to strengthen public health (Scott-Samuel and Springett, 2007), but they did introduce a range of initiatives such as neighbourhood renewal, Sure Start (to provide pre-school children with a better start in life), and a social exclusion unit, which were well intentioned, if not always effective. These have now mostly been discontinued. Despite the development of some positive interventions, the term 'health improvement' crept into the policy language, as did targets and the move to reducing lifestyle risk factors in what is described as the behavioural turn: health promotion focusing upon empowering healthy choices and moralizing about lifestyle (Brown, 2018). As Scott-Samuel and Springett (2007) comment, 'health improvement is a target' – it does not signify the values and processes of health promotion, which is a coherent ideology with sets of principles and methods of working.

Despite this gloomy picture, political discourse still notes the importance of prevention, as discussed in the NHS (2014, p. 3) Five Year Forward View which emphasizes the need for a radical upgrade 'in prevention and public health', yet investment is lagging:

> At least 80% of 20th century mortality reduction resulted from factors other than healthcare. Yet society remains persuaded that we are on the threshold of a new era in which medicine drives that progress—as it has been for at least 50 years, while non-clinical factors continued to make most of the running.
> (Milne, 2018, p. 1)

Despite some positive policy discourse in relation to public health, the focus in England has been upon structural reforms and efficiency savings under the name of austerity (Kings Fund, 2015), with public health remaining the poorer neighbour in terms of priority setting, as has frequently been the historical case (Warwick-Booth *et al.*, 2018b). Despite lack of investment in prevention, there is some possibility for 'street level bureaucrats' and dedicated health promoters to carry on activities successfully because cost effectiveness is not always a service cut, and in some areas the third sector continues to operate well to support health and wellbeing. The welcome support of key players such as Michael Marmot remains evident in his tireless work to promote the importance of the social determinants of health.

Many countries are in the same position as England, having made attempts to increase health promotion but, failing to appreciate the Ottawa Charter's central idea that the key sectors to promote health lie outside the health (care) sector, tend to send health (care) workers on courses. We will always need doctors to rescue the ill and diseased and it is vital that they are there. However, the failure to appreciate the social model of health seriously hampers the development of health promotion. It means that health promotion continues to be seen as an adjunct to the medical, health care enterprise. What is needed is paradigm shift so that the complex nature of health can be better understood and therefore be used to inform system change (Keshavarz Mohammadi, 2020). Health and associated health promotion are deeply political by nature, requiring an equity lens, yet political extremism has gained ground since 2016, leading to the prioritization of economic interests and the increased use of anti-democratic techniques (such as fake news) at the expense of democracy and health (Ackerman *et al.*, 2019). Finally, as Duncan (2013) argues, we need a deeper historical understanding of previous health promotion failures and how these link to conceptual, organizational and ideological difficulties so that we might better determine how to reorient health policy to achieve health promotion as it is outlined within the Ottawa Charter.

Refreshing the Theory Base

There is no dispute that health promotion requires a robust theory base. However, Keshavarz Mohammadi (2020) notes that 'the critical mass of scholarship and development in the health promotion is trailing behind' (p. 637). In this section we consider theoretical developments and directions for health promotion.

McQueen *et al.* (2007) have, arguably, led the debates on developing appropriate theory bases for health promotion in the 21st century. Mittelmark (2005) has expressed frustration that health promotion tends to be insular and is missing opportunities for theoretical development due to a lack of attention to the importance of communicating with other disciplines. He gives the example of community psychology as one where there are clear parallels between the two areas:

> With its longstanding emphases on person-environment fit in community settings, coping and social support, promotion of social competence, stimulation of citizen participation and empowerment, and organizing for community and social change, community psychology bears a striking resemblance to health promotion.
>
> (Mittelmark, 2005, p. 55)

Nelson and Prilleltensky's work (2010) in community psychology, where they see its mission as advancing the liberation and wellbeing of oppressed communities, would concur with this.

This statement suggests what Mittelmark, a key figure in contemporary health promotion, sees health promotion *as*. It also suggests that students of health promotion need to read in other disciplines and to look critically at what disciplines health promotion *does* draw on. The usual starting point for considering the multidisciplinary nature of health promotion is Bunton and MacDonald's (1992) seminal book (now in its second edition: Bunton and MacDonald, 2002). They provide discussion of the contribution to health promotion of sociology, psychology, education, epidemiology, economics, social policy, marketing and communications. At the point they wrote that book, there was a concerted effort to move health promotion in the direction of a social model of health (as opposed to a medical model) and thus there is a discernible lack of attention to the disciplines of medicine, nursing or social work: knowledge areas based on a personal relationship between professionals and clients/patients have tended to be less favoured within the health promotion academic community in the attempt to move health promotion more towards social policy and strategic level development. Further developments since then have included recent calls to 'strengthen salutogenesis as a theory base for health promotion' (Bauer *et al.*, 2019, p. 1) and, in the light of the Covid-19 pandemic, to renew focus on globalization and health scholarship (Labonté, 2020).

As discussed in Chapter 1, as a discipline that draws on other primary disciplines, health promotion is something of a 'hybrid' discipline, or, as Seedhouse (1997) describes it, a 'magpie profession'. Thus, health promotion has much in common with a range of areas with double-barrelled names: environmental psychology, political ecology, cultural epidemiology, social psychology, behavioural economics, which, according to Mittelmark (2005), would enrich health promotion.

The need for academic health promotion to extend beyond borders fits with all the thinking within the *practice* of health promotion that, as the determinants of health lie outside the health (sickness) service, there is a need to develop partnerships, inter-professional and inter-sectoral collaboration, and to liaise with sectors such as transport, housing, employment, education, agriculture, architecture, urban design, media – in short, with those sectors where health *originates*. It makes sense, therefore, that health promotion as an academic discipline needs to cross boundaries and to capitalize on the insights of any relevant disciplines. This leads to a discussion of whether health promotion is multidisciplinary and/or interdisciplinary.

Health promotion describes itself as eclectic and multidisciplinary (McQueen, 2001). Multidisciplinarity is usually taken to mean that several disciplines have something to offer in understanding a phenomenon; interdisciplinarity is taken to mean that disciplines borrow ideas from each other, in a transfer of insights. As Baldwin (2020, p. 260) argues, 'the complexities of the social systems in which health 'issues' are located require complex, collaborative, multi-strategy approaches' and the same can be said for health promotion's disciplinary nature. Given the complexity of the determinants of health in the complex world of the 21st century, however, there is a need perhaps to go further than this. Albrecht *et al.* (1998) call for a transdisciplinary paradigm in order to understand human health, where a unified conceptual framework can incorporate the diversity presented by different disciplines and thus help to understand the complexity of the world. How a transdisciplinary paradigm could be adopted in health promotion remains to be discussed and worked out. Nevertheless, health promotion, it is argued, must be nimble, dynamic and proactive (Baldwin, 2020; Fleming *et al.*, 2020). In keeping with this, Keshavarz Mohammadi (2020) has pointed out that 'complexity science' provides a different way for health promotion to address the challenges of practice given that it takes into account multiple pathways of causality and complex relationships that exist, in this instance, between the multiple factors that influence health. Keshavarz Mohammadi (2020) reiterates the fact that health is a complex phenomenon and, whilst this is a well-rehearsed contention, he emphasizes that health promotion must therefore be approached as such by taking on board ideas from complex adaptive systems theory. The said complexity of health is reflected in more recent moves towards 'whole systems' approaches, for example, to mental health (Peate, 2017) and obesity (Bagnall *et al.*, 2019).

A further challenge for the development of the theory base of health promotion is to ensure that it does not remain Eurocentric. MacDonald (1998) espoused his view over a decade ago, that health promotion *is* a Eurocentric phenomenon and more recently there have been calls to develop a critical public health in the global South (Colvin, 2011). Airhihenbuwa is one of the main critics who have pointed out how Western models of, for example, psychology do not serve well those societies that do not derive their values from individualistic norms, and he also suggests that health promotion has been mishandled in Africa by emphasizing, for example, individual empowerment, rather than understanding the collective and communitarian nature of those societies (Airhihenbuwa, 2007).

The role of lay knowledge has been debated in health promotion. In work on lay epidemiologies, the idea has been extended recently into notions of 'community epidemiologies', for example in the work of Salant and Gehlert (2008), on African-Americans' ideas about breast cancer risk. The authors argue that, when discussing breast cancer risk, whether in nostalgic memories about traditional ways of life in the South, or references to competing health risks and the sense of being victimized by outside forces, community played 'a central conceptual role in participants' responses' (p. 612). Others are more critical of this postmodern privileging of all accounts of health and illness, whether professional or not; Prior (2003), for example, acknowledges the experiential dimensions of lay knowledge, but points out the limitations of such knowledge and challenges the notion of lay 'expertise'. Allmark and Tod (2006) explore the ethical dilemmas for health professionals posed by a lay epidemiology that conflicts with medical advice but conclude: 'engaging with lay epidemiology is likely to increase the effectiveness of public health work, as well as helping ensure that it is ethically sound' (Allmark and Tod, 2006, p. 463). That position is endorsed by Henderson (2010, p. 5), who suggests that if health professionals privilege scientific knowledge over lay knowledge this risks 'misunderstanding the manner in which the experiences and belief of their clients impact health-seeking behaviour', and this will undermine their practice. This issue has become even more important with the rise of blogs and online forums for patients to share information and experiences; in their study of an online community of parents of children with heart defects, Bellander and Landqvist (2020, p. 519) point out that 'patient expert knowledge is a useful, relevant and often a most welcome source of information for people facing a medical problem'. Indeed, Pols (2014, p. 75) calls this knowledge '*knowing in action*'.

Challenging Oppression

The third of the roles of academic health promotion outlined at the start of this chapter was to challenge health inequities and oppressive practice, and to present critiques of systems of stratification and divisions, which limit the potential of people. Academics have provided a sociology *of* health promotion (Bunton *et al.*, 1996) and also made use of critical theory to challenge orthodoxies in order to bring about transformational change. Health promoters need to be self-reflexive, reflective practitioners who do not get lost in theory, but who use theory to better understand the complexities of real life and thus come up with robust means of bringing real health and social justice to people on the ground. A key aspect of health promotion is to develop anti-oppressive practice and thus to challenge oppression wherever it is encountered. What does the academic community within health promotion have to say about inequalities?

Jenny Douglas has provided consistent critiques of health promotion from a black perspective for many years (1995, 1997). She argues that the discourse of multiculturalism disguises the issues facing black and minority ethnic communities in Europe. More recently, Douglas (2018) notes that the racialized, gendered and classed experience of black women remains detrimental to their health over the life course, because of their enduring experiences of discrimination in education, employment, housing as well as health and social care. Douglas (2019) also argues that black women's activism in relation to health issues remains largely ignored by white feminist scholars, particularly in the UK. She has documented her own experiences as a Black female academic witnessing and experiencing racism whilst working in health promotion and public health (Douglas, 2017).

Hylton (2010) argues that critical race theory (CRT) has emerged as an effective framework to challenge racism in his chosen area of study (sport) but also within society more generally. This would be our conclusion too – that racist acts are not aberrational but are deeply embedded into global society; they are not simply acts of individual agency, but part and parcel of institutional life. It is therefore incumbent upon health promoters not only to examine 'whiteness' (especially for those who *are* white), in order to understand whiteness as a process and to see its role in upholding systems of power, but also to consider the institutional racism of their respective organizations and the structures of power within their national contexts.

Following these basic tenets of CRT, we also assert that the other forms of discrimination do exist; we do not feel we need to make a case to show that they do. Thus sexism, ageism, discrimination against people who are differently abled, who are gay, lesbian or transgendered, who are from particular classes, castes or ethnic groups, all flourish. There is also discrimination against people with particular health statuses, for example those who are obese, who have experienced mental ill health or other stigmatized illnesses, including HIV/AIDS.

Despite the presence of many in health promotion who would call themselves feminists, there is scant critical feminist critique of health promotion, such as that provided by Lesley Doyal (1995) or Wilkinson and Kitzinger (1994) of health in general. A notable contribution in health promotion is Moore's (2010) excellent feminist critique of the 'new health paradigm' in which she suggests a 'new feminist critique of health promotion'. Furthermore, in their attempt to 'ignite an agenda for women and health promotion', Pedersen *et al.* (2014, p. 140) state that:

> Health promotion, as a field, has paid only limited attention to gender inequity to date, but could be an active agent of change if gender equity became an explicit goal of health promotion research, policy and programmes.

They go on to suggest a framework for women's health promotion. There *are* clear feminist voices within health promotion, arguing that patriarchy is a major obstacle to women achieving their full potential, yet challenges remain in keeping issues on the agenda such as gender-based violence, traditions harmful to women (such as genital cutting), sexual harassment and forced marriage. Health promotors also need to continue to try to gain more attention for health conditions that predominantly affect women, including family planning, reproductive health and women's cancers, and to listen to women who report that their voices are often not heard by health professionals (Thomas and Warwick-Booth, 2019). A number of issues affecting the health and wellbeing of women and stopping them realizing their potential are seen as 'cultural' issues. In this light, it can be argued that 'multiculturism' has not served women well.

Meanwhile White *et al.* (2011) and EC (2011) draw attention to men's health and the need for particular attention to their poorer health status in key areas (White and Pettifer, 2007; Conrad and White, 2010) requiring health strategies designed specifically for men. Robertson and Baker (2017, p. 102) state that:

> …despite certain improvements in the practice of men's health promotion and in men's health outcomes, issues remain in terms of premature mortality, particularly for certain groups of men. We further suggest that many of the difficulties in improving and promoting the health of men further lie with a market-driven neoliberal policy context that engenders inequality through the inequitable distribution of and access to material resources and through individualistic approaches to health promotion that serve men from economically and socially disadvantaged locations least well.

Children and young people, too, are often neglected in health promotion. This might seem a surprising assertion when they feature so strongly in health promotion interventions; in industrialized countries, many examples can be found of attempts to curb teen use of alcohol, reduce teen pregnancies, encourage healthy eating, improve oral health, increase exercise rates and educate young people on how to become responsible, healthy adults. What we mean by neglect is that their voices are not heard and children and young people are seen as problematic, are pathologized and requiring to 'be educated'. Aceves-Martins *et al.* (2019) argue that there

★ My points in time.

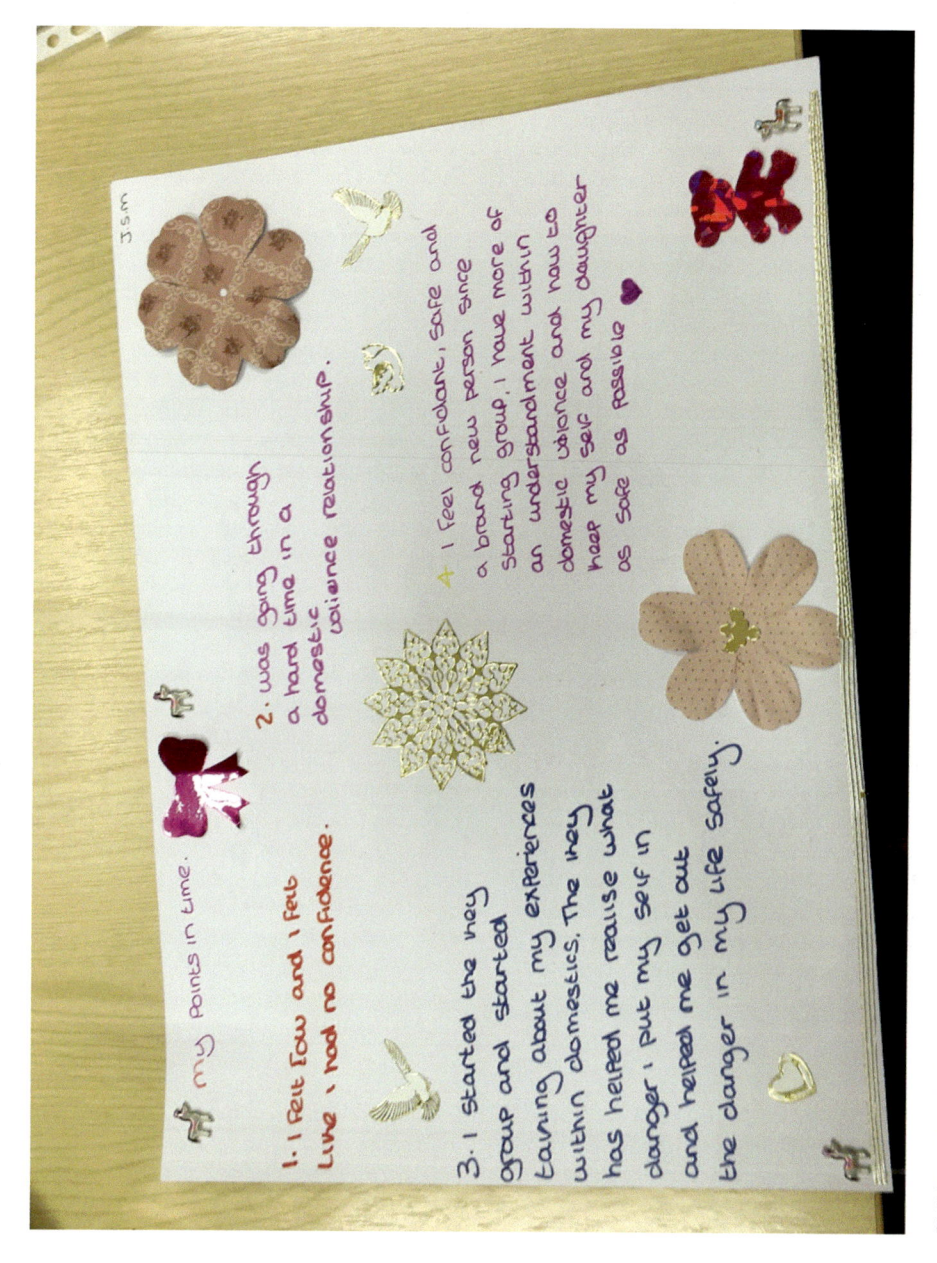

1. I felt low and I felt Lune, had no confidence.

2. Was going through a hard time in a domestic voilence relationship.

3. I started the iney group and started tauning about my experiences within domestics. The iney has helped me realise what danger I put my self in and helped me get out the danger in my life safely.

4. I feel confodant, safe and a brand new person since starting group, I have more of an understandment within domestic voilance and how to keep my self and my daughter as safe as possible

JSM

Children and young people – ensuring voices are heard using storyboards.

Towards the Future of Health Promotion 197

is little evidence related to involving youth in health-related programmes despite the potential to encourage positive interactions between health promotors and young adults during the development, implementation and evaluation of health promotion efforts intending to benefit youth. Furthermore, young people *do* face health issues that are problematic. Hagell *et al.* (2018) point out that significant proportions of young people today experience disadvantage that is detrimental to their longer term health outcomes. Young people's mental health has recently been receiving more attention, with UK research focusing upon experiences of both loneliness (Snape and Manclossi, 2018) and wellbeing (Pyle and Hassle, 2018) in younger age groups. However, what is viewed as 'problematic' or 'troublesome' by health professionals (or 'experts') is not necessarily seen as such by young people themselves. A recent example of this disconnect highlights the importance of establishing the meaning that young people give to their behaviour. Research with young women into risk-taking and health found that taking risks served a function and purpose; a space to escape from the pressures of everyday life (Cross *et al.*, 2011), and some well-intentioned health promotion interventions may be reinscribing young people into expected norms rather than supporting them to achieve their own goals (Cross and Warwick-Booth, 2018). We need to take such things into account when designing interventions that aim to reduce so-called 'risky' behaviours. This highlights the importance of consultation with, and the participation of, young people in health promotion efforts.

Children are often seen as 'captive audiences' for health education, particularly if they are in institutional and instructional contexts such as schools. There are good examples where children and young people are consulted or are full participants in deciding when and how to tackle their health issues (e.g. MacGregor *et al.*, 1998; Alderson, 2000). In terms of methods to include young people, Noreen Whetton was a pioneer. She developed the draw and write technique to find out what really quite young children (in primary school) felt and needed in terms of health issues. Later, Berry Mayall (1994) produced extraordinary insights from children in her work in primary schools in England. Not asking children and young people what they think and believe is common even in initiatives acclaimed as being 'bottom-up' and participative, but the methods are there to include them (Cross and Warwick-Booth, 2016; Warwick-Booth and Coan, 2020).

Although it is obviously essential to prepare children and young people for adult life, this is not the only reason for health promotion with young people – rather, they have the right to a happy and fulfilling childhood *now*. Therefore they have health promotion needs as children and young people *now* so that they can enjoy that childhood and process of growth into being healthy young people. Early years are an important social determinant of health (Marmot *et al.*, 2020).

Health promotion is surprisingly quiet about some of the issues affecting children in resource-poor countries. The literature reflects the concerns of adults and the global North, focusing on child survival, diseases and conditions; these are clearly important but there is a relative neglect of issues such as children's mental health, and 'social' issues such as abuse, lack of power, child rights, child labour and the use of children in conflicts, though work in these areas is gradually developing.

At the other end of the age spectrum, the voices of the aged have historically often been invisible. Cattan (2009a, 2010) critiqued ageism within society and within health promotion; her work on loneliness and mental health among elderly people living in the UK is not just poignant – it is a damning indictment of the way in which elders are perceived and subsequently treated in highly industrialized, capitalist economies (Cattan *et al.*, 2005). More recently, Golinowska *et al.* (2016) maintain that the elderly have long been neglected within health promotion activities, as medical needs are prioritized at the expense of social activities. However, some work is beginning to address these social issues, for example via the UK Campaign to End Loneliness amongst older populations groups. As people live longer and poorer countries go through demographic changes resulting in an increased 'grey population', healthy ageing needs to be a larger part of health promotion.

Vincente Navarro has perhaps been the most consistent voice writing from a neo-Marxist perspective and thus highlighting the important role of class. This perspective has gone somewhat out of fashion amidst political rhetoric describing 'classless' societies. He points out that 'race mortality differentials are large in the US, but class mortality differentials are even larger' (Navarro, 2009, p. 5). A young African American is 1.8 times more likely to die from a cardiovascular condition than a young white American, but a blue-collar (i.e. working class) worker is 2.8 times more likely than a white-collar businessman to die from a cardiovascular condition. The fact that 'class has almost disappeared from political and scientific discourse' (p. 7) being replaced by 'less conflictive categories' such as 'status', which are less threatening to the social order, disguises these inequities. He argues that ignoring the existence of class means that inequities within countries are glossed over, and there is a lack of recognition of the wealth of those at the 'top' of the poorest countries. The maldistribution of wealth and the class privileges embodied therein are drastically underestimated by the WHO, according to Navarro. In regard to the Commission of the Social Determinants of Health, he suggests that 'The Commission's studious avoidance of the category of power (class power as well as gender, race and national power) and how power is produced and reproduced in political institutions is the greatest weakness of the report'. Such class-blindness means that we see it that 'inequalities kill', whereas Navarro suggests that it is 'those who benefit from the inequalities that kill'. This standpoint conforms with Raphael's seventh SDH discourse described above, and if the analysis is located here, it has fundamentally different outcomes for how to address the SDH. This is not at all to suggest that Navarro is scathing of the report – he has suggested that its authors should receive the Nobel Peace Prize. *But* he feels that the report does not go far enough. McCartney *et al.* (2019) more recently argue that it remains important to explore the interrelationship between social class, and other social processes such as stigma linked to the characteristics of gender, ethnicity, sexuality, disability, age and religion. Other public health researchers highlight the role of social systems of power including racism, sexism, heterosexism, classism and others, in maintaining health inequalities (Gkiouleka *et al.*, 2018).

In keeping with our social model of health, it is unsurprising that we are critical of medical models of disability. That model has long been seen as insufficient to understand disability, and disabled writers, notably Oliver (1983, 1990), developed a social model of disability from the point of view of disabled people. This shifted the dominant paradigm away from individualized situations of impairment towards disabling environments and systemic barriers to living fulfilling lives as disabled people. Whereas the medical model assumes that disabled people have a 'problem', based on dependency, deviation from the norm, and that disability is a personal misfortune, and that exclusion is an appropriate way to 'deal with' disabled people, the social model assumes that the 'disability' is located in the structures – which may be physical, or attitudinal and social – that disable people who have particular needs due to an impairment. Although the disability movement coined the phrase 'Nothing about us without us', the voices of people with disabilities are also often relatively silent, especially if they are also elderly (Cattan *et al.*, 2009a, b, 2012). However, mechanisms to involve people with learning disabilities in health promotion research and interventions via co-production are gaining ground in the global North.

'Learning disability' is the term used in the UK to describe those with a significantly reduced ability to understand new or complex information or to learn new skills, and a reduced ability to cope independently. Learning disabled people thus have impaired intelligence and impaired social functioning, which has affected their development since childhood (Department of Health, 2001). NHS (2019) data suggest that 1 in 215 people have a learning disability in England, with people in this category having much lower life expectancy than individuals in the general population (women living 18 years less and men losing 14 years comparatively). As a group, they have been historically left out of health promotion initiatives, but research in this area is gaining ground. Southby (2019) argues that befriending can be a way for adults with learning disabilities to have new, beneficial experiences, because taking part in social activities can improve health. However, studies in this area are in their infancy; therefore health promoters need to know more about how befriending relationships work in such instances.

These categories – age, 'race', gender, dis/ability – are useful but they render invisible other forms of discrimination. 'Travellers', a term used to describe gypsies, those of Romany origin and travelling families, occupy one of the most discriminated against positions in Europe, with appalling health statistics. They are subjected to unfair laws, are excluded from the services provided to the rest of society and their mistreatment is condoned in ways that would be unacceptable even in conservative societies if they were simply black or women. Whilst locally targeted health interventions can be successful in supporting health improvements within Gypsy and Traveller communities, structural determinants and racism remain an issue (Warwick-Booth *et al.*, 2018a). Huge human rights gains have been made by gay and lesbian people in much of the industrialized world, but these are fragile and easily rescinded, and health outcomes are still poorer within LGBTQI+ communities. Homophobia is still a feature of all societies, and the deaths of gay activists in Africa and other locations show that people still lose their lives simply for being who they are and for standing up for their rights.

Whilst many writers tend to focus on single areas of discrimination, what is useful for us, in the messiness and complexity of the real world, is to see how these areas intersect and overlap, and how marginalization can be compounded. Thus, the black, working class, disabled woman living in a deprived area of London or the black, rich, upper class man living in a 'nice' neighbourhood in Kampala occupy social niches that defy easy analysis. To help with this analysis, feminist theory has described 'intersectionality' as the interaction between gender, race and other categories of difference. The concept of intersectionality allows a thorough examination of 'difference'. As Morris and Bunjun (2007) argue, multiple social categories create a unique social location, and not only does this influence a person's ability to navigate the social world, but it is *only* from this location that people can negotiate that world. Hankivsky *et al.* (2009) further suggest that intersectionality can provide a progressive research and policy paradigm, and thus a theoretical foundation for pursuing social justice, given that history, social and economic structures work in tandem to reinforce the status quo and thus prevent progress for marginalized groups such as women (Morris and Bunjun, 2007). The associated need to understand intersectionality (Heard *et al.*, 2019, p. 1) when working to promote health remains essential:

> Public health researchers are increasingly acknowledging intersectionality as an important theoretical approach, providing a framework for investigating health inequalities by highlighting intersections of individuals' multiple identities within social systems of power that compound and exacerbate experiences of ill health.

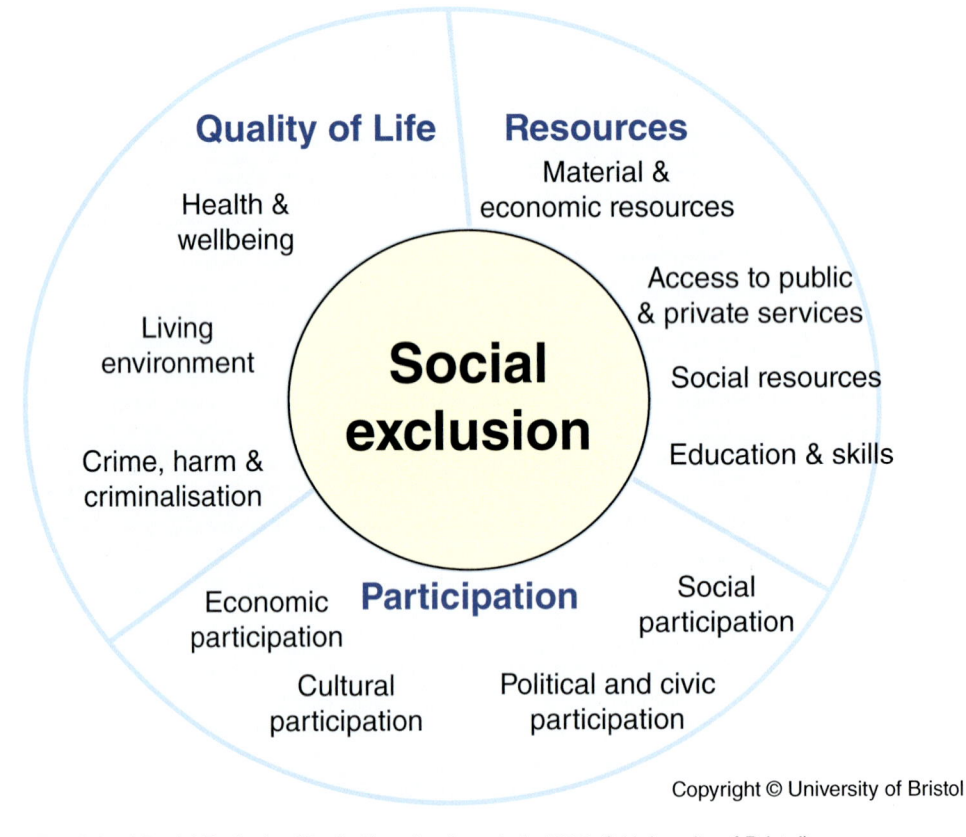

Fig. 6.1. The Bristol Social Exclusion Matrix (from Levitas *et al.*, 2007; © University of Bristol).

Marginality can lead to social exclusion, defined by Levitas *et al.* (2007, p. 9) as,

> ... a complex and multi-dimensional process. It involves the lack or denial of resources, rights, goods and services, and the inability to participate in the normal relationships and activities available to the majority of people in a society, whether in economic, social, cultural or political arenas. It affects both the quality of life of individuals and the equity and cohesion of society as a whole.

The Bristol Social Exclusion Matrix captures this diagrammatically (Fig. 6.1).

Combating oppression and social exclusion are clearly major challenges of the 21st century, with research illustrating that socially excluded older adults experience decreased quality of life and poorer health outcomes (Prattley *et al.*, 2020). We now turn to other challenges of the new century. We cannot present an exhaustive list, but we present here a few of the main problems as we see them.

Understanding the Challenges of the 21st Century

The fourth role of the academic community is to throw light on the 'big questions' facing the global community. Arguably, globalization, the environment and new public health issues are among these.

Globalization

Debate about the positive and negative impacts of globalization centres on its impact on health (McClean, 2003), and whether it is an important mechanism for addressing inequality. Wolf (2004) argues that globalization is *the* solution to poverty and inequality; it increases growth and wealth and as a result decreases poverty (Labonté, 2010). Many argue that globalization is a force for good, particularly for development (Warwick-Booth and Cross, 2018). Stiglitz (2006) similarly offered an optimistic perspective on globalization, suggesting that it *can* 'work'; however, there are those that highlight increasing global health inequalities associated with it. One of the 'particularly disturbing' aspects of globalization according to Khor (2001, p. 18) is increased inequality. He suggests that rapid liberalization has caused greater inequality by favouring certain income groups over others. He notes the increasing disparities between skilled and unskilled workers (in both the global North and South); the disparities between those with capital and those with just their labour; the rise of the new *rentier* class (i.e. those with unearned income) partly due to the rapid rise of debt servicing, which redistributes income from the poor to the rich; and the agricultural pricing system favouring traders rather than farmers, resulting in farmers becoming poorer. Not a great deal has changed since Khor wrote about this. More recently, for example, Baru and Mohan (2018) point to the rising inequities in access, availability and affordability of health care services due to the increasing commercialization of the sector in not only India but also several other countries in Asia, South America and Africa.

Kohr also argues that most developing countries are ill-equipped to cope with the forces of globalization and, furthermore, have seen a decline in their independent policy-making capacity, whilst having to accept the policies made by outside agencies. Given that the key economic players and most influential agencies driving globalization reside in the global North (such as the IMF, World Bank and WTO), power and control are vested here. In contrast, the global South lacks bargaining and negotiating strength. Elmawazini *et al.* (2019) refer to the wealth of literature that exists which links globalization with economic and health inequalities between regions and countries. They note the 'health gap' between richer and poorer countries but argue that, in the case of sub-Saharan Africa, it is economic and demographic structures that are the main determinants of this rather than globalization and that many of the health challenges faced in this region are preventable through local policy. One solution, they argue, is for African countries to spend more on primary healthcare and shift policy towards supporting *brain-gain* rather than *brain-drain* and that 'the need to create an enabling environment to encourage return-migration of highly skilled African in the diaspora cannot be over-emphasized' (Elmawazini *et al.*, 2019, p. 132).

Moghadam (2005) suggests that globalization has expanded gender equality, and that the globalization of politics and international NGOs has allowed women's movements to grow globally. According to Martell (2010), globalization exposes women to more education and information, leading to empowerment and greater equality. However, this has also been contested. Baru and Mohan (2018) argue that the neoliberal globalization agenda has particularly disadvantaged women and other marginalized groups given the alliances that have been made with conservative politics and religious fundamentalism. They point out how:

> these alliances have resulted in the control of women's bodies and contributed to the reversal of hard-won rights for heath and gender justice in many parts of the world. [For example] one of the most widespread consequences of religious interference to gender-based health inequities in the avoidable mortality and morbidity from unsafe abortion despite the availability of medical technology for safe termination of pregnancy... The criminalization of homosexuality is another example of how religious fundamentalist positions influence state policy to violate the right to privacy of individuals.
>
> (Baru and Mohan, 2018, p. 91)

The relationship between the processes of globalization and health are complex and go beyond what we are able to discuss here. Not only is there a large amount of literature arguing that globalization has exacerbated inequality, therefore worsening health for some, but there has also been a globalization of health trends, due to the globalization of unhealthy lifestyles and huge changes in patterns of nutrition (Shrecker, 2020). Globalized marketing has meant that products such as soft drinks like Coca-Cola can be found in the remotest villages, and marketing of formula feeding of babies is prevalent (Labbock and Nazro, 1995; MacDonald, 2006). Consumption of processed food and cigarettes has increased consistently in poorer countries (Graham, 2008) contributing to the rising burden of non-communicable diseases (Adebiyi *et al.*, 2016).

HIV, whilst seemingly a globalized disease, is experienced very differently by people in different parts of the world. It is particularly disproportionately experienced by those in sub-Saharan Africa, who, according to Kharsany and Karim (2016), accounted for more than 70% of the global burden of infection. Whilst there has been a substantial decrease in AIDS-related deaths in the past two decades, it is estimated that the majority of new infections (approximately two-thirds) are in young women in that region, which is indicative of an ongoing crisis. Whereas in the UK HIV has become almost a manageable, albeit long-term, condition, it remains a matter of life and death in Africa, particularly if funding for anti-retrovirals (ARVs) is reduced in the future.

The processes of globalization influence health outcomes, directly and indirectly, in many different ways including health systems, migration, trade and investment, and changing lifestyles to name a few (Labonté, 2018). It is argued that the challenges to reduce health inequalities associated with globalization are 'substantial' (Shrecker, 2020). However, it is also highlighted by many that, despite the forces of globalization, governments have a huge part to play in reducing health inequalities by tacking the underlying social determinants of health such as education, basic healthcare, employment, housing and social connectedness, and that this must be achieved by first and foremost by supportive public policy (Shrecker, 2016; Elmawazini *et al.*, 2019).

Globalization clearly raises key issues for the global governance of health, making it both necessary and possible. At a national conference in Health Inequities in India in 2018 the role of globalization and neoliberalism in determining political, economic and social relations between richer and poorer countries was considered at length. It was concluded that 'the twin process[es] of globalization and liberalization have been important drivers of health inequities' (Baru and Mohan, 2018, p. 91). In particular it was noted how neoliberalism has changed how non-governmental organizations work and how major foundations (such as the Bill and Melinda Gates Foundation) have significantly influenced the global health agenda, including what issues are prioritized and how health is governed.

Sustainable development, the environment and climate change

Globally agreed frameworks for health governance are perhaps overshadowed by the need for such agreements on how to tackle climate change and environmental issues. From the discussion of the development of health promotion in Chapter 1, it is clear that a concern with the environment, ecosystems and sustainability has been present from the outset. The Ottawa Charter stated, 'The protection of the natural and built environment and the conservation of natural resources must be addressed in any health promotion strategy' (WHO, 2009, p. 3). As Labonté (2018) argues, sustainable development has become the dominant theme of the post-2015 development agenda because ecological crisis and the impacts of climate change keep the environment as a high global priority. Baum (2009, p. 73) commented that 'lifestyles in rich countries carry a huge ecological footprint', arguing that the environment represents the key health issue of the 21st century. Yet climate change impacts most on the already vulnerable such as those who live in substandard housing or rely on subsistence farming (NIEHS, 2015). Ron Labonté argued more than two decades ago that 'Health professionals should not wait to be invited into sustainable development discussions. They must invite themselves' (Labonté, 1997, p. 267). More recently, Fortune et al. (2018) outline how 'health promotion and sustainable development share several core priorities such as equity, intersectoral approaches and sustainability...which have strong resonance' (p. 621). They argue that this is because the health inequities we face cannot be resolved simply by relying on the health sector for solutions. The Sustainable Development Goals (discussed in more detail in Chapter 3) are testimony to this. Just one of them (Goal 3) mentions health specifically, whilst the majority reference issues directly related to sustainability and sustainable development. However, despite the obvious synergy between health promotion and sustainable development, Jelsøe et al. (2018) contend that strategies in the two areas are not sufficiently integrated, which results in unintended consequences that can actually be detrimental to health, and to the environment. Jelsøe et al. (2018, p. 99) argue, therefore, that there are three key areas to address in future research:

> 'a) the duality of health promotion and sustainability and how it can be handled in order to enhance mutually supportive processes between them; b) the social dimension of sustainability and how it can be strengthened in the development of strategies for health promotion and sustainable development; and c) exploring and identifying policy approaches and strategies for integrating health promotion and sustainable development'.

Langer et al. (2015) argue that women are key to the sustainable development agenda. In their 2015 paper Langer et al. propose:

> 'a comprehensive model for sustainable development that takes account of women's roles in production and reproduction and their dual role as consumers and providers of health care, which affect all domains of sustainable development – societal, environmental, and economical...When women are valued, enabled, and empowered in each of these domains, gender equality and health can be achieved; and when women are healthy and have equity in all aspects of life, sustainable development will be possible' (p. 1168).

For more details please see Langer et al. (2015). The focus on sustainable development was reflected in the most recent International Union of Health Promotion and Education Conference on Health Promotion held in New Zealand in 2019, the theme of which was 'Waiora: promoting planetary health and sustainable development for all'. The conference sought to 'reorient health promotion efforts towards planetary health and sustainable development while including a focus on equity and social justice' (Ratima, 2019), issues that are the heart of health promotion efforts. We return to this conference later in this chapter.

New public health challenges

Globalization has led to the perception of 'global' health issues. For example, the increase in the prevalence of obesity during the last few decades has been so rapid that a new term has been coined – 'globesity' (Costa-Font and Mas, 2016). There has been a major shift from it primarily being a public health concern of the most affluent societies to now being seen in less industrialized countries and the World Health Organization states that most of the world's population now lives in countries where overweight and obesity kills more people than underweight (WHO, 2020). Figures suggest that globally in 2016 there were more than 1.9 billion overweight adults and, of these, at least 650 million people were obese (WHO, 2020). In 2019 there were an estimated 38.2 million children under the age of 5 years who were obese or overweight (WHO, 2020). Childhood obesity is an increasing issue in low- and middle-income countries (UNICEF, 2019).

This increasing prevalence in children raises concern about the creation of a growing health and economic burden for the next generation, particularly as there is evidence that obesity in childhood persists into adulthood (Llewellyn et al., 2016). Data from 'developing' or transition countries indicate that the association between a child's socio-economic status and the patterns of obesity are complex. As Poskitt (2014) argues, the prevalence of obesity and overweight in children varies between and within low- and middle-income countries depending on the environments the children live in – greater affluence, urbanization and more technology are all associated with overweight.

In countries undergoing epidemiological transition, there will be the 'old' problems of infectious diseases alongside the newer diseases created by changing lifestyles. Old and emerging infectious diseases are more of a threat than ever at a global level, not just in poorer regions. Since 2013, when the first edition of this book was published, we have witnessed outbreaks of Ebola in West Africa, SARS and avian flu in Asia, and the Zika virus in South America. At the time of writing, in early 2020, the world is experiencing a global pandemic from Covid-19, causing unprecedented disruption to every aspect of human life.

Mental health is receiving increasing attention as a global health issue. Whilst it is not a 'new' issue, it is only relatively recently that we are beginning to appreciate the impact of mental ill-health on global health experience and outcomes. It is now understood that common mental disorders and substance-use disorders are responsible for the largest proportion of the global burden of disease (Wainberg et al., 2017). This burden is further exacerbated by the lack of access to adequate mental health care services, particularly in low- and middle-income countries. In addition, climate change, civil unrest and conflict, terrorism and security threats, antibiotic resistance, and advancing technology all have the potential to create new (and potentially unanticipated) public health challenges (Warwick-Booth and Cross, 2018).

Epidemiological Transition and the 'Triple Burden'

Attention has turned recently to the effects on health of development, and as countries become more 'developed', they go through demographic as well as epidemiologic transitions. Whilst the data on these transitions are patchy in some regions, more data are becoming available. The results from the Global Burden of Disease Study 1990–2017 showed that sub-Saharan Africa is experiencing a rising burden of non-communicable diseases (NCDs) (Gouda et al., 2019). South Asia is also experiencing a rise in NCDs including cardiovascular disease, diabetes, cancer and chronic respiratory diseases and this is having a huge detrimental economic, as well as health, impact (Rijal et al., 2018). The combination of non-communicable and communicable (infectious) diseases (CDs; which less 'developed' countries experience more of) has historically been referred to as the 'double burden' of disease; however, many now argue that poorer regions face a 'triple burden' of disease – NCDs, CDs *and* disease/disability resulting from rapid urbanization, industrialization and globalization such as road traffic accidents, injuries in the work place, and mental ill-health (Ortiz and Abrigo, 2017). For example, in Brazil the health of the population generally improved between 1990 and 2016; however, an epidemiological transition towards NCDs occurred and, in addition, 'interpersonal violence grew as a health concern' (Marinho et al., 2018). On publication of the results from its Second National Burden of Disease Study, which examined mortality trends over a 15 year period from 1997–2012, South African academics highlighted again how the poor health of the nation was related to a 'quadruple' burden of disease – HIV/AIDS, NCDs, CDs and injuries (Pillay-van Wyk et al., 2016).

The Sustainable Development Goals highlighted NCDs as a significant issue with the aim of reducing the incidence of NCD mortality by a third by the year 2030; however, the emphasis was on the domestic financing of efforts to address this but some have questioned the feasibility and sustainability of this approach (Allen, 2017). Whilst these 'newer' diseases are undoubtedly important – and under-resourced (Ozgediz and Riviello, 2008) – there is a need to reflect on whether this concern shifts too much attention away from the key heal issues of less developed countries. Non-communicable diseases account for approximately 71% of all deaths globally and it is predicted that, by the year 2030, they will take over communicable, maternal, neonatal and nutritional diseases combined as the leading cause of death in sub-Saharan Africa (Bigna and Noubiap, 2019). However, it is important not to forget that the more common causes of death in poorer countries are the same – diarrhoea, malaria, acute respiratory infections and so on. Certainly, the emerging NCDs require urgent attention but so do these other main killers. Too many children in Africa do not survive long enough to go on to become the adults at risk of NCDs, and it is estimated that, globally, one in three people do not have safe water or enjoy the dignity of having adequate toilets (WHO, 2019). This focus on disease here makes the point that diseases are an essential aspect of health promotion endeavour, as they can devastate people's lives. We take up the theme later of newer approaches to positive health in the final section of this chapter. We now turn to discuss what particular role universities can play in taking forward the development of health promotion.

The Role of Universities

Universities play vital roles in knowledge exchange and innovation, and in thinking about the environment, sustainability and health (Orme and Dooris, 2010). Innstrand and Christensen (2018, p. 68) state that 'universities provide an ideal setting to promote health and wellbeing to students, staff and the wider community through their education, research, knowledge exchange and institutional practices'. At least four roles for universities can be outlined:

1. Carrying out health promotion research, which makes a difference.
2. Capacity building for health promotion.
3. Engaging with communities.
4. Developing as health-promoting universities and thereby modelling a settings approach.

Health Promotion Research

Health promotion research itself is essential to the continued development of the discipline and given the complexities of health-related challenges, the need for a strong evidence base underpinning practice has always been present (Green, 2000). Lahtinen et al. (2005) wrote a useful paper contributing to an understanding of the distinctive nature of health promotion research, and of how to assess its quality. Although presented as a 'Finnish approach', it has far wider relevance. They suggest that there are three factors that mark health promotion research out from research in other disciplines. First, health promotion research is 'research on action' aiming to make changes for better health, either at individual, organizational or environmental levels. It is concerned with processes of change, rather than merely providing detailed 'state of the art' or descriptive accounts of phenomena. Health promotion research, implicitly, is therefore concerned with making a difference for the better. Secondly, health promotion research is multidisciplinary (Lahtinen et al., 2005, p. 3). Whilst not rejecting intra-disciplinary research, health promotion research does maintain openness and 'makes simultaneous use of several different scientific disciplines, such as theology, biomedicine, behavioural sciences, pedagogy, nursing science, social sciences and economics' (Lahtinen et al., 2005, p. 4). The third feature is the way in which health promotion research incorporates the value base of health promotion. Health promotion research must 'practice what it preaches' and therefore explicitly incorporate participation, inclusion, empowerment, transparency, sustainable development and emphasize 'the importance of working with people in respectful partnership, in contrast to a style in which "experts" know best' (Lahtinen et al., 2005, p. 4). More recently, Woodall et al. (2018) build upon this work to argue that health promotion research has four distinct features, akin to those noted by Lahtinen. First, health promotion research offers application to real world contexts. Secondly, health promotion research is built upon values, derived from the Ottawa Charter, therefore it encompasses participation and respect. Woodall et al. (2018) also point out that health promotion research involves the relinquishing of professional control and the associated co-production of knowledge (third distinct feature). Finally, the fourth distinct feature is that health promotion research has an expansive methodological toolkit available for researchers to draw upon. Woodall et al. (2018) also conclude that optimism can be held about the future of health promotion research.

Much of the research that we conduct within the Centre for Health Promotion Research at Leeds Beckett illustrates health promotion values, offers application to real-world contexts (for example via evaluating the success of interventions, and by adding to the growing health promotion evidence base) and works with community members to co-produce knowledge (Newell and South, 2009). South (2014) argues that understanding the nature of participation is essential because of the associated implications of this for contemporary health promotion research.

The 'Finnish approach' has seven health promotion research criteria, followed by seven criteria for general research quality. The first seven relate to health promotion relevance, values, innovation, discourse, practice, action and context. Taken together, these seven areas ensure that health promotion research is related to the body of ideas, values and priority areas outlined by the epistemic community, is appropriate to the context and ensures action. The general quality criteria relate to scientific quality, defined scope, anticipated outcomes, operationalization, feasibility, process evaluation, and documentation and dissemination. These latter seven ensure that health promotion research is well designed and scientifically sound and the results are properly fed back into the arena to inform future practice.

Capacity Development

As well as research, universities and other HEIs have teaching as a core function, and a major role in educating health workers in their initial training as well as in continuing professional development and 'life-long learning'. Three universities in England were asked in 1972 to develop courses for specialist health educators, later described as health promotion specialists. Leeds Beckett, formerly Leeds Metropolitan, was one of these three universities. Warwick-Booth *et al.* (2018b) argue, however, that the demand to train a 'health promotion' workforce is no longer what it was in the UK, with reductions in workforce budgets for health promotion education potentially stagnating both the learning and development of practitioners, although this is not the case in other countries.

Professional development is one of the eight 'tracking indicators' proposed by the Bangkok conference for national capacity building in health promotion. Professional development requires national level education and training programmes, and a professional association. Another of the eight is performance monitoring, encompassing national level research and evaluation, plus information systems to monitor and report on relevant indicators to health promotion policies and priorities (Catford, 2005). The UK Public Health Skills and Knowledge Framework (PHE, 2016, 2019a, b) outlines the core skills and competencies required for the public health workforce, listed in Box 6.1. Online resources include a mapping tool to enable education and training providers to map learning units or modules against the framework.

The need to invest in the training and education of health promotion practitioners and other workers so that they have the required competencies and skills to address complex health issues within rapidly changing social and political contexts is clear (Warwick-Booth *et al.*, 2018b). The importance of learning is central to tackling the many global health challenges discussed in preceding chapters as it underpins workforce development (Welter *et al.*, 2017) and serves to improve population

---

Box 6.1. Public Health Skills and Knowledge Framework.

- A1 Measure, monitor and report population health and wellbeing; health needs; risks; inequalities; and use of services.
- A2 Promote population and community health and wellbeing, addressing the wider determinants of health and health inequalities.
- A3 Protect the public from environmental hazards, communicable disease and other health risks, while addressing inequalities in risk exposure and outcomes.
- A4 Work to, and for, the evidence base, conduct research, and provide informed advice.
- A5 Audit, evaluate and re-design services and interventions to improve health outcomes and reduce health inequalities.
- B1 Work with, and through, policies and strategies to improve health outcomes and reduce health inequalities.
- B2 Work collaboratively across agencies and boundaries to improve health outcomes and reduce health inequalities.
- B3 Work in a commissioning-based culture to improve health outcomes and reduce health inequalities.
- B4 Work within political and democratic systems and with a range of organizational cultures to improve health outcomes and reduce health inequalities.
- C1 Provide leadership to drive improvement in health outcomes and the reduction of health inequalities.
- C2 Communicate with others to improve health outcomes and reduce health inequalities.
- C3 Design and manage programmes and projects to improve health and reduce health inequalities.
- All workers should work within ethical and professional boundaries while promoting population health and wellbeing, and addressing health inequalities.

(Public Health England, 2019a, b)

health (Koh, 2010). Strengthening the capacity of academic health promotion globally is vital, as it will provide a solid scientific base for the development of knowledge-based practice and the facility to critically determine current and future health promotion needs (Barry, 2008). Whilst some contexts (e.g. the UK) are challenging, contextually, in relation to the provision of health promotion education because of the political nature of health, current policy direction and marketization, this does not ultimately diminish need (Warwick-Booth *et al.*, 2018b), so the need to build health promotion capacity remains present.

Hawe *et al.* (1998) described capacity building as the 'invisible work' of health promotion, and then define it as an approach to the development of sustainable skills, structures, resources and commitment to health improvement in health and other sectors to prolong and multiply health gains many times over (Hawe *et al.*, 2000). Aluttis *et al.* (2014) offer a framework of several domains of capacity building for public health drawn from the wider literature; organizational structure and resources; partnerships; workforce; knowledge development as well as leadership and governance, all underpinned by country specific context. Bergeron *et al.* (2017) also provide a menu of theories, models and frameworks to support capacity building and point out that their usage should be intentional, explicit and referenced.

Carrington and Detragiache (1999) asked the question back in the 1990s as to whether the universities and training institutions of Africa were servicing the demands of *developed* countries, due to the outpouring of health professionals trained in Africa leaving to work in developed nations. However, in health promotion, with a lack of capacity to educate health promotion workers in many countries of the global South, health promotion courses are accessed in those countries of the global North where courses are run. Studying overseas is an expensive way of gaining qualifications. Distance learning is an alternative, but also comes with challenges. Technological developments such as the proliferation of open-access online courses (MOOCs) have increased access to health promotion education for many and can potentially address some of the training difficulties experienced within economically poorer areas of the world (Liyanagunawardena and Aboshady, 2017). Yet, many countries do not yet enjoy a level of internet connectivity that makes online learning possible and health promotion education remains in danger of being Eurocentric (Dixey, 2013).

Although students learn enormously by studying overseas (Dixey, 2001), they usually return to their post in an unchanged organization, and can then face bureaucratic inertia, and/or a lack of opportunity to act on their learning. If new learning is not translated into practice, demoralization can ensue. The same is true where a student studies in their country, is enthused with new ideas but returns to find colleagues who are 'stuck in their ways'. Cross *et al.* (2020) illustrate that peer support has value as an approach in the context of Ghana. They found that a peer-mentoring scheme as part of a postgraduate qualification evaluated well because it benefitted both mentees and mentors. The relationships that developed between those involved is argued to bode well for building a community of experts in health promotion as a starting point in tackling Ghana's health and development agenda. Edwards and Collinson (2002) suggest that for employees to feel empowered at work, they need to have clear broad objectives, they need the right of access to the means of achieving the objectives, they need to be enabled to use their own initiative, and they need 'participatory power' – the right to challenge and debate goals and methods. These conditions are not always present in many of the contexts in which health workers (as potential health promoters) work, especially in countries where it is not the norm to challenge senior colleagues. Furthermore, rather than educating one or two workers per year (by sending them overseas on expensive courses), the aim needs to be to create a critical mass of health promotion practitioners capable of driving change from the 'middle ground'. The middle ground is that which can close the implementation gap by facilitating dialogue between strategic direction and local action – between the policy makers at 'the top' and local communities on the ground (Attwood *et al.*, 2003). Health promotion rests on the idea of putting communities at the centre of change, in the belief that top-down, programmatic approaches to change do not work. The same is true when attempting to change the approach to health promotion within any country wishing to change the way it tackles health issues – it is not likely that change imposed from above will be successful.

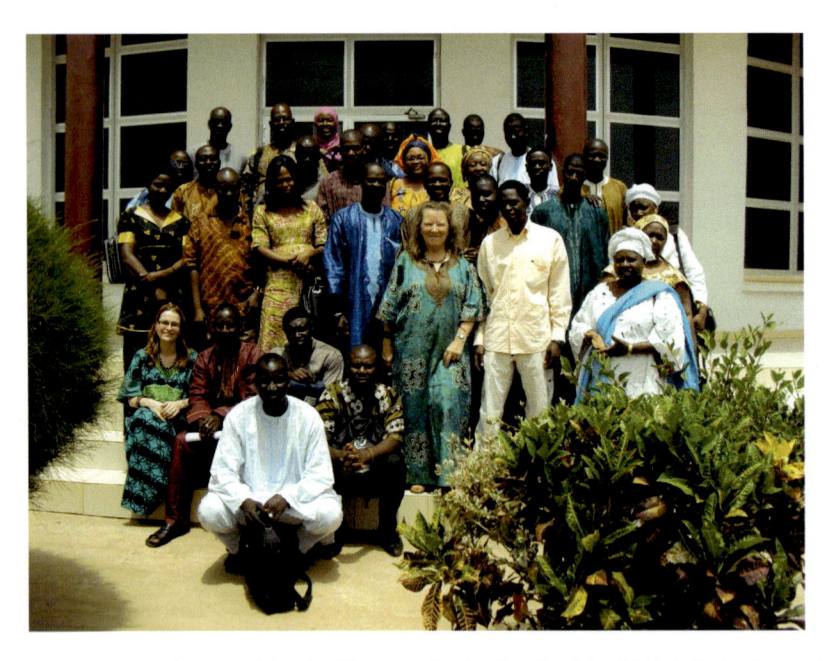

Leeds Beckett postgraduate students studying health promotion in The Gambia, 2011 (with Louise and Sally).

An approach to capacity building is thus needed that attempts to address the implementation gap by tackling 'grassroots delivery mechanisms'. There is a lack of a *community* of practice capable of effecting change. Lave and Wenger (1998), who developed the concept of communities of practice, felt that such communities are built through 'apprenticeship' – learning how to be a member, participating and gradually taking on the professional identity, language and practices of that community, and thus enabling a new identity of public health/health promotion worker. According to Attwood *et al.* (2003), communities of practice are useful to individuals but, more importantly, 'are collectively valuable as repositories of knowledge and learning' (p. 147). One aim therefore must be to create communities of practice, with learning shared in multidisciplinary groups, helping to break down professional competitiveness (Nyamwaya, 2003) and encourage communication across disciplines (Attwood *et al.*, 2003). However, communities of practice can be hugely variable in terms of how they are used because they are complex, as well as multifaceted and operate according to a range of different models (Ranmuthugala *et al.*, 2011).

Given the lack of capacity in some parts of the world, the challenges facing many universities (Warwick-Booth *et al.*, 2018b), including those in the global South (Bourne, 2000) and the expenses facing students, some universities have responded by delivering work in partnership in those parts of the world in need of infrastructure and capacity building (Jackson *et al.*, 2007; Dupere, 2007; Dixey and Green, 2009). However, criticisms have been highlighted in such approaches, in terms of power differentials and coloniality, therefore educational capacity building projects need to work to decolonize them (Adriansen and Madsen, 2019).

Engaging with Communities

Universities, even in the current neoliberal climate, are important resources for the communities that surround them. Universities in higher-income countries are wealthy institutions with all kinds of physical, social and knowledge capital. Knowledge transfer partnerships and Community Campus Partnerships are examples of ways in which universities engage with communities. Cynics argue that such mechanisms are developed in the hope of financial gain for institutions. However, we would hope that there are other reasons, some based on altruism and others on tackling inequalities, and widening participation that universities espouse.

Two examples of our engagement with communities are, first, a long-term relationship with the

Hamara Centre in Leeds. Hamara is an example of a thriving and energetic NGO making a valuable contribution to the lives of ethnic minorities in Leeds, including asylum seekers and refugees, plus providing a service to the traditional, local white neighbourhoods. Secondly, we have worked in partnership with institutions in some African countries (The Gambia, Tanzania and Zambia) to provide both education and research support such as technical advice, bid writing and evaluation work. This demonstrates working both locally and globally.

Hamara, a name that means 'ours' in Urdu, is a voluntary sector organization based in Leeds, UK, which is working to improve the health and well-being of minority ethnic communities across the city, but particularly the South Asian community in the locality where the centre is based. Hamara is involved in range of activities around women's empowerment, older people's health, youth activities and inter-faith work as well as providing a community gym and café in the Centre itself. University staff in the Centre for Health Promotion Research have forged strong links with Hamara, with collaborative activities spanning more than a decade. In the first instance, assistance was provided in designing and analysing a community health needs assessment that helped secure funding to develop the centre, as well as collaborative evaluation of the centre itself and some of its funded interventions. Both organizations have continued to identify opportunities for dialogue and joint working, with the value of partnership working evident in that the university team brought skills such as facilitation and report writing, while Hamara offered the facilities of the centre, a culturally appropriate setting that many service users were familiar with, and organizational support.

This long-term partnership has been of benefit to both organizations. Access to academic skills in research, critical thinking and programme planning and evaluation have enhanced the capacity of Hamara to secure funding and to develop as an organization committed to addressing health inequalities. From a university perspective, the partnership has brought better understanding of the health issues facing minority ethnic communities, it has given staff experience of working with a grassroots community organization, new research opportunities have been identified and the university is seen to demonstrate respect for the diversity of languages, faiths and cultures in the city. Overall, the work with Hamara provides an example of how community–campus partnerships need to be built over time, and are ultimately based on good communication, mutual learning and relationships founded on trust.

Our second example involves negotiating the tricky waters of North–South relationships. Despite the focus on sustainable 'partnerships' in the discourse of development, and its emphasis in funding calls suggesting that donor agencies value partnerships, there is little literature on the processes and operationalization of such types of collaboration (Jentsch, 2004). Brehm (2001) suggests that whilst the financial power is held by the 'Northern' partner, there is little hope that a partnership can mean true equality and the sharing of responsibilities. Manji (2006), likewise, is sceptical about there being sufficient trust between North and South partners for true partnerships to develop, though some of the ingredients of successful partnerships have been noted (Dixey and Green, 2009).

Our role as an HEI formed a valuable addition to a partnership between Dar-es-Salaam Institute of Technology in Tanzania and Chainama College in Lusaka, Zambia, which had both been tasked with providing training support to community-based organizations and small and medium enterprises who had been awarded contracts for collecting waste from households in their respective communities. Our role was to develop participative methodologies to support research on the effects of gender, empowerment and income generation. As outsiders, we were able to suggest research questions that were 'taken for granted' by our African colleagues, and also to bring in novel ways of asking those questions and writing up the research.

The fourth role of universities, to model a settings approach by working towards becoming a health-promoting university, will not be explored fully here. Dooris has written about settings, including university settings (Dooris, 2001; Dooris and Martin, 2002; Doherty and Dooris, 2006, 2010). The idea was taken up in Germany (Stock et al., 2010), China (Tian et al., 2003), and Norway (Innstrand and Christensen, 2017). It has been argued to be global in more recent literature, though major challenges remain in adapting the Ottawa Charter principles into meaningful action within large, complex and culturally diverse organizations (Dooris et al., 2019).

Towards the Future of Health Promotion

Understanding 'healthworlds'

As has been discussed elsewhere in this book, and in keeping with the social model of health, health promotion efforts should aim to privilege lay 'voices' and perspectives. In order for this to happen, voices must be 'heard'. Often lay opinion is not in tandem with public health and health promotion opinion. Robertson (1998) has commented that

> 'Health promotion makes room for the stories which individuals and communities tell about their everyday experience of health, which legitimizes them as being important to our understanding of health as statistics on morbidity and mortality rates'.

Some of this 'room' was made in Chapter 1; in moving towards greater room for lay involvement in creating health, and lay epidemiologies, we show the importance of a 'constructionist epistemology' – in other words, knowledge (in this case, understandings of 'health') is constructed by interactions between people in the real world. These meanings are not 'given' but alter and develop over time. These meanings are what health promoters need to start with, not try to change or suggest that they are 'wrong'. Fox and Ward (2006, p. 476) point out that 'health must be acknowledged to be a highly contextualized outcome of the lived body/self and its relation with the material and psychosocial environment'. Radley and Billig (1996) make a similar point when they stress that ideas about health and illness 'articulate a person's situation in the world and, indeed, articulate that world in which the individual will be held accountable to others' (p. 221). A recent contribution to this perspective is that of Germond and Cochrane (2010) in their use of the concept of 'healthworlds'. They write:

> The healthworld relates to people's conceptions of health, to their health-seeking behaviour, and to their conditions of health. Individuals' healthworlds are shaped by, and simultaneously affect, their social shared healthworld constituted by the collective search for health & well-being. (p. 309)

They also point out that, while healthworlds may be patterned in a coherent way at a community level, often people utilize differing healing systems and explanations for health. This suggests that a real danger is to overemphasize such beliefs and practices as 'determined'. Biographical factors and changing circumstances mean that people may change their ideas, and this element of agency is important to bear in mind. Fried et al. (2015) also comment on agency in their study of healthworlds in tuberculosis treatment and antiretroviral therapy in South Africa; they conclude that health care providers and health systems should foster 'individual agency while respecting patients' collectively mediated healthworlds' (p. 632).

Another issue commented on by Calnan and Williams (1991) is that of the salience of health; health concerns were often not primary factors in people's behaviour; indeed, health tends to be taken for granted unless it fails. And even if people see the advice they receive as important and apt, they may not be able to act on it, given their circumstances. The impact of resources on health has been the focus of many studies on lay perceptions of factors in health, as we saw in Chapter 1.

People often have a clear idea of the social determinants of health, whilst also seeing health as linked to individual lifestyle choices. For instance, in their study of post-soviet citizens, Abbott et al. (2006) highlight the focus on the environment and poverty in people's accounts of the causes of illness: 'Informants' talk about their lives suggested a complex understanding of health that recognizes the influence of factors over which they have little control' (p. 234). Yet when respondents discussed responsibility for health, they emphasized the role of the individual in terms of coping, strength of will and behaviour. Similarly, Blaxter (1997) found that whilst people identified many factors important in health and illness, what they stressed as most important was behaviour. Both these two studies suggest that people in deprived and difficult circumstances are the most likely to stress behaviour as important in preventing illness, whereas middle class respondents were the most likely to see structural factors such as poverty as important in health and illness (Blaxter, 1997). Blaxter's (1997) explanation for this is that accounts of health and illness are strongly linked to identity and thus those whose lives are indeed most affected by lack of income and other structural factors do not want to talk about their risk status, and instead stress not giving in to illness and the moral responsibility to cope. Similar findings were reported by Popay et al. (2003), where those in deprived circumstances were reluctant to attribute ill health to those circumstances, even when their accounts of their own lives and health suggested how important they were. Smith and Anderson (2018) set out to address these findings in their own meta-ethnography of 17 qualitative studies on lay perspectives on socio-economic health inequalities in Britain. They found that people in disadvantaged circumstances in fact had a good understanding of the links between material hardship and ill-health, as well as the psychosocial pathways through which such factors impacted on health, for instance through stress. Yet they found that, despite this: 'people living in disadvantaged circumstances are often reluctant to explicitly acknowledge health inequalities, a finding that we suggest can be understood as an attempt to resist the stigma and shame of poverty and poor health and to (re)assert individual agency and control' (Smith and Anderson, 2017, p.146).

Garthwaite and Bambra (2017) also explore perspectives on health inequalities, focusing on the views of people from socio-economically contrasting areas of Stockton-on-Tees, UK, in an age of austerity. Like Smith and Anderson, they found that those in the most deprived areas recognized factors like income, housing and stress as important for health inequalities; yet they too found lifestyles and behaviour entered into people's accounts, as this quote from one respondent in a more deprived area shows:

> 'I think it's cos them in Hartburn have jobs and they have loads of money. They've got good work and they've got good living. And I think some of these in the Town Centre they just go around getting drunk, being homeless. It's a lifestyle choice, it gets them out of it for a couple of days, y'know?'
> (Garthwaite and Bambra, 2017, p. 271)

They also point out that their findings indicate a certain amount of fatalism in people's accounts, which the authors find understandable – indeed realistic – given the circumstances of people's lives in more deprived areas.

This work on people's perceptions and understandings of health tell us that people see health and its social determinants in complex ways. They are thus likely to react to health communication, messages about risk and healthy lifestyles, in complex ways too. Health promotion has begun to embrace the idea of complexity theory (Pisek and Greenhalgh, 2001; Walby, 2007) and insert it into its theory and practice (McQueen, 2000; Campbell, 2011), but there remains to be a proper marrying of the sociology of lay health beliefs and health promotion theory. What we have to be clear about in health promotion is that the relativist and critical standpoint adopted logically leads to seeing health as based on historical, contextual and subjective exigencies, and thus leads to better understanding of the complexities of 'health'. The health beliefs literature, however, does resonate with some of the new agendas for health, particularly in the emerging ideas of wellbeing and happiness, and this is explored in the next section.

Wellbeing and Happiness – New Paradigms for the 21st Century?

Recent times have seen a move towards a new paradigm of health, with the concepts wellbeing, happiness and wellness emerging in the health discourse. The New Economics Foundation has launched its Happy Planet Index and the government of Bhutan has launched a measure of Gross National Happiness (GNH) to replace GNP (Gross National Product). These moves key into the zeitgeist where hypercapitalism is being scrutinized, and the claims that economic growth necessarily leads to 'development' and 'progress' are questioned. These developments in the 21st century are logical extensions of, and accelerate, changes that began to emerge in the last century. The 20th century saw major breaks with how things used to be seen in the past – a series of 'paradigm shifts' occurred, which transformed science and ways of thinking. In a nutshell, these changes could be seen as a reaction against the Enlightenment notions of rationality and positivism, where 'science' was split off from 'emotions', where 'objectivity' was prized over the 'merely' subjective. As Outram (2006, p. 6) suggests, the Enlightenment was where:

> Man gained control over nature, and then over other human beings, by controlling them 'rationally' through the use of technology … Enlightenment in this view is ultimately totalitarian in the sense that it abandons the quest for meaning and simply attempts to exert power over nature and the world. The Enlightenment relies on 'rationality', reasoning that is free from superstition, mythology, fear and revelation, which is often based on mathematical 'truth', which calibrates ends to means, which is often therefore technological, and expects solutions to problems which are objectively correct.

For some, the logical end of this process (of Enlightenment) was the Nazi extermination camps, where people were 'treated as mere objects to be administered' (Outram, 2006, p. 7).

The new ways of looking at the world challenged the idea that there was one universal truth waiting to be discovered; quantum theory suggested that matter was not solid or static and Einstein presented his ideas about relativity, turning upside down ideas about space and time. Rather than reality being 'objective', and available to all, it began to be seen that 'reality' depends on where you happen to be standing. The newer, more interactive understanding of reality placed the observer centrally – developing the notion that we bring about our own reality. This systemic or interactive (or ecological) view replaced a linear view of how things work, with a circular view – that systems maintain stability by feedback, and that every system is connected to other systems in a process of reciprocal determinism. As Gerhardt (2004, p. 9) puts it:

> How one person behaves affects how another behaves and his or her behaviour then influences the original person in a circular process. Cause and effect depend on your vantage point, on where you start in the loop, and how much information you include or exclude. There is not one truth, but several possible truths.

The ideas of many possible truths resonates with postmodern ideas of the importance of listening to multiple voices, of the reintegration of the emotional, the subjective, the lived experience, not only into social science but also into the popular imagination, and the valuing of the plurality of cultures, faiths and ways of life that make up our globalizing world. In certain disciplines such as psychology, it has led to the development of critical psychology, which challenges the dominant stress on cognitions and the ability to measure quantitatively people's attitudes, feelings and emotional states. In geography, the paradigm shift can be exemplified by the move into understanding how people perceive the world, with their own 'mental maps' based on gender, ethnicity, age and ability – these are more 'real' than the actual physical manifestation of the geography on the ground as drawn by 'objective' map makers. It has brought about a major new field of qualitative research based on phenomenology, social interactionism and other methods, which attempt to understand the world from the point of view of the people who inhabit that world. In terms of understanding health, it led to the seminal work of the late Mildred Blaxter, whose work on lay beliefs of health has challenged the dominant medical ways of understanding 'health'. Thus, whereas the Enlightenment scientists saw emotion as getting in the way of seeing the world 'properly', the 20th century began to see a real reintegration of the importance of the emotional and subjective, such that in the 21st century this has become a more dominant paradigm. It is not surprising, perhaps, that it was in the immediate post-war period that the WHO's radical definition of health emerged, questioning, as it does, the purely medical, scientific concept of health, and establishing the importance not only of holistic health, but of the inter-subjective state of emotional, social and mental health. This was precisely when the role of technology as a means to bring about human health and happiness was beginning to be questioned.

This worldview challenges the notion of 'experts' – now the people who are the experts on their health are those living with their own bodies, with their own homes and neighbourhoods, and not the outside professionals who do not share the same lived experiences. Thus 'experts by experience' has become a common catchphrase. The challenge for health promotion 'experts' was discussed in Chapter 5.

A politics of wellbeing has emerged. Wellbeing is in the UN Declaration on the Right of Development: '… development is a comprehensive economic, social, cultural and political process, which aims at the constant improvement of the wellbeing of the entire population on the basis of their active, free and meaningful participation in development and the fair distribution of benefits' (UN, 1986). This is all related to what it means to be human, to live well, and to have a 'good' life (Atkinson et al., 2019). Tomlinson and Kelly (2013) note the trend, internationally, to using a wider range of indicators to measure progress and development suggesting that this is occurring for several reasons. Firstly, a 'growing disillusionment with economic growth as the basis for improvements in happiness'; secondly, 'awareness of climate change and the realisation that much economic growth is environmentally destructive and socially useless'; thirdly, the demand for measures of happiness is being driven by a focus on mental health rather than ill-health; and finally, 'behavioural economists are supporting happiness measures as feedback on the health, wealth and happiness outcomes of deliberately designed choice architectures' (p. 152). Whilst there is latterly a political swerve towards wellbeing and happiness, Tomlinson and Kelly (2013) note how academic interest in wellbeing and happiness significantly predates this and the attendant growth in sub-disciplines such as positive psychology. They refer to this the 'new science of happiness' (Tomlinson and Kelly, 2013, p. 139) and point to the launch of the *Journal of Happiness Studies* in 2000 by way of example (an interdisciplinary journal devoted to the scientific study of subjective wellbeing).

Increased attention has been paid to what defines a good life in the recent past, particularly in policy circles in the UK, but also beyond (Atkinson et al., 2019). As stated, this has resulted in a growing focus on happiness and wellbeing, and the development of measures of subjective wellbeing. In response to this interest the What Works Centre for Wellbeing (UK) was set up in 2015 in order to collate understand, collaborate and collate evidence on how to improve wellbeing (see: www.whatworkswellbeing.org). The key aim of the What Works for Wellbeing agenda is to promote wellbeing in public policy based on robust evidence (Bache, 2019). In some senses, the UK is only just catching up with other countries on this. In the global South, for example, Bhutan has used its Gross National Happiness measure rather that Gross National Product to influence social and economic policy since 1972, whilst in 2019, according to the Happy Planet Index, Costa Rica was the happiest country in the world.

It does appear that what makes most people happy is the quality of their relationships with friends, family and work colleagues, and the most important factor is belonging to the local community (Anielski, 2007). We can appreciate that if people are well connected, with strong personal relationships, are physically active, aware and taking notice of what is happening, feel they are learning, are able to give and be generous, then they have higher levels of wellbeing. Altruism ('doing something for others without a motive of self-interest or self-gain and where one does not have a stake in the outcome of the act') is positively linked to better health (Kumar and Dixit, 2017, p. 481). In their study of older people in India, Kumar and Dixit (2017) found that altruism and happiness both predicted self-reported levels of health. This makes the focus on social capital within health promotion, and the importance to health of 'connectedness', seem well placed. Anielski (2007), though, suggests that social capital is only one aspect of capital. If social capital represents relationships, there are four other important types of capital – human capital (people), natural capital (natural resource and the environment), built capital (the built environment) and financial capital (money). That 'natural capital' has a bearing on health has been well documented, and features largely in people's own accounts of what makes them feel alive; time spent in and with nature positively impacts on wellbeing and is especially known to improve children's physical, socio-emotional and cognitive health and development (Tillmann et al., 2019). White (2017), among others, has also pointed out the importance of the environment for wellbeing, particularly for rural communities in low- and middle-income countries.

A wealth of activity in this area is trying to develop scales to measure happiness and feelings of wellbeing, for example, the 'Happiness Measures' index (Fordyce, 2005). Clearly, there are some theoretical and methodological issues with exploring these dimensions of human existence in a positivist and reductionist way, and using more exploratory, qualitative methods is arguably more appropriate. However, happiness surveys do consistently demonstrate a clear statistical relationship between happiness and health – and significantly, this is stronger than the relationship between happiness and wealth (Graham, 2008). In addition, happiness is strongly and independently related to mental health (this among other factors such as optimism, life satisfaction and resilience) (Beida et al., 2017). Some indexes of wellbeing, including that used by the UK, have been criticized for not taking well enough into account factors outside the individual that might impact on subjective wellbeing such as climate change, and the socio-political context, for example. Canada, in contrast, has a much more comprehensive Index of Wellbeing that encompasses eight domains – living standard, health, environment, democratic engagement, time use, education, community vitality, and leisure and culture; and, interestingly, the index has no subjective measures of wellbeing (see www.ciw.ca). In addition, Atkinson et al. (2019) argue that individual subjectivity is inherently linked with community wellbeing, which is not always accounted for in such measures.

White (2017) is critical of the attention given to happiness and wellbeing, suggesting that it indicates that 'all may not be well' and that it reflects 'the erosion of the social in late capitalist modernity' (p. 121). She goes on to argue that the focus on individual definitions of wellbeing in policy worsens this erosion. Drawing on research findings from more 'collectivist' rather than 'individualist' societies such as Bangladesh, India and Zambia, White (2017) argues that *relational* wellbeing is a more important indicator than individual wellbeing as it is crucial for social inclusion and societal change. This is a most compelling argument – we have already pointed out the benefits of social capital and community to health (see Chapter 2). Please see White (2017) for a fuller discussion.

This new discourse is in danger of being a Eurocentric/North Atlantic phenomenon. Beida *et al.* (2017) notes the predominance of research in the global North, which not only limits the generalizability of findings but does not adequately consider cultural, environmental and historical differences. However, 'Southern' voices have been calling for a changed conception of 'development' from that espoused by the global North for some time, and the fact that Bhutan is leading the way in switching from measures of economic growth towards measures of happiness suggests that these ideas are not luxuries promulgated by richer countries. Sen's notion of development as freedom is a major strand of the development discourse, based on the idea that development can be measured by the removal of 'unfreedoms', which are those things that leave people with little choice and no ability to exercise their 'reasoned agency' (Sen, 1999, p. xii). Sen's idea of the 'capability framework' (Sen, 1980) can be used to measure quality of life; it 'suggests that quality of life should be measured by focussing on people's capabilities, namely their real opportunities to lead the life that they have reason to value'. Implicitly, it

> ... criticizes approaches to the measurement of quality of life exclusively based on resources, such as income, or, in the case of health-related quality of life, health status, and mental states, such as satisfaction, happiness, and desire fulfilment.
>
> (Giuntoli, 2010)

None of these approaches provides comprehensive accounts of quality of life – another important factor for wellbeing. A longitudinal study in Ireland demonstrated how quality of life is dependent on several factors, not just physical health and ageing, and that loneliness and social participation are notably important for older people's quality of life (Ward *et al.*, 2019). Both Sen (1993) and Nussbaum (2000) stress the importance of freedom to quality of life, to capability and thus to health. The opportunities and liberties available to individuals allow them to function as full human beings, rather than merely subsisting. These opportunities, which enable greater control and choice, have clear implications for empowerment.

New Models of Health?

This discussion raises the issue of whether models of health conventionally adopted by the epistemic health promotion community adequately fulfil the needs of the new century, given that definitions of health are subjective, culture-bound and change over time. One of the key dimensions which is mentioned in students' discussions of Labonté's model (presented in Chapter 1) is the lack of a spiritual circle. Likewise, it has been noted that a notion of positive health should necessarily include a spiritual dimension (Green *et al.*, 2019). There is increasing recognition in some circles that spiritual health is an integral part of human health and experience (Nunes *et al.*, 2018) and there have been recent calls for WHO to include spiritual health in its definition (Chirico, 2016). Vader (2006) appeals to the public health community to take spiritual health seriously if health improvements are to occur (see Box 6.2). Whilst an agreed definition of spiritual health does not exist (Ghaderi *et al.*, 2018) the concept is at the forefront of many cultures' and faith-systems' understandings of health; for example, for Aboriginal Australians '… Health does not just mean the physical well-being of the individual but refers to the social, emotional, spiritual and cultural well-being of the whole community. This is a whole of life view and includes the cyclical concept of life-death-life' (National Health and Medical Research Council, 1996).

The post-Enlightenment reintegration of the emotional into everyday life affects the way we build our models of health. For example, O'Donnell's (2009) definition of health, which has been adopted by the *American Journal of Health Promotion* (http://www.healthpromotionjournal.com/), includes spiritual, emotional, intellectual and social health in an outer wheel, with physical health at the centre.

There have been attempts to define spiritual health and there are calls to design health promotion interventions that promote it (Charzynska, 2015). Perhaps this is one of the ways in which the

> **Box 6.2. A comment on spiritual health.**
>
> Just as the physical, mental and social dimensions are interrelated and interact, we can also assume that there will be interactions between spirituality, spiritual health, and the other dimensions of health. Belief in and commitment to the transcendental and the metaphysical, no doubt because of its intimate link to the very sense and purpose of existence, is probably the most powerful motivator of human behavior and behavior change known today. Its manifestations can be either positive and constructive, or unbelievably destructive. Harnessing forces for constructive human behaviour change is, and always has been, one of the stumbling blocks and major challenges of public health professionals. By ignoring the spiritual dimension of health, for whatever reason, we may be depriving ourselves of the leverage we need to help empower individuals and populations to achieve improved physical, social, and mental health. Indeed, unless and until we do seriously address the question – however difficult and uncomfortable it may be – substantial and sustainable improvements in physical, social and mental health, and reductions in the health gradient within and between societies, may well continue to elude us.
>
> (Vader, 2006, p. 457)

concepts developed in the last century no longer fully and adequately serve the needs of the 21st – the most quoted definition of health is still that proposed by the WHO in 1946. Apart from the lack of mention of spiritual health, many see the WHO's idea as utopian and unachievable, given the stress on a 'complete' state of physical, mental and social health. However, it is still important to assert that health is *not* merely about *not* being ill or diseased. It is much more than that. The WHO's definition also implicitly suggests that health is a dynamic process of development, where we can become all that we want to be.

Some view spiritual health as one aspect of mental health and Chapman (2019) notes how the terms 'positive health' or 'wellbeing' are often used in place of 'spiritual health'. Chapman (2019, p. 1082) states that

> the quality of our lives and our ultimate well-being as human beings require[s] much more than simply avoiding certain health risks and adopting healthy lifestyle practices. It seem[s] to me that providing permission and pathways for people to grapple with the 'whys' and the purpose of their life [is] as important [...] after all, what is really the ultimate source of motivation for the adoption of healthful practices, but a sense of hopefulness and the fulfilling of our perceived destiny as human beings?

Such perspectives support the case for a greater policy focus on wellbeing and mental health (Barry, 2009).

Spiritual health includes the dimensions of fulfilment, meaning and wellbeing, and despite the decline of organized religion in many 'developed' countries in particular, Inglehart's research on changes in 43 countries shown that 'Spiritual concerns are not vanishing: on the contrary, we find a consistent cross-national tendency to spend more time thinking about the meaning and purpose of life' (Ingelhart, 1997, p. 328). Research in India shows how strongly spirituality is linked to subjective wellbeing (McIntyre *et al.*, 2020). Perhaps this is one area where lay perspectives need to be incorporated rather more into definitions of what it means to be a healthy, well-integrated and happy person in contemporary times!

Thinking Afresh and Developing New Paradigms

The discussion in this chapter and the previous ones, about the disciplinary base of health promotion, shows how in a number of areas of study, there has been a rejection of simple, linear models of human behaviour. This is very evident in communication theory and in the psychology of behaviour change. New ways of conceptualizing behaviour change suggest that what is more important than concentrating on the 'choices' individuals make, is rather to focus on how shared social practices are initiated, sustained and become normalized. This would shift the area of focus from health behaviours to health practices, and from behaviour change to practice change, and implicitly from individualized 'choices' to the social construction of daily life. The field of behavioural science has expanded exponentially since the publication of Thaler and Sunstein's book *Nudge: Improving Decisions about Health, Wealth and Happiness w*as published in 2008. As of May 2020, there are nearly 300 behavioural science teams in government, businesses and other organizations around the world (Nesterak, 2020), many of which are currently occupied with finding evidence-based solutions to supporting the significant changes in behaviour required to tackle the Covid-19 pandemic.

In Chapter 4 we considered digital technology and health in some detail. Aside from debates about whether technology is a force for good or not, the implications of technological advances for public health must be taken into account in what has been termed the Fourth Industrial Revolution (Schwab, 2016) characterized by 'the range of new technologies that are fusing the physical, digital and biological worlds, impacting all disciplines, economies and industries, even challenging ideas about what it means to be human' (p. 1). Add to this the big issues of our time – climate change, increasing health and social inequalities, environmental degradation and even the threat of human extinction – and it is clear to see the need for a major change in mindset. Concepts such as social justice also need rethinking, as argued by people like Sir Michael Marmot, Professor Clare Bambra and Professor Danny Dorling. Dorling (2011) has set out to redefine 'injustice'. He argues that 'the five tenets of injustice are that: elitism is efficient, exclusion is necessary, prejudice is natural, greed is good and despair is inevitable'.

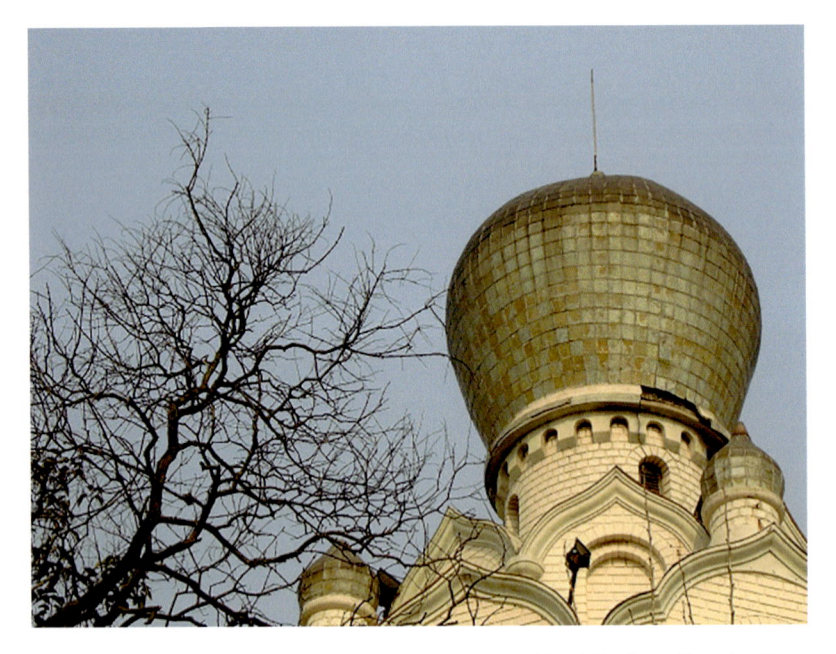

Religion is part of everyday life for many people, contributing to their spiritual life (from Creative Commons source – the foreign religion in shanghai city by iris_kayak is licensed under CC BY-ND 2.0).

Finally, Gregg and O'Hara (2007a) have attempted to outline the value base of health promotion in the 21st century and to suggest a model that fits the zeitgeist, in their Red Lotus model. First, they produced a useful overview of the values and principles found in current health promotion practice, showing the continuum of values spanning conventional health promotion and the newer, holistic, ecological and salutogenic health promotion (Table 6.1).

After presenting the challenges of working with those values in practice, they go on, in a second paper, to present a new model of health promotion for 'holistic, ecological and salutogenic health promotion practice', which they call the 'red lotus model' (Gregg and O'Hara, 2007b). Having argued that existing health promotion planning models do not explicitly use values and principles systematically, they show how their model enables incorporation of the central values in each stage of the planning cycle for health promotion activities. They suggest that there are three domains: the philosophical, ethical and technical, and these are presented here (Tables 6.2, 6.3 and 6.4).

Table 6.1. The continuum of values and principles evident in current health promotion practice (Gregg and O'Hara, 2007a, pp. 8–9).

Focus of value or principle	Holistic, ecological, salutogenic health promotion value or principle	Description of each end of the values and principles continuum	Conventional health promotion value or principle
Worldview	Organic	Seeing the world as a living, breathing, dynamic whole as opposed to seeing the world as an unchanging, static machine	Mechanistic
Epistemology	Constructionist, Subjectivist	Acknowledging that all people are connected and that collectively they construct knowledge and understanding about their world, as distinct from believing that there is only one truth that is ascertained by an objective observer	Objectivist
Science	Ecological	Using the science of ecology, which recognizes that people exist in multiple ecosystems, from the individual level, to the family group, community and population level. All parts within the whole system affect each other, and the whole is greater than the sum of the parts. Ecological science incorporates the tenets of connectedness, complementarity, uncertainty and non-locality. This principle is distinct from reductionism or positivism, in which understanding about the whole comes from simply understanding each part	Reductionist, positivist
Health paradigm	Holistic	Understanding that health is a complex concept that includes aspects of wellbeing that relate to the whole person, rather than seeing heath as an absence of disease or 'unhealthy' behaviours, as reflected in the biomedical and behavioural health paradigms	Biomedical, behaviourist
Emphasis	Health and wellbeing	Emphasizing factors that create and support health, wellbeing, happiness and meaning in life, as distinct from emphasis on risk factors for disease	Rates of disease and risk behaviours
Motivation for health	Health as a resource for living, sense of purpose and enjoyment of life	Recognizing that health provides a sense of purpose and enables greater enjoyment of life and is not an end in itself. This is distinct from believing that fear about the consequences of unhealthy behaviours are the primary motivators for people to develop long-term sustainable changes	Fear about consequences of unhealthy behaviours
Assumptions about people	People are naturally healthy	Assuming that when left to their own devices, people will do the best they can for themselves, their families and their communities, given their circumstances and available resources. This is distinct from assuming that left to their own devices, people will naturally adopt 'unhealthy' lifestyles	People are naturally unhealthy
Health promotion strategies	Participatory processes that enable and empower people	Using participatory processes that enable and empower people to connect with their inner wisdom and gain control over their lives and the determinants of their health. This is distinct from using disempowering interventions that target 'at risk' people and educations and their 'unhealthy' behaviours	Target 'at risk' people with behaviour change strategies
Population focus	Determined by equality	Prioritizing work with communities that are most marginalized, vulnerable, disadvantaged and often regarded as 'hard to reach' based on considerations of equity. This is distinct from working with more visible groups or whole populations, or the less vulnerable and more accessible populations	Whole groups or populations

Continued

Table 6.1. Continued.

Focus of value or principle	Holistic, ecological, salutogenic health promotion value or principle	Description of each end of the values and principles continuum	Conventional health promotion value or principle
Power	Participatory, egalitarian	Facilitating participatory and egalitarian processes that assist with the redistribution of power, rather than processes that have their foundations in patriarchy and domination	Patriarchal, dominator
Change processes	Active participation of people affected by the issue	Ensuring that people most affected by an issue are an integral part of all components of a health promotion change process that addresses the issue, as distinct from being targeted as recipients of decisions made external to them	Passive recipients of external decisions
	Processes do not impinge on personal autonomy	Ensuring that all relevant parties consent to health promotion change processes and acknowledging and respecting that not all people will choose the same actions, rather than processes that expect all people to adopt the same actions, irrespective of their own processes	Universal processes that restrict personal autonomy
	Maximum beneficence	Actively considering what the benefits of any health promotion change process may be to the full range of beneficiaries, as distinct from processes that only consider a limited range of beneficiaries	Limited beneficence
	Non-maleficence is a priority consideration	Actively considering what the potential harms of any health promotion change process may be; who may be harmed by the change processes and in what way; taking steps to minimize or avoid this harm; communicating risks involved in a truthful and open manner. This is distinct from change processes that do not assess the full range of potential harms due to a belief that health promotion processes will result in positive health outcomes	Scope of maleficence not fully considered
Basis for practice	Practice based on evidence of need and effectiveness, and sound theoretical foundations	Ensuring that needs assessment process incorporate the perspectives of all stakeholders, and that health promotion practice is based on sound evidence of need, evidence of effectiveness, and appropriate theoretical foundations. This is distinct from practice that is based on a selective use of evidence and/or political motives	Practice based on selective use of evidence, or on political imperatives
Strategy approach	Multiple strategies	Using multiple strategies incorporating all action areas of the Ottawa Charter, as opposed to reliance on one or two strategies, particularly legislation and regulation, and developing personal skills for behaviour change	One or two strategies
Governance and decision making	Collaborative models of governance and decision making	Using models of governance and decision making that facilitate active and meaningful participation by all stakeholders, as distinct from non-democratic governance and decision making	Health worker led and/or imposed from outside
Professional role	Ally	Working with a person as an ally and a resource, who is on tap for the community, as distinct from working on top of people as an outside expert who assumes they know what's best for the community	Expert
Evaluation objects of interest	Sustainable changes to determinants of health	Ensuring that evaluation focuses on assessing the sustainable changes in the range of factors that enable people to increase control over the determinants of their health, as distinct from evaluating changes in rates of 'unhealthy' behaviours and diseases	Behaviour changes and disease rates

Table 6.2. Values and principles in the philosophical domain (Gregg and O'Hara, 2007b, p. 14).

Value	Principle	Explanation
Organic worldview	The existence of an organic universe	Seeing the world as a living, breathing, dynamic whole
Constructionist epistemology	The construction of knowledge through interactions within and between health promotion practitioners and communities	Acknowledging that all people are connected and that collectively they construct knowledge and understanding about their worlds
Ecological science	The science underpinning health promotion is ecological	Using the science of ecology, which recognizes that people exist in multiple ecosystems, from the individual level, to the family group, community and population level. Health is determined by complex interactions between people (including their biological status, such as age, gender and genetics, state of health and wellbeing, socio-economic status, attitudes, values, beliefs and behaviours) and their social, economic, political, built and natural environments. All parts within the whole system affect each other, and the whole is greater than the sum of the parts. Ecological science incorporates the tenets of connectedness, complementarity, uncertainty and non-locality
Holistic health paradigm	The concept of health includes interrelated dimensions of spiritual, mental, social and physical health and wellbeing	Understanding that health is a complex concept that includes aspects of wellbeing that relate to the whole person or communities of people
Salutogenic focus	Focusing on the creation of health	Emphasizing factors that create and support health, wellbeing, happiness and meaning in life
Health is purposeful	The motivation for health is as a resource for living	Recognizing that health provides a sense of purpose and enables greater enjoyment of life and is not an end in itself
Assumption of positive intentions	Assume that people have a natural desire to do the best for themselves, their families and their communities	Assuming that when left to their own devices, people will do the best they can, given their circumstances and available resources
Empowering health promotion strategies	Participatory processes that enable and empower people	Using participatory processes that enable and empower people to connect with their inner wisdom, and gain control over their lives and the determinants of their health

These three tables contain a huge number of ideas and as such embrace some of the complexity we have mentioned previously, providing links between principles and practice. We cannot do justice here to the full use of the symbolism of the red lotus flower, and we suggest that you read the paper to appreciate this. We also do not present Gregg and O'Hara's work as the only or 'best' way of conceptualizing the values of health promotion, but as one device to enable readers to think about the important issue of the values and principles base of health promotion.

Final Thoughts

Health promoters see in the world around them systemic inequalities in the capabilities (Sen, 1993) of entire continents, nations and the communities and individuals, to lead lives with value and meaning to themselves. If health is about living a meaningful life, then this is surely our primary concern and starting point. In a world of global plenty, where resources are not an issue (but the distribution of them is), then our engagement must be with an attempt to re-shape the lived-experience of those struggling in the margins between mere existence and a meaningful life. Socio-economic and political inequalities restrict people's freedoms and capabilities, capacity for self-determination and independence and ability to develop their personhood. They cannot be, in Maslow's terms, self-actualized beings.

A global ethic is at the heart of health promotion, where universal norms and values are shared.

Table 6.3. Values and principles in the ethical domain (Gregg and O'Hara, 2007b, p. 15).

Value	Principle	Explanation
Equity-based priority communities	Prioritize action with the most vulnerable or disadvantaged communities	Prioritizing work with communities that are the most marginalized, vulnerable, disadvantaged and often regarded as 'hard to reach' based on considerations of equity
Equitable distribution of power	Power is distributed equitably between stakeholders	Facilitating participatory and egalitarian processes that assist with the redistribution of power
Ethical change processes	Change processes enable active participation of people affected by the issue	Ensuring that people most affected by an issue are an integral part of all components of a health promotion change process that addresses the issue, as distinct from being targeted as recipients of decisions made external to them
	Processes do not impinge on people's personal autonomy	Ensuring that all relevant parties consent to health promotion change processes and acknowledging and respecting that not all people will choose the same actions
	Beneficence is a priority consideration	Actively considering what the benefits of any health promotion change process may be and who may be the beneficiaries
	Non-maleficence is a priority consideration	Actively considering what the potential harms of any health promotion change process may be, who may be harmed by the change processes and in what way. Taking steps to minimize or avoid this harm. Communicating risks involved in a truthful and open manner
Evidence-based practice	Practice is based on evidence of need and effectiveness, and sound theoretical foundations	Ensuring that needs assessment processes incorporate the perspectives of all stakeholders, and that health promotion practice is based on sound evidence of need, evidence of effectiveness, and appropriate theoretical foundations

Table 6.4. Values and principles in the technical domain (Gregg and O'Hara, 2007b, p. 16).

Value	Principle	Explanation
Comprehensive actions	Portfolio of multiple strategies is used to address complex issues	Using multiple strategies incorporating all action areas of the Ottawa Charter
Democratic governance	Collaborative models of governance and decision making	Using models of governance and decision making that facilitate active and meaningful participation by all stakeholders
Practitioner is a resource	Work with communities as an ally	Working with communities as an ally and a resource on tap for communities
System-level evaluation	Evaluate sustainable changes to systems that support people to increase control over their health	Ensuring that evaluation focuses on assessing the changes in the range of factors that enable people to increase control over the determinants of their health

These are outlined in the many declarations and statements produced over the years by the health promotion community. Dower has elaborated on the idea of a global ethic suggesting it includes '… a norm of global responsibility according to which agents have responsibilities to promote what is good anywhere in the world (or, as often as not, to oppose what is bad)' (Dower, 2003, p. 18). Promoting what is good and living well together as a global community sits well not only with our moral intuitions but also with Rawls' famous phrase, 'the justice of fairness' (Rawls, 1971). Health promoters thus embody a personal ethic with global scope and a will to act to make the world a 'better place', invoking Karl Marx's famous maxim that the point is not only to understand the world, but to change it. Health promoters clearly go further than, say, traditional epidemiologists, whose role is to describe the world (of disease and illness), whereas a fundamental part of the role of the health promoter is to change the world. This stance was reflected in the most recent global conference on health promotion. The 23rd World Conference on Health Promotion hosted by the International Union of Health Promotion and Education (IUHPE) took place in New Zealand in 2019 and resulted the Rotorua Statement – WAIORA: Promoting Planetary Health and Sustainable Development for All. Waiora is an indigenous concept that expresses the interconnections between health and the natural environment, and the need for sustainable development. The statement calls for urgent action on planetary health, and the need to put people and the planet at the heart of decision making (IUHPE, 2019a). It argues that sustainable development for all is necessary in order to achieve environmental, social and health justice for everyone, now and in the future. Four key areas were identified as needing immediate action: (i) ensure health equity throughout the life course, within and among countries, and within and across generations; (ii) make all urban and other habitats inclusive, safe, resilient, sustainable and conducive to health and wellbeing for people and the planet; (iii) design and implement effective and fair climate change adaptation strategies; and (iv) build collaborative, effective, accountable and inclusive governance systems and process at all levels to promote participation, peace, justice, respect of human rights and intergenerational health equity (IUHPE, 2019a). The accompanying Indigenous Peoples' Statement for Planetary Health and Sustainable Development (IUPHE, 2019b) forefronts the interactive relationships between humankind, our planet and the material and spiritual realms. This ended with the following – 'We call on the health promotion community and the wider global community to make space for and privilege Indigenous people's voices and Indigenous knowledges in taking action with us to promote the health of Mother Earth and sustainable development for the benefit of all' (IUHPE, 2019b, p. 2).

Following McGregor (2004, pp. 98–99), it is essential that health promoters have 'an engagement in how we are involved in reproducing power imbalances, oppression, and difference between ourselves and others'. This political awareness necessarily moves us away from the language of 'helping' and towards 'working alongside', 'joining together' in an empathic identification with others (Peterson, 2007). In addition, as Fleming (2020) argues, 'it is important to ensure that the discourse about health issues and the politics of health focus on the social determinants of health' (p. 3).

Health promoters with their personal ethic of social justice and equity may appear to be relentlessly optimistic about the role of health promotion as a means to save the world from health injustices. Health promotion is a profession of hope and it does place at its centre a hopeful view of people and the enduring qualities of what it means to be human. The social determinants of health are well known and tackling the major ones is relatively straightforward; other areas are less tangible and thus more difficult, but Barry (2009) has argued for example in the case of mental health, that we have robust evidence from systematic reviews about the effectiveness of interventions tackling social determinants. The use of policy to tackle the social determinants is also becoming a refined science (Exworthy, 2008). We thus have no excuse for not taking action – we know what to do.

However, optimism needs to be tempered with realism, and we have to be realistic about what *can* be achieved. We can perhaps pause here to reflect on what are the most important things for health promoters to do, in the absence of being able to do everything. What then are the most important things on the health promoter's 'to do list'?

To Do List

- Recognize that networks are stronger than hierarchies, and work to build coalitions, networks and means of enabling the marginalized to access these too.
- Remind the major global players that whilst the discourse on health has moved into newer ways of conceptualizing health and development to include less easily measured factors such as happiness, satisfaction and wellbeing, there are many whose basic needs are not being met. There is therefore still a need for focus on the basic social indicators of development such as life expectancy at birth, maternal mortality, literacy rates, access to safe water and so on.
- Given that social capital is crucial to communities taking charge of their own affairs, work to maintain and build social capital in innovative and creative ways.
- Develop the evidence base on the success of attempts to tackle social determinants and how these affect health.

- Develop settings as a practical means of 'doing' health promotion, thus creating enabling environments for true transformation, whilst also recognizing that there are interstitial spaces where often the most marginalized live their lives.
- Continue to develop methods for authentic participation.

Summary

This book summarizes our thinking on health promotion and is presented as *one* contribution to the field. It's important the readers find other views and also follow up ideas that we have only been able to skim over here. Fields of endeavour apart from health promotion also struggle with the goals of empowerment, equality, justice, and are also contemplating how to deal with challenges of the 21st century, such as complexity, globalization and social capital. These fields might include education, criminal justice, social work, sport, development, and so provide rich and relevant avenues for further reading. Much of our work is fuelled by the sense of injustice exemplified by the obscene levels of wealth in the global North and the continuing, pernicious and crippling levels of poverty in parts of the global South, in tandem with the inequalities seen *within* countries. The result is that people cannot become all they are capable of becoming; they live in conditions which are not dignified, and their human rights are not respected. If health promotion is essentially about enabling people to take control of the determinants of their health, we can only too plainly see that many people, perhaps the majority in global terms, are not in charge of their own destinies. Those destinies are determined, rather, by those in charge of global markets. There is a groundswell movement towards challenging those powers and creating a global world where health and human happiness are prioritized. We need to put a halt to unsustainable development and learn lessons from those middle-income countries that have developed decent living standards and good levels of health for their populations. Nothing short of a transformation is needed in the way that global priorities are set, and in the way that power and wealth are distributed. There do appear to be openings for such transformations with more room to hear the voices of civil society in calling for different ways of measuring wellbeing, happiness and development, and in challenging the power of the corporations, governments and other powerful interests who wish to subjugate and silence those voices. Never has this been more apparent than in the effect that the Covid-19 pandemic is having at the time of writing. The pandemic is causing many of us to pause, to question the nature of the world we find ourselves in and the lives we are leading. It remains to be seen whether these opportunities for creating a more just world will materialize, but health promotion, as a movement for health justice, needs to keep creating a place for itself at the global debating table, whilst continuing to practice at grassroots level to bring small but significant changes to people's lives.

Note

[1] A previous version of this chapter was written by Rachael Dixey.

Further Reading

Costello, A. (2018) *The Social Edge: The Power of Sympathy Groups for Our Health, Wealth and Sustainable Future.* Thornwick, UK.

Green, J., Cross, R., Woodall, J. and Tones, K. (2019) *Health Promotion: Planning and Strategies.* 4th edition. Sage, London.

Haworth, J. and Hart, G. (2012) *Well-Being: Individual, Community and Social Perspectives.* Palgrave Macmillan, London.

Lueddeke, G.R. (2020) *One Health, One Planet, One Future.* Routledge, London.

Marmot, M. (2015) *The Health Gap: The Challenge of an Unequal World.* Bloomsbury, London.

Smith, S. (2011) *Equality and Diversity – Value Incommensurability and the Politics of Recognition.* The Policy Press, London.

References

Abbott, P.A., Turnov, S. and Wallace, C. (2006) Health world views of post-soviet citizens. *Social Science & Medicine* 62, 228–238.

Aceves-Martins, M., Aleman-Diaz, A.Y., Giralt, M. and Solà, R. (2019) Involving young people in health promotion, research and policy-making: practical recommendations. *International Journal for Quality in Health Care* 31, 2, 147–153.

Ackerman, M., Moyses, S.T., Franco de Sa, R.N.P., MenPromotion Internationaldes, R., Nogueira, J.A.D., Zancan, L., Manoncourt, E. and Wallerstein, N. (2019) Democracy and health promotion. *Health Promotion International* 34 (S1), i1–i3, doi: 10.1093/heapro/daz016

Adebiyi, A.O., Ogunniyi, A., Adediran, B.A., Olakhinde, O.O. and Siwoke, A.A. (2016) Cognitive impairment among the ageing population in a community in Southwest Nigeria. *Health Education & Behaviour* 43, 93S–99S.

Adriansen, H.K. and Madsen, L.M. (2019) Capacity-building projects in African higher education: issues of coloniality in international academic collaboration. *Learning and Teaching* 12, 1–23.

Airhihenbuwa, C.O. (2007) 2007 SOPHE Presidential Address: On being comfortable with being uncomfortable: centering an Africanist vision in our gateway to global health. *Health Education Behaviour* 34, 31.

Ajayi, J.E.A., Lameck, K.H., Goma, G. and Ampah, J. (1996) *The African Experience with Higher Education*. Association of African Universities, Accra, Ghana.

Albrecht, G., Freeman, S. and Higginbotham, N. (1998) Complexity and human health: the case for a transdisciplinary paradigm. *Culture, Medicine and Psychiatry* 22, 55–92.

Alderson, P. (2000) School students' views on school councils and daily life at school. *Children and Society* 14, 121–134.

Allen, L.N. (2017) Financing national non-communicable disease responses. *Global Health Action* 10(1), doi:10.1080/16549716.2017.1326687

Allmark, P. and Tod, A. (2006) How should public health professionals engage with lay epidemiology? *Journal of Medical Ethics* 32, 460–463.

Alston, P. (2018) *Statement on Visit to the United Kingdom, by Professor Philip Alston, United Nations Special Rapporteur on extreme poverty and human rights*. Available at: https://www.ohchr.org/EN/NewsEvents/Pages/DisplayNews.aspx?NewsID=23881&LangID=E (accessed 2 October 2019).

Aluttis, C., van den Broucke, S., Chiotan, C., Costongs, C., Michelsen, K and Brand, H. (2014) Public health and health promotion capacity at national and regional level: a review of conceptual frameworks. *Journal of Public Health Research* 3, 199.

Amunyunzu-Nyamongo, M. and Nyamwaya, D. (eds) (2009) *Evidence of Health Promotion Effectiveness in Africa*. African Institute for Health, Nairobi.

Anielski, M. (2007) *The Economics of Happiness: Building Genuine Wealth*. New Society Publishers, Grabiola Island, Canada.

Anugwom, E.E. (2020) *Health Promotion and Its Challenges to Public Health Delivery System in Africa*, doi: http://dx.doi.org/10.5772/intechopen.91859

Arsenijevic, J. and Groot, W. (2020) Health promotion policies for elderly: some comparisons across Germany, Italy, the Netherlands and Poland. *Health Policy*. Available at: https://doi.org/10.1016/j.healthpol.2020.01.013 (accessed 11 February 2020).

Atkinson, S., Bagnall, A., Cororan, R. South, J. and Curtis, S. (2019) Being well together: individual subjective and community wellbeing. *Journal of Happiness Studies*, doi: org/10/1007/s10902-109-00146-2

Attwood, M., Pedler, M., Pritchard, S. and Wilkinson, D. (2003) *Leading Change. A Guide to Whole Systems Working*. The Policy Press, Bristol, UK.

Bache, I. (2019) How does evidence matter? Understanding 'what works' for wellbeing. *Social Indicators Research*, 142, 1153–1173.

Bagnall, A.-M., Radley, D., Jones, R., Gately, P., Nobles., J., Van Dijk, M. Blackshaw, J., Montel, S. and Sahota, P. (2019) Whole systems approaches to obesity and other complex public health challenges: a systematic review. *BMC Public Health* 19(8), doi: 10.1186/s12889-018-6274-z

Baldwin, L. (2020) Sustaining the practice of health promotion. In: Fleming, M. and Baldwin, L. (eds) *Health Promotion in the 21st Century*. Allen & Urwin, London, pp. 245–262.

Barry, M. (2008) Capacity building for the future of health promotion. *Global Health Promotion* 15, 56–58.

Barry, M. (2009) Addressing the determinants of positive mental health: concepts, evidence and practice. *International Journal of Mental Health Promotion* 11, 4–17.

Baru, R.V. and Mohan, M. (2018) Globalisation and neoliberalism as structural drivers of health inequities. *Health Research Policy and Systems* 16 (Suppl 1): 91 doi.org/10.1186/s12961-018-0365-2

Bauer, G.F., Roy, M., Bakibinga, P., Contu, P., Downe, S., Eriksson, M., Espnes, G.A. et al. (2019) Future directions for the concept of salutogenesis: a position article. *Health Promotion International* 1–9, doi: 10/1093/heapro/daz057

Baum, F. (2009) Envisioning a healthy and sustainable future: essential to closing the gap in a generation. *Global Health Promotion Supplement* 1, 72–80.

Baum, F. and Fischer, M. (2014) Why behavioural health promotion endures despite its failure to reduce health inequities *Sociology of Health & Illness* 36, 213–225.

Baum, F. and Sanders, D. (1995) Can health promotion and primary health care achieve Health for All without a return to their more radical agenda? *Health Promotion International* 10, 149–160.

Beida, A., Hisrchfeld, G., Schönfeld, P., Brailovskaia, J., Zhang, X.C. and Margraf, J. (2017) Universal happiness? Cross-cultural measurement invariance of scales assessing positive mental health. *Psychological Assessment* 29 (4), 408–421.

Bellander, T. and Landqvist, M. (2020) Becoming the expert constructing health knowledge in epistemic communities online. *Information, Communication & Society* 23 (4), 507–522, doi: 10.1080/1369118X.2018.1518474

Bergeron, K., Abdi, S., Decorby, K., Mensah, G., Rempel, B. and Manson, H. (2017) Theories, models and frameworks used in capacity building interventions relevant to public health: a systematic review. *BMC Public Health* 17, 914, doi: 10.1186/s12889-017-4919-y

Bigna, J.J. and Noubiap, J.J. (2019) The rising burden of non-communicable diseases in sub-Saharan Africa. *The Lancet* 7 (10), e1295–e1296.

Blaxter, M. (1997) Whose fault is it? People's own conceptions of the reasons for health inequalities. *Social Science & Medicine* 44, 747–56.

Brehm, M.V. (2001) *Promoting Effective North–South NGO Partnerships*. Occasional paper series Number 35. INTRAC, Oxford, UK.

Brown, R.C. (2018a) Resisting moralisation in health promotion. *Ethical Theory and Moral Practice* 21, 997–1011.

Brown, R.C. (2018b) Resisting moralisation in Health Promotion. *Ethical Theory and Moral Practice* 21, 997–1011.

Bourne, R. (ed.) (2000) *Universities and Development*. Association of Commonwealth Universities, London.

Buckley, J. and O'Tuama, S. (2010) 'I send the wife to the doctor' – men's behaviour as health consumers. *International Journal of Consumer Studies* 34, 587–595.

Bunton, R. and MacDonald, G. (1992) *Health Promotion: Disciplines and Diversity*. Routledge, London.

Bunton, R. and Macdonald, G. (2002) *Health Promotion: Disciplines, Diversity and Developments,* 2nd edition. Routledge, London.

Bunton, R., Nettleton, S. and Burrows, R. (1996a) *The Sociology of Health Promotion: Critical Analyses of Consumption, Lifestyle and Risk*. Routledge, London.

Bunton, R., Nettleton, S. and Burrows, R. (1996b) *The Sociology of Health Promotion: Critical Analyses of Consumption, Lifestyle and Risk*. Routledge, London.

Calnan, M. and Williams, S. (1991) Style of life and the salience of health. *Sociology of Health and Illness* 13, 506–516.

Campbell, C. (2011) Embracing complexity: towards more nuanced understandings of social capital and health. *Global Health Action* 4, 1–3.

Campbell, C. and Scott, K. (2011) Retreat from Alma Ata?: the WHO's report on task shifting to community health workers for AIDS care in poor countries. *Global Public Health* 6, 125–138.

Carrington, W. and Detragiache, E. (1999) How extensive is the brain drain? *Finance and Development, A quarterly magazine of the IMF* 36, 2.

Carruth, L. (2014) Camel milk, amoxicillin, and a prayer: Medical pluralism and medical humanitarian aid in the Somali Region of Ethiopia. *Social Science & Medicine* 120, 405–412.

Cattan, M. (2009a) Loneliness, interventions. In: Reis, H. and Sprecher, S. (eds) *The Encyclopedia of Human Relationships*. Sage, London.

Cattan, M. (ed.) (2009b) *Mental Health and Well-being in Later Life*. McGraw-Hill/Open University Press, Maidenhead, UK.

Cattan, M. (2010) *Preventing Social Isolation and Loneliness among Older People*. VDM Publishing, Saarbrücken, Germany.

Cattan, M. (2012) Mental health issues for older people. In: Reed, J., Clarke, C. and MacFarlane, A. (eds) *Nursing Older Adults*. Open University Press/McGraw-Hill, Maidenhead, UK.

Cattan, M., White, M., Bond, J. and Learmouth, A. (2005) Preventing social isolation and loneliness among older people: a systematic review of health promotion intervention. *Ageing and Society* 25, 41–67.

Catford, J. (2005) The Bangkok conference: steering countries to build national capacity for health promotion. *Health Promotion International* 20, 1–6.

Catford, J. (2010) Editorial: Implementing the Nairobi Call to Action: Africa's opportunity to light the way. *Health Promotion International* 25, 1–4.

Chapman, L. (2019) Spiritual health revisited. *American Journal of Health Promotion* 33 (7), 1028–1084.

Charzynska, E. (2015) Multidimensional approach toward spiritual coping: construction and validation of the spiritual coping questionnaire. *Journal of Religious Health* 54 (5), 1629–1646.

Chen, H., Tu, S.P., The, C.Z., Yip, M.P., Choe, J.H., Hislop, T.G., Taylor, V.M. and Thompson, B. (2006) Lay beliefs about hepatitis among North American Chinese: implications for hepatitis prevention. *Journal of Community Health* 31, 94–112.

Chirico, F. (2016) Spiritual well-being in the 21st century: it's time to review the current WHO's health definition? *Journal of Health and Social Sciences* 1, 11–16.

Colvin, C.J. (2011) Think locally, act globally: developing a critical public health in the global South. *Critical Public Health* 21, 253–256.

Conrad, D. and White, A. (2010) *Promoting Men's Mental Health*. Radcliffe Publishing, Oxford, UK.

Costa-Font, J. and Mas, N. (2016) 'Globesity'? The effects of globalization on obesity and caloric intake. *Food Policy* 64, 121–132.

Cross, R. and Warwick-Booth, L. (2016) Using storyboards in participatory research. *Nurse Researcher* 23 (3), 8–12, doi: 10.7748/nr.23.3.8.s3

Cross, R. and Warwick-Booth, L. (2018) Neoliberal salvation through a gendered intervention: a critical analysis of vulnerable young women's talk. *Alternate Routes: A Journal of Critical Social Research* 290. Available at: http://www.alternateroutes.ca/index.php/ar/article/view/22449 (accessed 2 June 2020).

Cross, R., Milnes, K., Rickett, B. and Fylan, F. (2011) Risking a stigmatised identity: a discourse analysis of young women's talk about health and risk. *Qualitative Methods in Psychology* 12, 22–29.

Cross, R., Lowcock, D., Fiave, J., Agyeniwah, S. and Annan, G.K. (2020) 'Feeling part of a network of learning in health promotion': an evaluation of a postgraduate peer-mentoring scheme in Ghana. *Innovations in Education and Teaching International* 57, 175–185, doi: 10.1080/14703297.2019.1625799

Department of Health (DOH) (2001) *The Expert Patient: A New Approach to Chronic Disease Management for the 21st Century*. DOH, London.

Department of Health (2011) *Local Government's New Public Health Functions*. Department of Health, London.

Department of Health (2012a) *New Focus for Public Health – The Health and Social Care Act 2012 Factsheet B4*. Department of Health, London.

Department of Health (2012b) *The Health and Social Care Act 2012 – An Overview. Factsheet A1, updated 30 April 2012*. Available at: https://assets.publishing.service.gov.uk/government/uploads/system/uploads/attachment_data/file/138257/A1.-Factsheet-Overview-240412.pdf (accessed 25 August 2020).

Dixey, R. (2001) The experience of postgraduate study in the UK. *Africa Health* 2001, 6–7.

Dixey, R. (2013) After Nairobi: can the international community help to develop health promotion in Africa? *Health Promotion International* 29, 185–194.

Dixey, R. and Green, M. (2009) Sustainability of the health care workforce in Africa: a way forward in Zambia. *The International Journal of Environmental, Cultural, Economic and Social Sustainability* 5, 301–310.

Doherty, S. and Dooris, M. (2006) The healthy settings approach: the growing interest within colleges and universities. *Education and Health* 24, 42–43.

Dooris, M. (2001) The 'health promoting university': a critical exploration of theory and practice. *Health Education* 101, 51–60.

Dooris, M. and Martin, E. (2002) Developing a health promoting university initiative within the context of intersectoral action for sustainable public health: reflections from the University of Central Lancashire. *Promotion & Education* Supplement 1 – Special Edition, 16–24.

Dooris, M., Powell, S. and Farrier, A. (2019) Conceptualizing the 'whole university' approach: an international qualitative study. *Health Promotion International*. ISSN 09574824.

Dorling, D. (2011) *Injustice: Why Social Inequality Persists*. The Policy Press, Bristol, UK.

Douglas, J. (1995) Developing anti-racist health promotion strategies. In: Bunton, R., Nettleton, S. and Burrows, R. (eds) *The Sociology of Health Promotion*. Routledge, London.

Douglas, J. (1997) Developing health promotion strategies with black and minority ethnic communities which address social inequalities. In: Sidell, M., Jones, L., Katz, J. and Peberdy, A. (eds) *Debates and Dilemmas in Promoting Health*. Macmillan Press, Basingstoke, UK.

Douglas, J. (2017) The struggle to find a voice on Black women's health: from the personal to the political. In: Gabriel, D. and Tate, S.A. (eds) *Inside the Ivory Tower – Narratives of Women of Colour Surviving and Thriving in British Academia*. Trentham Books, London, pp. 91–107.

Douglas, J. (2018) The politics of black women's health in the UK: intersections of "race," class, and gender in policy, practice, and research. In: Jordan-Zachery, J.S. and Alexander-Floyd, N.G. (eds) *Black Women in Politics: Demanding Citizenship, Challenging Power, and Seeking Justice.* SUNY series in African American Studies/SUNY series in New Political Science. State University of New York Press, Albany, New York, pp. 49–68.

Douglas, J. (2019) Black women's activism and organisation in public health – struggles and strategies for better health and wellbeing (2019-06). *Caribbean Review of Gender Studies* 13, 51–68.

Dower, N. (2003) *An Introduction to Global Citizenship*. Edinburgh University Press, Edinburgh, UK.

Doyal, L. (1995) *What Makes Women Sick: Gender and the Political Economy of Health*. Rutgers University Press, New Brunswick, New Jersey.

Duncan, P. (2013) Failing to professionalise, struggling to specialise: the rise and fall of health promotion as a putative specialism in England, 1980–2000. *Medical History* 57, 377–396.

Dupere, S. (2007) Views on the international influence of Canadian health promotion. In: O'Neil, M., Pederson, A., Dupere, S. and Rootman, I. (eds) *Health Promotion in Canada: Critical Perspectives*. Canadian Scholars Press Inc., Toronto.

Easterly, W. (2009) How the Millennium Development Goals are unfair to Africa. *World Development* 37, 26–35.

EC (2011) *The State of Men's Health in Europe: Extended Report*. The European Commission, DG Sanco, Luxembourg. Available at: https://ec.europa.eu/health/sites/health/files/state/docs/men_health_extended_en.pdf (accessed 25 August 2020).

Economic Commission for Africa (2005) *Economic Report on Africa 2005: Meeting the Challenges of Unemployment and Poverty in Africa*. Economic Commission for Africa, Addis Ababa.

Edwards, P. and Collinson, M. (2002) Empowerment and managerial labor strategies: pragmatism regained. *Work and Occupations* 29, 272. doi: 10.1177/0730888402029003002

Elmawazini, K., Manga, P., Nwankwo, S. and AlNaser, B. (2019) Health gap between developed and developing countries: Does globalization matter? *Economic Change and Restructuring* 52, 123–138.

Exworthy, M. (2008) Policy to tackle the social determinants of health: using conceptual models to understand the policy process. *Health Policy and Planning* 23, 318–327.

Fleming, M. (2020) The importance of health promotion principles and practice. In: Fleming, M. and Baldwin, L. *Health Promotion in the 21st Century,* Allen & Urwin, London, pp. 1–12.

Fleming, M., Parker, E. and Baldwin, L. (2020) The changing nature of health promotion. In: Fleming, M. and Baldwin, L. *Health Promotion in the 21st Century,* Allen & Urwin, London, pp. 16–36.

Fordyce, M.W. (2005) A review of research on the happiness measures: a sixty second index of happiness and mental health. *Social Indicators Research Series* 26, 373–399.

Fortune, K., Posada, F.B., Buss, P., Galvão, L.A.C., Contreras, A., Murphy, M. *et al.,* (2018) Health promotion and the agenda for sustainable development, WHO Region of the Americas. *Bull World Health Organ,* 96, 621–626.

Fox, N. and Ward, K. (2006) Health identities: from expert patient to resisting consumer. *Health: An Interdisciplinary Journal for the Social Study of Health, Illness and Medicine* 10, 461–479.

Fried, J., Harris, B., Eyles, J. and Moshabela. M. (2015) Acceptable care? Illness constructions, healthworlds, and accessible chronic treatment in South Africa. *Qualitative Health Research* 25(5), 622– 635.

Garthwaite, K. and Bambra, C. (2017) 'How the other half live': Lay perspectives on health inequalities in an age of austerity. *Social Science & Medicine* 187, 268–275.

Gerhardt, S. (2004) *Why Love Matters; How Affection Shapes a Baby's Brain.* Routledge, London and New York.

Germond, P. and Cochrane, J. (2010) Healthworlds: conceptualising landscapes of health & healing. *Sociology* 44, 307–324.

Ghaderi, A., Tabatabaei, S.M., Nedjat, S. Javadi, M. and Larijani, B. (2018) Explanatory definition of the concept of spiritual health: a qualitative study in Iran. *Journal of Medical Ethics and History of Medicine* 11, 3–7.

Giuntoli, G. (2010) Understanding quality of life through Sen's capability framework: an application to people living with HIV/AIDS. PhD thesis, The Australian National University, Canberra.

Gkiouleka, A., Huijts, T., Beckfield, J. and Bambra, C. (2018) Understanding the micro and macro politics of health: intersectionality in health promotion inequalities, intersectionality and institutions: a research agenda. *Social Science & Medicine* 200, 92–98.

Golinowska, S., Groot, W., Baji, P. and Pavlova, M. (2016) Health promotion targeting older people. *BMC Health Services Research* 16, 5, 345.

Gouda, H.N., Charlson, F., Sorsdahl, K., Ahmazada, S., Ferrari, A.J., Erskine, H. *et al.* (2019) Burden of non-communicable diseases in sub-Saharan Africa, 1990–2017: results from the Global Burden of Disease Study 2017. *The Lancet* 7 (10), e1375–e1387.

Graham, C. (2008) Happiness and health: lessons – and questions – for public policy. *Health Affairs* 27, 72–87.

Green, J. (2000) The role of theory in evidence-based health promotion practice. *Health Education Research* 15, 125–129.

Green, J., Cross, R., Woodall, J. and Tones, K. (2019) *Health Promotion: Planning and Strategies.* 4th edn. Sage, London.

Gregg, J. and O'Hara, L. (2007a) Values and principles evident in current health promotion practice. *Health Promotion Journal of Australia* 18, 7–11.

Gregg, J. and O'Hara, L. (2007b) The Red Lotus Health Promotion Model: a new model for holistic, ecological and salutogenic health promotion practice. *Health Promotion Journal of Australia* 18, 12–19.

Gwyther, K., Swann, R., Casey, K, Purcell R, and Rice, S.M. (2019) Developing young men's wellbeing through community and school-based programs: a systematic review. *PLoS ONE* 14(5): e0216955. https://doi.org/10.1371/journal.pone.0216955

Hagell, A., Shah, R., Viner, R., Hargreaves, D., Varnes, L. and Heys, M. (2018) The social determinants of young people's health: identifying the key issues and assessing how young people are doing in the 2010s. Health Foundation Working Paper. Health Foundation, London.

Hall, J. and Taylor, R. (2003) Health for all beyond 2000: the demise of the Alma-Ata Declaration and primary care in developing countries. *The Medical Journal of Australia* 178, 17–20.

Hankivsky, O., Cormier, R. and Merich, D.D. (2009) *Intersectionality: Moving Women's Health Research and Policy Forward.* Women's Health Research Network, Vancouver.

Hawe, P., King, L., Noort, M., Gifford, S. and Lloyd, B. (1998) Working invisibly: health workers talk about capacity building in health promotion. *Health Promotion International* 13, 285–295.

Hawe, P., King, L., Noort, M., Jordens, C. and Lloyd, B. (2000) Indicators to help with capacity building in health promotion. NSW Health Department, Sydney.

Heard, E., Fitzgerald, F., Wigginton, B. and Mutch, A. (2019) Applying intersectionality theory in health promotion research and practice. *Health Promotion International* 1–11, doi: 10.1093/heapro/daz080.

Henderson, J. (2010) Expert and lay knowledge: a sociological perspective. *Nutrition and Dietetics* 67, 4–5.

Hylton, K. (2010) How a turn to critical race theory can contribute to our understanding of 'race', racism and anti-racism in sport. *Sociology of Sport* 45, 335–354.

Ingelhart, R. (1997) *Modernisation and Postmodernisation: Cultural, Economic and Political Change in 43 Societies.* Princeton University Press, Princeton, New Jersey.

Innstrand, S.T. and Christensen, M. (2018) Healthy Universities. The development and implementation of a holistic health promotion intervention programme especially adapted for staff working in the higher educational sector: the ARK study. *Global Health Promotion* 27, 68–76.

IUHPE (2019a) *Rotorua Statement - WAIORA: Promoting Planetary Health and Sustainable Development for All. IUHPE.* Available at: www.iuhpe.org (accessed 26 May 2020).

IUHPE (2019b) *Waiora – Indigenous Peoples' Statement for Planetary Health and Sustainable Development. IUHPE.* Available at: www.iuhpe.org (accessed 26 May 2020).

Jackson, S.F., Ridde, V., Valenti, H. and Gierman, N. (2007) Canada's role in international health promotion. In: O'Neil, M., Pederson, A., Dupere, S. and Rootman, I. (eds) *Health Promotion in Canada: Critical Perspectives*. Canadian Scholars Press Inc., Toronto.

Jelsøe, E., Thualagant, N., Holm, J., *et al.* (2018) A future task for health-promotion research: integration of health promotion and sustainable development. *Scandinavian Journal of Public Health* 46 (Suppl 20), 99–106.

Jentsch, B. (2004) Making southern realities count: research agendas and design in North-South collaborations. *International Journal of Social Research Methodology* 7, 259–269.

Jones, R. (2019) Climate change and Indigenous Health Promotion. *Global Health Promotion* 26, 3, 73–81.

Keneally, T. (2011) *Three Famines: Starvation and Politics*. Perseus, Reading, Massachusetts.

Keshavarz Mohammadi, N. (2020) One step back toward the future of health promotion: complexity-informed health promotion. *Health Promotion International* 34, 635–639.

Kharsany, A.B.M. and Karim, Q.A. (2016) HIV Infection and AIDS in sub-Saharan Africa: current status, challenges and opportunities. *Open AIDS Journal* 10, 34–48.

Khor, M. (2001) *Rethinking Globalisation: Critical Issues and Policy Choices*. Zed Books, London and New York.

Kickbusch, I., Allen, L. and Franz, C. (2016) The commercial determinants of health. *The Lancet Global Health* 4, e895–e896. https://doi.org/10.1016/S2214-109X(16)30217-0

Kings Fund (2015) Has the government delivered a new era for public health? Available at: https://www.kingsfund.org.uk/projects/verdict/has-government-delivered-new-era-public-health (accessed 25 August 2020).

Koh, H.K. (2010) A 2020 vision for healthy people. *New England Journal of Medicine* 362, 1653–1656, doi: 10.1056/NEJMp1001601

Kumar, A. and Dixit, V. (2017) Altruism, happiness and health among elderly people. *Indian Journal of Gerontology* 31 (4), 480–496.

Labbock, M. and Nazro, J. (1995) *Breastfeeding: Protecting a Natural Resource*. Institute for Reproductive Health, Washington, DC; cited in Macdonald, T. (2005) *Third World Hostage to First World Health*. Radcliffe Publishing, Oxford, UK.

Labonté, R. (1997) Econology: integrating health and sustainable development: guiding Principles for decision making. In: Sidell, M., Jones, L., Katz, J. and Peberdy, A. (eds) *Debates and Dilemmas in Promoting Health: A Reader*. Open University Press, Basingstoke, UK, pp. 260–270.

Labonté, R. (2010) Health promotion, globalisation and health. In: Douglas, J., Earle, S., Handsley, S., Jones, L., Lloyd, C.E. and Spurr, S. (eds) *A Reader in Promoting Public Health*. Sage, London, pp. 235–245.

Labonté, R. (2018) Reprising the globalization dimensions of international health. *Globalization and Health* 14, 49, doi: 10.1186/s12992-018-0368-3

Labonté, R. (2020) Globlization and health scholarship in a time of pandemic: from critical past to uncertain future. *Globalization and Health* 16, 31, doi: org/10.1186/s12992-020-00563-6

Labonté, R., Sanders, D., Msathole, T., Crush, J., Chianda, A., Dambisya, Y., Runnels, V., Packer, C, Mackenzie, A., Tomblin Murphy, G. and Bourgeault, I.L. (2015) Health worker migration from South Africa: causes, consequences and policy responses. *Human Resources for Health* 13, 92. Available at: http://human-resources-health.biomedcentral.com/articles/10.1186/s12960-015-0093-4 (accessed 11 May 2016).

Lahtinen, E., Koskinen-Ollonqvist, P., Rouvinen-Wilenius, P., Tuominen, P. and Mittelmark, M. (2005) The development of quality criteria for research: a Finnish approach. *Health Promotion International* 20, 306–315.

Langer, A., Meleis, A., Knaul, F.M., Atun, R., Aran, M. Arreola-Ornelas, H. *et al.* (2015) Women and Health: the key for sustainable development. *The Lancet* 386, 1165–1210.

Lave, J. and Wenger, E. (1998) *Communities of Practice: Learning, Meaning, and Identity*. Cambridge University Press, Cambridge, UK.

Lessa, I. (2006) Discursive struggles within social welfare: restaging teen motherhood. *British Journal of Social Work* 36, 283–298.

Levitas, R., Pantazis, C., Fahmy, E., Gordon, D., Lloyd, E. and Patsios, D. (2007) *The Multidimensional Analysis of Social Exclusion*. A Research Report for the Social Exclusion Task Force. Available at: https://dera.ioe.ac.uk/6853/1/multidimensional.pdf (accessed 25 August 2020).

Liyanagunawardena, T.R and Aboshady, O.A. (2017) Massive open online courses: a resource for health education in developing countries *Global Health Promotion*, doi: 10.1177/1757975916680970

Llewellyn, A., Simmonds, M., Owen, C.G. and Woolacott, N. (2016) Childhood obesity as a predictor of morbidity in adulthood: a systematic review and meta-analysis. *Obesity Reviews* 17(1), 56–67.

Local Government Information Unit (2012) *A Dose Of Localism – The Role of Councils in Public Health*. Local Government Information Unit, London.

Lupton, D. (1992) Discourse analysis – a new methodology for understanding the ideologies of health and illness. *Australian Journal of Public Health* 16, 145–150.

MacDonald, T.H. (1998) *Rethinking Health Promotion, A Global Approach*. Routledge, London.

MacDonald, T. (2006) *Health, Trade and Human Rights*. Radcliffe Publishing, Oxford, UK.

MacGregor, A., Currie, C. and Wetton, N. (1998) Eliciting the views of children about health in schools through the draw and write technique. *Health Promotion International* 13, 307–318.

Manji, F. (2006) Collaboration with the South: agents of aid or solidarity? In: Eade, D. (ed.) *Development, NGOs and Civil Society*. Oxfam, Oxford, UK.

Marinho, F., de Azeredo Passos, V.M., Malta, D.C., França, D.M.X., Araújo, V.E.M., Bustamante-Teixeira, M.T. et al., (2018) Burden of disease in Brazil, 1990–2016: a systematic subnational analysis for the Global Burden of Disease Study 2016. *The Lancet*, 392 (10149), 760–775.

Marmot, M., Allen, J., Boyce, T., Goldblatt, P. and Morrison, J. (2020) *Health Equity in England: The Marmot Review Ten Years On*. Institute of Health Equity, London.

Martell, L. (2010) *The Sociology of Globalization*. Polity, Cambridge, UK.

Mayall, B. (1994) *Negotiating Health: Primary School Children at Home and School*. Cassell, London.

McCartney, G., Bartley, M., Dundas, R., Katikireddi, V.S., Mitchell R., Popham, F., Walsh, D. and Wami, W. (2019) Theorising social class and its application to the study of health inequalities. *SSM Population Health* 100315. https://doi.org/10.1016/j.ssmph.2018.10.015

McClean, S. (2003) Globalization and health. In: Orme, J., Powell, J., Taylor, P., Harrison, T. and Grey, M. (eds) *Public Health for the 21st Century: New Perspectives on Policy, Participation and Practice*. Open University Press, Maidenhead, UK.

McGregor, C. (2004) Care(full) deliberation: a pedagogy for citizenship. *Journal of Transformative Education* 2, 90–106.

McIntyre, E., Saliba, A. and McKenzie, K. (2020) Subjective wellbeing in the Indian general population: a validation study of the Personal Wellbeing Index. *Quality of Life Research* 29, 1073–1081.

McQueen, D.V. (2000) Perspectives on health promotion: theory, evidence, practice and the emergence of complexity. *Health Promotion International* 15, 95–97.

McQueen, D.V. (2001) Strengthening the evidence base for health promotion. *Health Promotion International* 16, 261–268.

McQueen, D.V., Kickbusch, I., Potvin, L., Peliakn, J.M., Balbo, L. and Abel, T. (eds) (2007) *Health and Modernity: The Role of Theory in Health Promotion*. Springer, New York.

Mercer, H. (2020) A consensus-building strategy of health promotion in the Americas *Global Health Promotion* 27, 1, 3–5.

Milne, E. (2018) The transfer of public health to local authorities suggests alternatives are possible. *BMJ* 361, k2330, doi: 10.1136/bmj.k2330

Misan, G.M.H., Oosterbroek, C. and Wilson, N.J. (2017) Informing health promotion in rural men's sheds by examination of participant health status, concerns, interests, knowledge and behaviours. *Health Promotion Journal of Australia* 28, 207–216.

Mittelmark, M. (2005) Global health promotion: challenges and opportunities. In: Scriven, A. and Garman, S. (eds) (2005) *Promoting Health: Global Perspectives*. Palgrave Macmillan, Basingstoke, UK.

Moghadam, V. (2005) *Globalizing Women: Transnational Feminist Networks*. Johns Hopkins University Press, Baltimore, Maryland.

Moore, S. (2010) Is the healthy body gendered? Toward a feminist critique of the new paradigm of health. *Body & Society* 16, 95–118.

Morris, M. and Bunjun, B. (2007) *Using Intersectional Feminist Frameworks in Research: A Resource for Embracing the Complexities of Women's Lives*. Canadian Research Institute for the Advancement of Women, Ottawa.

Naples, N. (2003) *Feminism and Method: Ethnography, Discourse Analysis, and Activist Research*. Routledge, New York.

National Health and Medical Research Council (1996) *Promoting the Health of Indigenous Australians. A Review of Infrastructure Support for Aboriginal and Torres Strait Islander Health Advancement*. Final report and recommendations, NHMRC, Canberra, part 2, 4.

Navarro, V. (2009) What we mean by social determinants of health. *Global Health Promotion* 16, 5–16.

Nelson, G. and Prilleltensky, I. (2010) *Community Psychology: In Pursuit of Liberation and Well-being*. Palgrave Macmillan, Basingstoke, UK.

Nesterak, E. (2020) *Imagining the Next Decade of Behavioral Science. Behavioral Scientist*. [Internet] Available at: www.behavorialscientist.org (accessed 21 May 2020).

Newell, C. and South, J. (2009) Participating in community research: exploring the experiences of lay researchers in Bradford. *Community, Work and Family* 12, 75–89.

NHS (2014) *Five Year Forward View*. Available at: https://www.england.nhs.uk/wp-content/uploads/2014/10/5yfv-web.pdf (accessed 3 June 2020).

NHS (2019) *Health and Care of People with Learning Disabilities, Experimental Statistics: 2017 to 2018 [PAS]* Available at: https://digital.nhs.uk/data-and-information/publications/statistical/health-and-care-of-people-with-learning-disabilities/experimental-statistics-2017-to-2018 (accessed 2 June 2020).v

NIEHS (2015) *Climate Change and Human Health*. National Institute of Environmental Health Sciences, North Carolina.

Nunes, S., Fernandes, H., Fisher, J. and Fernandes, M.G. (2018) Psychometric properties of the Brazilian version of the lived experience component of Spiritual Health and Life-Orientation Measure (SHALOM). *Psicologia: Reflexäo e Critcia* 31(2), doi:10.1186/s4115-018-0083-2

Nussbaum, M.C. (2000) *Women and Development: The Capabilities Approach*. Cambridge University Press, Cambridge, UK.

Nyamwaya, D. (2003) Health promotion in Africa: strategies, players, challenges and prospects. *Health Promotion International* 18, 85–87.

O'Donnell, M.P. (2009) Definition of health promotion 2.0: embracing passion, enhancing motivation, recognizing dynamic balance, and creating opportunities. *American Journal of Health Promotion* 24, iv.

Oliver, M. (1983) *Social Work and Disabled People*. Macmillan, Basingstoke, UK.

Oliver, M. (1990) *The Politics of Disablement*. Macmillan, Basingstoke, UK.

Orme, J. and Dooris, M. (2010) Integrating health and sustainability: the higher education sector as a timely catalyst. *Health Education Research* 25, 425–437.

Ortiz, D.A.P. and Abrigo, M.R.M. (2017) The triple burden of disease. *Philippine Institute for Development Studies* XVII, 2, 1–2.

Outram, D. (2006) *The Enlightenment*, 2nd edition. Cambridge University Press, Cambridge, UK.

Ozgediz, D. and Riviello, R. (2008) The 'other' neglected diseases in global public health: surgical conditions in sub-Saharan Africa. *PLoS Med* 5(6): e121.

Peate, I. (2017) Mental health provision: Time for a whole-system approach. *British Journal of School Nursing* 12 (10), doi: 10.12968/bjsn.2017.12.10.494

Peckham, S., Gadsby, E., Jenkins, L., Coleman, A., Bramwell, D. and Perkins, N. (2017) Views of public health leaders in English local authorities – changing perspectives following the transfer of responsibilities from the National Health Service to local government *Local Government Studies* 43, 5, 842–863.

Pederson, A., Rootman, I. and O'Neill, M. (2005) Health promotion in Canada: back to the past or towards a promising future? In: Scriven, A. and Garman, S. (eds) *Promoting Health: Global Perspectives*. Palgrave Macmillan, Basingstoke, UK.

Pedersen, A., Greves, L. and Poole, N. (2014) Gender-transformative health promotion for women: a framework for action. *Health Promotion International* 30, 140–150.

Pescosolido, B.A., Manago, B. and Olafsdottir, S. (2019) The global use of diverse medical systems. *Social Science & Medicine*. https://doi.org/10.1016/j.socscimed.2019.112721 (accessed 25 August 2020).

Peterson, C. (2007) *Hearing from Students: How Transformative Education Really Changes Lives*. NAFSA, Seattle, Washington.

Petterson, B. (2011) Some bitter-sweet reflections on the Ottawa Charter commemoration cake: a personal discourse from an Ottawa rocker. *Health Promotion International* 26, S2, ii173-ii179.

Pisek, P.E. and Greenhalgh, T. (2001) The challenge of complexity in health care. *British Medical Journal* 323, 625–628.

Pols, J. (2014) Knowing patients: turning patient knowledge into science. *Science, Technology and Human Values* 39(1), 73–97.

Popay, J., Bennett, S., Thomas, C., Williams, G., Gatrell, A. and Bostock, L. (2003) Beyond 'beer, fags, egg and chips'? Exploring lay understandings of social inequalities in health. *Sociology of Health and Illness* 25, 1–23.

Porter, C. (2006) Ottawa to Bangkok: changing health promotion discourse. *Health Promotion International* 22, 72–79.

Poskitt, E.M. (2014) Childhood obesity in low- and middle-income countries. *Paediatric International Child Health* 34, 239–249.

Potvin. L. and Jones, C.M (2011) Twenty-five years after the Ottawa Charter: the critical role of health promotion for public health. *Revue Canadienne De Sante Publique* 102, 4, 244–248.

Prattley, J., Buffel, T., Marshall, A. and Nazroo, J. (2020) Area effects on the level and development of social exclusion in later life. *Social Science and Medicine* 246, 112722. https://doi.org/10.1016/j.socscimed.2019.112722

Prior, L. (2003) Belief, knowledge and expertise: the emergence of the lay expert in medical sociology. *Sociology of Health and Illness* 25, 41–57.

PHE (Public Health England (2016) Public health skills and knowledge framework (PHSKF) https://www.gov.uk/government/publications/public-health-skills-and-knowledge-framework-phskf (accessed 5 June 2020).

PHE (2019a) Public Health Skills and Knowledge Framework: August 2019 Update. https://www.gov.uk/government/publications/public-health-skills-and-knowledge-framework-phskf/public-health-skills-and-knowledge-framework-august-2019-update (accessed 5 June 2020).

PHE (2019b) *Public Health Skills and Knowledge Framework Sub-functions Explained*. Public Health England, London.

Pyle, E. and Hassle, C. (2018) Children's well-being and social relationships, UK: 2018. Office for National Statistics, London.

Radley, A. and Billig, M. (1996) Accounts of health and illness: dilemmas and representations. *Sociology of Health and Illness* 18, 220–240.

Ranmuthugala, G., Plumb, J.J., Cunningham, F.C., Georgiou, A., Westbrook, J.I. and Braithwaite, J. (2011) How and why are communities of practice established in the healthcare sector? A systematic review of the literature. *BMC Health Services Research* 11, 273. https://doi.org/10.1186/1472-6963-11-273

Raphael, D. (2003) Barriers to addressing the societal determinants of health: public health units and poverty in Ontario, Canada. *Health Promotion International* 18, 397–405.

Raphael, D. (2011) A discourse analysis of the social determinants of health. *Critical Public Health* 21, 221–236.

Ratima, M. (2019) Leadership for planetary health and sustainable development: health promotion community capacities for working with Indigenous peoples in the application of Indigenous knowledge. *Global Health Promotion* 26, 3–5.

Rawls, J. (1971) *A Theory of Justice*. Harvard University Press, Cambridge, Massachusetts.

Rijal, A., Adhikari, T.B., Khan, J.A.M., Berg-Beckhoff, G. (2018) The economic impact of non-communicable diseases among households in South Asia and their coping strategy: a systematic review. *PLoS ONE* 13 (11), e02057245.

Robertson, A. (1998) Shifting discourses on health in Canada: from health promotion to population health. *Health Promotion International* 13, 155–166.

Robertson, S. and Baker, P. (2017) Men and health promotion in the United Kingdom. *Health Education Journal* 76(1), 102–113, https://doi.org/10.1177/0017896916645558

Robertson, S., Gough, B., Hanna, E., Raine, G., Robinson, M., Seims, A. and White, A. (2018) Successful mental health promotion with men: the evidence from 'tacit knowledge'. *Health Promotion International* 33(2), 334–344.

Robertson, S., White, A., Gough, B., Robinson, R., Seims, A., Raine, G. and Hanna, E. (2015) *Promoting Mental Health and Wellbeing with Men and Boys: What Works?* Leeds Beckett University: Centre for Men's Health, Leeds, UK.

Salant, T. and Gehlert, S. (2008) Collective memory, candidacy and victimisation: community epidemiologies of breast cancer risk. *Sociology of Health and Illness* 30, 599–615.

Sampson, U.K.A., Amunyunzu-Nyamongo, M. and Mensah, G.A. (2013) Health promotion and cardiovascular disease prevention in sub-Saharan Africa. *Progress in Cardiovascular Diseases* 344–355.

Sanders, D., Stern, R., Struthers, P., Ngulube, T.J. and Onya, H. (2008) What is needed for health promotion in Africa: band-aid, live aid or real change? *Critical Public Health* 18, 509–519.

Sawyerr, A. (2002) *Challenges Facing African Universities: Selected Issues*. Paper presented to the 45th Annual Meeting of the African Studies Association, 5–8 December, Washington, DC.

Schwab, K. (2016) *The Fourth Industrial Revolution*. World Economics Forum, New York.

Scott-Samuel, A. and Springett, J. (2007) Hegemony or health promotion? Prospects for reviving England's lost discipline. *Journal of the Royal Society of Health* 127, 211–214.

Scott-Samuel, A. and Wills, J. (2007) Health promotion in England: sleeping beauty or corpse? *Health Education Journal* 66, 115–119.

Secretary of State for Health (2012) *Health and Social Care Act 2012*. The Stationery Office, London.

Seedhouse, D. (1997) *Health Promotion: Philosophy, Prejudice and Practice*. John Wiley & Sons, Chichester, UK.

Seidler, Z.E, Dawes, A.J., Rice, S.M., Oliffe, J.L. and Dhillon, H.M. (2016) The role of masculinity in men's help seeking for depression: A systematic review. *Clinical Psychology Review* 49 (2016) 106–118.

Sen, A. (1980) Equality of what? In: McMurrin, S.M. (ed.) *Tanner Lectures on Human Values*. University of Utah Press, Salt Lake City, Utah. Reprinted in Sen, A. (1982) *Choice, Welfare and Measurement*. Blackwell, Oxford, UK, pp. 353–369.

Sen, A. (1993) Capability and well-being. In: Nussbaum, M. and Sen, A. (eds) *The Quality of Life*. Oxford University Press, Oxford, UK.

Sen, A. (1999) *Development as Freedom*. Taylor and Francis, New York.

Shrecker, T. (2016) Globalization, austerity and health equity politics: taming the inequality machine, and why it matters. *Critical Public Health* 26, 4–13.

Shrecker, T. (2020) Globalization and health: political grand challenges. *Review of International Political Economy* 27, 26–47.

Smith, K.E. and Anderson, R. (2018) Understanding lay perspectives on socioeconomic health inequalities in Britain: a meta-ethnography. *Sociology of Health & Illness* 40(1),146–170, doi:10.1111/1467-9566.12629

Snape, D. and Manclossi, S. (2018) *Loneliness in Children and Young People*. Office for National Statistics, London.

South, J. (2014) Health promotion by communities and in communities: Current issues for research and practice. *Scandinavian Journal of Public Health* 42(Suppl 15), 82–87.

Southby, K. (2019) An exploration and proposed taxonomy of leisure: befriending for adults with learning disabilities *British Journal of Learning Disabilities* 47, 223–232.

Sparks, M. (2011) Building healthy public policy: don't believe the misdirection. *Health Promotion International* 26, 259–262.

Stiglitz, J. (2006) *Making Globalisation Work: The Next Steps to Global Justice*. Allen Lane, London.

Stock, C., Milz, S. and Meier, S. (2010) Network evaluation: principles, structures and outcomes of the German working group of health promoting universities. *Global Health Promotion* 17, 25–32.

Thomas, C. and Warwick-Booth, L. (2019) *The State of Women's Health in Leeds: Women's Voices. Final Report*. Leeds Beckett University, Leeds, UK.

Tian, X., Zhou, L., Mao, X., Zhao, T., Song, Y. and Jagusztyn, M. (2003) Beijing health promoting universities: practice and evaluation. *Health Promotion International* 18, 107–113.

Tillmann, S., Button, B., Coen, S.E. and Gilliland, J.A. (2019) 'Nature makes people happy, that's what it sort of means': children's definitions and perceptions of nature in rural Northwestern Ontario. *Children's Geographies* 17(6), 705–718.

Tomlinson, M.W. and Kelly, G.P. (2013) Is everybody happy? The politics and measurement of national wellbeing. *Policy & Politics* 41(2), 139–157.

UN (1986) Declaration on the Right to Development. Available at: http://www2.ohchr.org/english/law/rtd.htm (accessed 3 November 2012).

UNICEF (2019) Children, food and nutrition: growing well in a changing world. UNICEF, New York.

Vader, J.P. (2006) Spiritual health: the next frontier. *European Journal of Public Health* 16, 457.

Veary, J., Luginaah, I., Magitta, N., F., Shilla, D.J. and Oni, T. (2019) Urban health in Africa: a critical global public health priority. *BMC Public Health* 19, 340. https://doi.org/10.1186/s12889-019-6674-8

Viens, A.M. and Vass, C. (2020) Frameworks and guidance to support ethical public health practice. *Journal of Public Health* 42, 203–207.

Wainberg, M.L., Scirza, P., Shultz, J.M., Helpman, L., Mootz, J.J., Johnson, K.A., Neria, Y., Bradford, J.E., Oquendo, M.A. and Arbuckle, M.R. (2017) Challenges and opportunities in global mental health: a research-to-practice perspective. *Current Psychiatry Reports* 19, 8, doi: 10.1007/s11920-017-0780-z

Walby, S. (2007) Complexity theory, systems theory, and multiple intersecting social inequalities. *Philosophy of the Social Sciences* 37, 449–470.

Ward, M., McGarrigle, C.A. and Kenny, R.A. (2019) More than health: quality of life trajectories among older adults – findings from the Irish Longitudinal Study of Ageing (TILDA). *Quality of Life Research* 28, 429–439.

Warwick-Booth, L and Coan, S. (2020) *Using Creative Qualitative Methods in Evaluating Gendered Health Promotion Interventions. Technical Report*. Sage Research Methods Cases (online resource), doi: https://doi.org/10.4135/9781529707281

Warwick-Booth, L. and Cross, R. (2018) *Global Health Studies: A Social Determinants Perspective*. Polity Press, Cambridge, UK.

Warwick-Booth, L., Woodward, J., O'Dwyer, L. and Di Martino, S. (2018a) *An Evaluation of Leeds CCG Gypsy and Traveller Health Improvement Project*. Leeds Beckett University, Leeds, UK.

Warwick-Booth, L., Woodall, J.R., Cross, R.M., Bagnall, A. and South, J. (2018b) Health promotion education in changing and challenging times: reflections from the UK. *Health Education Journal*, doi: https://doi.org/10.1177/0017896918784072

Welter, C.R., Jacobs, B., Jarpe-Ratner, E., Naji, S. and Gruss, K. (2017) Building capacity for collective action to address population health improvement through communities of practice: a distance based education pilot. *Pedagogy in Health Promotion* 3, 1S, 21S–27S.

White, A.K. and Pettifer, M. (2007) *Hazardous Waist: Tackling Male Weight Problems*. Radcliffe Publishing, Oxford, UK.

White, A., McKee, M., Richardson, N., Madsen S.A., de Sousa, B., de Visser, R., Hogston, R., Makara, P. and Zatoński, W. (2011) Europe's men need their own health strategy. *British Medical Journal* 343, d7397.

White, S.C. (2017) Relational wellbeing: re-centring the politics of happiness, policy and self. *Policy & Politics* 45, 121–136.

WHO (World Health Organization) (1978) *Declaration of Alma-Ata, International Conference on Primary Health Care, Alma-Ata, USSR, 6–12 September 1978*. WHO, Geneva. Available at: http://www.who.int/publications/almaata_declaration_en.pdf (accessed 3 November 2012).

WHO (2006) *Working Together for Health*. WHO, Geneva.

WHO (2009) *Milestones in Health Promotion: Statements from Global Conferences*. WHO, Geneva.

WHO (2018) The health and well-being of men in the WHO European Region: better health through a gender approach. WHO, Geneva.

WHO (2019) 1 in 3 people globally do not have access to safe drinking water. Available at: www.who.org (accessed 13 May 2020).

WHO (2020) Key Facts: Obesity and Overweight. Available at: www.who.org (accessed 18 May 2020).

Wilkinson, S. and Kitzinger, C. (1994) *Women's Health – Feminist Perspectives*. Taylor & Francis, London.

Wolf, M. (2004) *Why Globalization Works: The Case for the Global Market Economy*. Yale University Press, New Haven, Connecticut.

Woodall, J., Warwick-Booth, L., South, J., and Cross, R. (2018) What makes health promotion research distinct? *Scandinavian Journal of Public Health* 46 (Suppl 20), 118–122.

Index

Note: bold page numbers indicate tables; italic page numbers indicate figures.

Abbott, P.A. 20, 21, 22, 210
ABCD (Assets Based Community Development) 62, *64*, 67
Abercrombie, N. 87
Aboriginal peoples 32, 214
academic health promotion 187, 193–195, 201
access 17, 44, 54, 122, 126, 201, 204
accountability 3, 54, 156, 172
Aceves-Martins, M. 196–198
action learning/research 148, 162
activism 121, 167–168, 171, 200
    health 65–66, *66*, 67, 170, 192, 196
addiction 122, 134, 135
Adelaide conference (WHO, 1988) 11–12, 13–14, **15**
Adeleye, O.A. 94
ADEPT model 98
advertising 122, 128, 129, 164
    see also marketing
advocacy 11, **15**, 43, 75, 90–94, 162, 176
    criticisms of 93
    defined 90–91
    four models/two dimensions of 91–92
    health promoters' role in 93–94
    and lobby groups 92–93
    and social marketing 128
    types of 91, **91**
Afghanistan 16
Africa 21, 117–118, 186, 190, 195, 200, 210
    community development/empowerment in 6, 25
    Ebola in 96, 204
    foreign aid to 5–6
    and globalization 201, 202
    health worker crisis in 191–192
    HIV/AIDS in 16, 202, 204
    infant/child mortality in 16, 204
    NCDs in 7, 204
    NGOs/civil society in 61, 156, 171
    training/education in 177, 207, 209
    women in 16, 61
    see also specific countries
African-Americans 28, 53, 195, 198–199
age factor 22, 47, 113, 116
ageing population 12, 189
agency 27, 41, 67, 169, 210
agenda setting 3, 75, 82, 87, 92
agents 118, **172**, 173

agriculture 80, 113, 173, 194, 203
Ai Wei Wei 121
aid 5–6, 51, **97**, 173
air quality 77, *77*, 80
Airhihenbuwa, Collins 175, 195
Albrecht, G. 194
alcohol 6, 12, 58, 165, 189, 196
    and lobby groups/media campaigns 92, 117
    and motivational interviewing 135
    and policy 7, 76, 80, 83, 173
Algeria 113
Alidu, L. 22
Allah Nikkhah, H. 30
Allegrante, John 175
Allen, M. 166
alliances *see* partnerships
Allmark, P. 195
allotments/greenhouses 58, 62, *63*
Alma Ata Conference (WHO, 1978) 10, 186–187, 189, 191
    Declaration of 14, **15**, 42, 56, 66, 187, 190
Alston, P. 81, 86
Altogether Better programme (UK) 25
altruism 213
Aluttis, C. 207
Anderson, R. 210–211
Anielski, M. 213
anthropology 20
anti-oppressive practice 195–201
Antonovsky, A. 9, 10, 18, 50
Anugwom, E.E. 191–192
Appiah, K.A. 112
Archer, M. 168
Aristotle 1
Arnott, D. 98
Arnstein, S. 56
Arsenijevic, J. 190
ART (antiretroviral therapy) 65
artificial intelligence (AI) 121, 127
asbestos 165–166
Asia 16, 25, 177, 201, 204
see also specific countries
asset-based approach 33
    and communities 48, 49, 50, 62, *64*, 67, 176
Assets Based Community Development (ABCD) 62, *64*, 67
Astana Declaration (2018) 56, 66
Asthana, S. 161

asthma 123, 125
asylum seekers/refugees 16, 122, 178
Atkinson, S. 213
Attree, P. 54
Attwood, M. 173, 178, 179, 208
Aubel, Judi 52
austerity policies 80–81, 84–86, 193, 211
Australia 3, 21, 48, 160, 189
    Aboriginal peoples 32, 214
autism 117, 123
autonomy 30, 32, 134, 163, 164, **220**
Ayran, G. 119

Backett, K. 21
Bagnall, A.M. 43, 60, 119
Baim-Lance, A. 51
Baistow, K. 29
balance, lay concepts of 20–21, 189
Baldwin, L. 194
Bamako initiative 57
Bambra, C. 79, 161, 211, 216
Bangkok Conference/Charter (WHO, 2005) 13, 75, 155, 190, 206
Bangladesh 53, 177, 214
Bantaba approach (Gambia) 120–121
Barić, L. 151, 155
Barnes, B. 27
Barnes, M. 95
Barrett, E. 87, 172
Barry, J. 93
Barry, M. 176, 221
Baru, R.V. 201–202
Baum, F. 3, 43, 151, 202–203
Baxter Magdola, M. 112
Beattie, A. 172
Becker, C. 18
behaviour change 14, **15**, 23, 44, 54, 76, 137, 215, **218**
    and digital technology 121, 122, 124, 125
    and fear/shock tactics 166–167
    and health communication 106, 109, 119, 132
    and social marketing 128, 129
behaviour change theory 124, 132–138
    and beliefs/perceptions 132–133
    and COM-B model 137–138
    Covid-19 case study 137, 138
    critiques of 136–138
    Health Action Model 132, 133, 136, 138
    Health Belief Model 128, 132, 133, 138
    and intention 136
    and motivation 133
    and motivational interviewing *see* motivational interviewing
    Planned Behaviour Theory 132, 133, 136, 138
    Protection Motivation Theory 132, 133, 136, 138
    and stages of change 135–136, 155
    Transtheoretical Model 132, 133, 135, 138

behavioural science 215–216
Bellander, T. 195
Bergeron, K. 207
Berne, Eric 114
Bhutan 211, 213, 214
Bichmann, W. 59
Big Data 107, 125–126, 137
Bill & Melinda Gates Foundation 6, 91, 96, **97**, 202
Billig, M. 210
Black Lives Matter 26, 92
Black Report (1980) 5, 192
Blaxter, M. 17, 20, 22, 210, 212
Blinkhorn, A. 155
Blitstein, J.L. 127
BMA (British Medical Association) 92, 98
BMI (body mass index) 175
Bolivia 113
Bornstein, D. 90
bottom-up processes
    and community participation/development 57, 65
    and health communication 106, 119–121, 123, 128
    and policy 89, 90, 94
    and top-down processes 3, 43, 55, 148, 149, 171, 172–175, **172**, *174*
Bourdieu, P. 44, 47, 126, 189–190
Branscum, P. 135
Brazil 53, 58, 111, 204
breast cancer 108, 119, 195
breastfeeding 65
Brehm, M.V. 94–95, 209
Britain (UK) 7, 14, 20, 21, 22–23, 50, 168, 177, 189, 190
    Altogether Better programme in 25
    austerity policies in 81, 84–86
    and Brexit 96–97
    children/young people in 198
    CHWs in 53
    community-centred approaches in 60, 66, 67
    Conservative government of 84, 88
    Covid-19 crisis in 51, 121
    digital technology in 124, 126
    evidence-based practice in 158, 160
    happiness/wellbeing in 213
    Health Act (2007) 98
    health education in 206
    health inequities in 2, 4, 5, 14, 16, 211
    health policy in 80
    Health and Social Care Act (2012) 192
    lobbying in 92
    New Labour government 94, 193
    NHS in *see* NHS
    older people in 198
    partnership working in 94
    policy actors in 87
    Public Health Skills and Knowledge Framework 188–189
    racism in 196

settings approach in 151
social marketing in 129
social policy in 79
Thatcher government 192
see also England; Scotland; Wales
British Medical Association (BMA) 92, 98
bronchial conditions 58
Brown, K.F. 7
Brown, R.C. 76
Brownson, R.C. 160
Bunjun, B. 200
Bunton, R. 24, 194
Burke, B. 25, 27
Burke, Edmund 165
Bury, M. 23

Cairney, P. 98
Calnan, M. 17, 210
Campbell, C. 65, 110, 186
Campbell Library of Systematic Reviews 160
Canada 10, 21, 32, 53, 92, 98, 160, 165, 190, 213
cancer 7, 53, 123, 177, 196, 204
    breast 108, 119, 195
capability 24, 214
capacity building 32, 91, 155, 206–208
capitalism 3, 5, 156
    new 190
Capstick, S. 20, 23
car accidents 58, 204
cardiovascular diseases 191, 198–199, 204
carers 51
Carey, G. 80
Caribbean 16
Carlisle, S. 91, 95
Carrington, W. 207
Carruth, L. 189
Carter, M. 175
Catford, J. 191
Cattan, M. 198
Cattaneo, L. 25
Chapman, A. 25
Chapman, L. 215
charities 96, **97**, 170
Chau, J.Y. 127
chemotherapy 119
Chen, H. 189
Chibanda, Dixon 52
Chicago (USA) 58
Child-to-Child initiative 169–170
childbirth 51
children/infants 23, 77, 79, 119, 123, 153
    agency of 169
    and grandmothers 52
    and mortality 8, 16, 53, 59, 81, 167, 204
    neglected in health promotion 196–198, *197*
    and obesity 90, 164, 203
    and parents 79, 122, 175, 177, 195
    and women's health/rights 11
China 21, 51, 52, 78, 121, 164, 209
choice 7, 11, 27, 28, 79, 164, 215
    architecture 129, 130, 212
    and health communication 108, 109, 111, 116, 124, 128
    and health literacy 130
    and intervention ladder 166
    political 13, 81
Christensen, M. 225
chronic disease 23, 51, 126
Chuah, F.L.H. 59–60
CHWs (community health workers) 51–56
    activist role of 53
    defined 53
    and health professionals 55
    issues with 54–56
Cinderby, S. 50
citizenship 4, 149, *149*, 167–171
    and Child-to-Child initiative 169–170
    and community activism 167–168
    and NGOs 167, 170–171
    participative 168
    and solid waste management 168–169
civil society 3, 13, 42, 43, 148, 155, 167, 222
    see also NGOs
class 5, 22, 23, 44, 62, 199
climate change 3, 76, 83, 186, 190, 202–203, 204, 212, 216
co-production 48, 51, 67, 123, 162, 205
coalitions 92, 95, 156
Cochrane Collaboration 160
Cochrane, J. 210
coherence, sense of 18, 50
Coleman, J.S. 44, 47, 48
collaborative working *see* partnerships
Collinson, M. 207
COM-B model 137–138
Commission on Social Determinants of Health *see* CSDH
communication theories 106, 107–109, *109*, 118, 127, 194, 215
    see also health communication
communitarianism 93, 168, 195
communities 41–67, 148–149
    and communication 106, 110, 113, 116, 117, 119–120, 121
    and Covid-19 crisis 51
    defined/use of term 41–42
    empowerment *see* community empowerment
    and happiness 49–50
    'hard-to-reach' groups 53, 119, 121, 153, **217**, **220**
    and health activism 65–66, *66*
    and health professionals 25–26, 148, 173–175
    healthy/health-enabling 1, 41, 43, 49–50, 65
    indigenous 16, 21, 32, 190, 214, 221
    and lay perspective 50–56

communities (*continued*)
    and mapping *43*, 48, 58, *64*, 168
    and networks *see* networks
    online 124, 195
    and Ottawa Charter 10, 11, 14
    and outsiders 6
    and participatory approaches 41, 43, 50
    and policy **78**, 95
    of practice 208
    and public health crises 50, 51, 66
    and resilience 41, 42, 48, 49, 50, 65
    and social capital *see* social capital
    and trust 44, 45, 46–47
    and universities 208–209
    and WHO 42
    see also neighbourhoods
community activism 61, 167–168
'Community Arts for Health' projects 119
community commissioning 48
community development 31, 32, 41, 43, 56–57, 60–65, 67, 159, 172
    and ABCD 62, *64*
    in Africa 25
    defined/founding values of 60–61
    and Freire 61–62
    and health improvement 62–65
    and neoliberalism/big business 65
    and social capital 48, 61
    and storytelling 62, 64
    sustainable 54, 171
community empowerment 6, 27–29, 41, 42, 43, 66, *174*
    and activism 65
    and bottom-up/top-down processes *174*
    and community development 61
    and community participation 56, 57–58
    continuum 29, *29*, 60
    and education 106
    and grassroots organizations 3, 59, 173
    mediated/socio-political 60
    and Nairobi Call to Action 13
    and Ottawa Charter 11
community engagement 14, 54, 60, 62, 63, 65, 95, 208–209
community health champions 149
community health workers *see* CHWs
community participation 43–44, 50, 56–60, *57*, 93, 148–149, 167, 190
    community development approach 56–57
    continuum/spidergram of 59, *60*
    and empowerment 56, 57–58, 59, 60
    evaluating, challenges in 59–60
    and Grandmother Project 52
    health planning approach 56
    ladder/spectrum of 56, *57*
    medical approach 56
    and participatory budgeting (PB) 58–59, 66
    and Tostan (Senegal) approach 60, 61
community psychology 194

Community-Led Total Sanitation movement 167
competence 25, 55, 59, 132, 148, 149, 176, 178
    community 28, 194
complexity 29, 195, 211, **217**, 222
Conner, M. 138
conscientization 25, 26, 62, 113, 120
conservatism 47, **85**, 86, 88, 93, 190
constructionism 158–159, 210, **219**
control 19, *19*, 21, 42, 43, 67, 110, 128
    and digital technology 122, 123, 124
Cook, A. 94
COPD (chronic obstructive pulmonary disease) 23
Copenhagen discussion paper (WHO, 1986) 31
Corcoran, N. 131
Cornish, F. 110
coronary heart disease 23, 172
cost-benefit analysis 128, 133
Costa Rica 213
counselling 106, 111, 115
    and health coaching 134–135
Covid-19 pandemic 2, 17, 23, 51, 66, 77, 86, 96, 165, 194, 204, 222
    and behaviour change 137, 138, 216
    and digital communication 121, 125
    evidence base for 162
    inconsistent messages for 106
Craig, J.V. 161
Craig, R.L. 90
Crammond, B.R. 80
Crawford, R. 21, 22, 124
Cribb, A. 163
critical awareness/dialogue 25, 26, 62, 112, 195
Cross, R. 25, 132, 162, 207
Crossley, N. 168
Crow, D. 84
crowdsourcing 125
CRT (critical race theory) 196
CSDH (Commission for Social Determinants of Health, 2008) 2–3, 78, 176, 199
Cuba 16
cultural aspects 17, 21, 32, 52, 84, 163, 164, 165, 196
    and health communication 116
Curibata Declaration (2016) 86
Curtis, V. 166–167
Cyril, S. 25

Dahlgren, G. 2, 82, 125
Dalrymple, J. 25, 27
data security 107, 123
databases 160
Davies, R. 48
Davison, C. 21, 23
De Vos, P. 57
de-Graft Aikins, A. 23
death *see* mortality
Deaton, Angus 5–6

Deeming, C. 83
dementia 123
democracy 12, 31, 164, 190, 193
    and activism 121
    and community participation 58
    and education 4, 111, 115, 169
    ethical aspects of 164
    and policy 86, 87, 88, 92, 93, 95, 172
demographic trends 12–13
Denman, S. 150
Denmark 23, 124
depression 27, 52, 122, 189
Detragiache, E. 207
developing world 2, 5–6, 12, 52, 161–162, 189
    and aid 5–6, 51, 97, 173
    and globalization 201–202
    and obesity 203
    triple burden of disease in 204
development 5–6, 7, 211, 212, 214
    sustainable *see* sustainability
DeVerteuil, G. 65
Dewey, J. 110–111
Dhooge, Y. 26
d'Houtaud, A. 22
diabetes 23, 122, 123, 204
diarrhoea 2, 8, 167, 204
diet/nutrition 1, 6, 21, 122, 135, 159, 202
    and community fruit/vegetable growing 58, 62, 63
    healthy eating guidelines 92, 116, 159, 175, 196
    and policy 11
dieticians 138, 175, 177
digital technology 106, 117, 121–127, 149, 216
    and Big Data 107, 125–126, 137
    challenges for health of 126–127
    and Covid-19 pandemic 121, 125
    and digital divide 126, 137
    and eHealth literacy 131
    and health promotion principles 123–124
    and health service management 124–125
    and individualistic approach to health 124
    and security/privacy 107, 122, 123, 125–126
    telehealth/telecare platforms 123
    video games/virtual reality 123
    wearables 122, 123, 127
    see also mobile phones; social media
Dillard, J.P. 166, 167
disability 87, 116, 126, 172, 199
discourse analysis 189–190
disease *see* infectious diseases; NCDs
Dixey, R. 164, 165, 191
Dixit, V. 213
doctors *see* health professionals
dog bites 58
Doherty, B. 93
domestic violence 28
Dooris, M. 150, 152, 153, 155
Dorling, Danny 216

Douglas, Jenny 195–196
Douglas, R. 95
Dower, N. 220
Dowling, B. 94
Downie, R.S. 154, 164–165
Doyal, L. 196
drama/theatre 62, 115, 116, 117, 120, 121
Draper, A. 59
drugs 58, 166
Duncan, P. 17, 163, 190, 193
Durie, M. 32

E2Pi (Evidence to Policy initiative) 162
Eade, D. 170
Ebola 96, 204
ecological strategies 10, 12, 32, 33, 212, 216, **217**, **218**
    and Ottawa Charter 150, 190
    and settings approach 151, 152, 155
    and social capital 43
    see also environment; sustainability
economic determinants of health 43, 49, 78, 125, 190
    see also austerity policies
economic growth 3, 211, 212
economic recession 79, 80–81, 84–86
education 1, *12*, 31, 110–112, 124, 162, 178, 194, 202
    acquisition metaphor of 109–110, 112
    adult 111
    'banking' approaches to 110, 127–128
    health *see* health education
    humanistic 106, 111, 113
    and inequality 27, 28, 196
    and Ottawa Charter 10, 11
    and social change 111–112
    and social policy 7, 80, 88
    as transmission of knowledge 109, 112
    in UK, decline of 5
    see also training
Edwards, P. 207
Eggermann, M. 20
eHealth *see* digital technology
El Ansari, W. 55
Elmawazini, K. 201
Elwell-Sutton, T. 14
employment 1, 2, 4, 7, 78, 79, 88, 167, 196, 202
empowerment 24–30, 52, 90, 186, 190, 192, 205
    and advocacy 91, 93
    and citizenship *see* citizenship
    community *see* community empowerment
    as core value 31, 32, 33, 48
    and education 110
    and epistemology 159
    evaluation of 157
    and health communication 106, 107, 109, 111, 112, 115, 119, 120
    and health literacy 130, 132
    individual 27–28, 56, 61, 124, 195

empowerment (*continued*)
    and organizational change 155
    as outcome/process 29–30, *29*
    and participation 29, 30, *30*, **219**
    and policy 91, 93, 94, 95, 99
    and social marketing 128, 130
    and women 201, 203, 209
enablement 10, 11, **15**, 50
England 190, 199, 206
    community development in 62
    community participation in 56
    demise of health promotion in 192–193
    health inequality in 2, 5, 16, 78–79
    health trainers in 53–54
Enlightenment 211, 212
entrepreneurs 90
environment 33, 43, 125, 202–203, 216
    and Healthy Cities initiative 42, 66, 153, 178, 192
    and lobbying 93
    and policy 84, **85**, 88
    and pollution 3, 7, 77, *77*, 80, 125
    social 42, 44, 47, 210
    supportive 12, 13, 14, 188
    see also climate change; ecological strategies; sustainability
epistemology 157–159, 210, **217**, **219**
equilibrium, lay concept of 20–21, 189
equity 1–3, 4–5, 7, **15**, 191, 221
    and communities 42, 54, 61
    as core value 10, 11, 31, 123
    and policy 80, 86, 92
    and transformational change 148
    see also health inequalities; social justice
Eraut, M. 176
ethical change processes 33, **220**
ethics 149, 163–167, 195, **220**
    and communication 108–109, 119, 129–130
    and customary/reflective ethics 163
    and digital technology 123, 125, 127
    and doing no harm 163, 164
    and health care ethics 163
    and imposing health values 164–165
    and manipulating behaviour 166–167
    and not acting/doing nothing 165–166
    and policy 76–77
    political aspects of 1, 5, 7
    and rationing 165
    and right to intervene 165
    and voluntarism/autonomy/informed choice 164
Ethiopia 177, 189
ethnicity 1, 11, 14, 20, 23, 47, 126, 171, 199, 209
    see also African-Americans; indigenous peoples
Etkin, J. 122
Eurocentrism 25, 138, 191, 195, 207, 214
Europe 16, 42, 81, 151, 165, 166, 168, 199
    see also specific countries
European Union 16

evaluation 153–155, 162–163, **172**, *174*, 176
    black box of 159
    and communication 107
    defined 157
    epistemological/methodological issues in 157–159, 162
    and evidence-based practice 149, 156–157
Evans, L. 175
Evidence to Policy initiative (E2Pi) 162
evidence-based practice 31, 156–162, 165, 216, **220**, 221
    appraising evidence in 161
    epistemological/methodological issues in 157–159
    and evaluation 149, 156–157
    and forms of evidence 159, **159**
    framing questions in 160
    hierarchical approach to 158
    and local context 161
    obtaining evidence in 160–161
    and policy-making 82–83, 98, 161–162
    and practitioners 160, 161
    quality of evidence in 162
    and RCTs 59, 158, 159
    steps/skills in 160
Ewles, L. 165
experts 83, 107, 109, 148, 205, 212

Facebook 121, 125, 153
Fag Ends project (Liverpool, UK) 55–56
families 45, 47, 51
family planning 120, 196
Fankanta initiative (Gambia) 120
Farquhar, S.A. 53
fast food 8, 117
FCTC (Framework Convention on Tobacco Control, 2005) 76
'Feed the World' campaigns 115
feedback 108, *109*, 112, 113, 117, 120, 124, 212
feeder disciplines 24
female genital mutilation 61, 163, 164, 196
feminism 27, 62, **85**, 195, 196, 200
Field, M.G. 22
financial crisis 84–86
Finnish approach 205–206
Fiore, Q. 115
Fisher, W.F. 170
Fitbit 122, 125
Five Year Forward View (NHS) 65, 124–125, 193
Fleming, M. 13, 32, 221
Floridi, L. 125
Floyd, George 26
food advertising 77
food safety 80
food security 8
foreign aid 5–6
Fortune, K. 203
Fox, N. 210

France 22
Frankel, S. 23
Fraser, C. 113
Fraser, H. 93
Freire, Paulo 25, 26, 27, 61–62, 110, 111, 127–128, 173
French, J. 128
Fresbach, S. 166
Friel, S. 3
Friendship Bench 52
Frosh, S. 168
Fukuyama, F. 46, 47, 48

Gabe, J. 24
Gagliani, M. 76
Gale, N.K. 54
Galea, G. 151
Galer-Unti, R.A. 93
Galway Consensus 175–178
    and competence-based approach 176
    eight domains of 176
    and Public Health Skills and Career Framework 177–178
    and three levels of health promoters 176–177
Gambia *43*, 80, 120–121, *208*, 209
Gambling, T.S. 109
Garthwaite, K. 211
Garvin, T. 107, 109, 110, 112
Gates, Bill 6, 91
Gavens, I. 83
Gehlert, S. 195
Geldof, Bob 115
gender 14, 17, 22, 195–196, 199, 209, 212
    and globalization 201–202
    and health communication 113, 116
    and help seeking behaviours 189
    and inequality 29, 44, 47
    and lay beliefs 23
    see also men's health; women
Gerhardt, S. 212
Germany 190, 209
Germond, P. 210
Ghana 23, 64, 191, 207
Gilmore, A.B. 88
Gilson, L. 98
Giuntoli, G. 214
Glenton, C. 55
global burden of disease 16, 189, 202, 204
global governance 75, 94, 202
globalization 93, 96, 117, 186, 201–202, 203, 204, 222
GMP (Grandmother Project) 52
GNH (Gross National Happiness) 211, 213
Golinowska, S. 198
Golubchikov, O. 65
Gonzales-Salgado, I. 98
Gordon, R. 128
governments 1, 4, 6, 31, 87–88, 123, 148, 155, 167, 202
    and Covid-19 pandemic 137
    see also policy
Grace, Victoria 25
grandmothers 50, 52
Grant, A.M. 18, 19
grassroots organizations 3, 59, 90, 117, 171, 173, 208, 209, 222
Green, J. 28, 108, *109*, 128, 138, 151, 162
Green, L.W. 150
green space 48, 50
Greenpeace 87, 92
Gregg, J. 33, 164, 216, 219
Greve, H. 51
Griffiths, J. 128, 155
Groot, W. 190
Gross National Happiness (GNH) 211, 213
Grunfeld, E.A. 22
Guareschi, P. 58–59
gun culture/control 79, 165
Gunn, L. 78–79, 89
Gutiérez, L. 29
Gwyther, K. 189
Gypsy/Traveller communities 16, 199–200

Hagell, A. 198
Hale, J. 166, 167
Hall, J. 186
Hall, S.M. 81
Halliday, J. 161
Hamara Centre, Leeds (UK) 209
Hancock, T. 151
Hankivsky, O. 200
happiness 17, 18–20, 49–50, 211–214, **217**
    measurements of 211, 213, 214, 222
    and social/natural capital 213
'hard-to-reach' groups 53, 119, 121, 153, **217**, **220**
Harris, T.A. 114
Hart, R. 56
Harvey, D. 1
Hawe, P. 207
health 17–24
    and balance/equilibrium 20–21
    and control 19, *19*, 21
    defined 17, 18, 20, 214
    as happiness/wellbeing 18–20, *19*
    lay perspectives on 20–24, 210–211
    measurement/indices of 9, 17
    prerequisites of 10
    and salutogenesis 10, 17–18
Health Action Model 132, 133, 136, 138
health activism 65–66, *66*, 67, 170, 192, 196, 200
Health in All Policies *see* HiAP
health behaviours *see* behaviour change
Health Belief Model 128, 132, 133, 138, 211
health campaigns 89, *97*, 108, 115, 117, 120, 121, 127, 166–167
    see also advocacy; social marketing

health care systems 1, 6, **9**, 31, 41, 191, 192, 202
    access to 17
    and CHWs 52, 53, 56
    cost of 10
    and policy 75, 81
    reorienting 176, 177, 189, 203
    strengthened by health promotion 13, 14, **15**
health coaching 134
health communication 106–138, 211
    and behaviour change theory *see* behaviour change theory
    bottom-up/participatory approaches 119–121
    channel/message components in 115
    and communication theories 107–109
    and culture 116
    and digital technology *see* digital technology
    ethical questions with 108–109
    and empowerment 106, 107, 109, 111, 112, 115, 119, 120
    evaluation of 107
    and feedback 108, *109*, 112, 113, 117, 120, 124
    four components in 112–117, **113**
    and health literacy *see* health literacy
    inconsistent messages in 106
    and interpersonal skills 107, 113
    and Johari window 113, 114
    and lay knowledge 117
    and mass media 115, 116, 117–118
    and non-verbal communication 115
    and patient education 107
    and peer education 118–119
    receiver component in 116–117
    sender component in 113–115, **113**
    and social marketing *see* social marketing
    and theatre/drama 62, 115, 116, 117, 120, 121
    as top-down/one-way process 106–107, 109–110, 127, 138
    and transactional analysis 113–114
    two-way 107
    see also health education
health education 6, 11, 14, 99, 106, 107, 109–112, 138
    assumptions in 109, *110*
    and empowerment 109, 111
    and health literacy 130
    one-way 109–110
    two-way 110–112
    see also health communication
Health For All movement 192
health impact assessments 96
health improvement officers 177
health inequalities 3, 4–5, 7, 14–17, 78–79, 186, 195, 216
    and communities 42, 43, 44, 54, 56
    and data collection 16
    and digital technology 107, 126
    and global health policy 96
    and health literacy 130
    lay perspectives on 211
    and settings approach 152–153
    and social marketing 128
    structural causes of 79
    see also anti-oppressive practice
health literacy 106, 126, 127, 130–132, 188
    clinical/public health approaches to 131–132
    defined 130, 132
    and digital technology 131
    measurement of 131
    three levels of 130
health planning 42, 56, 57, *60*, 82, 108, 132, 157, 171
    three domains of 216
health policy 80–82, 178
    global 96–98, **97**
    and other policy areas 80–81, *81*, 88
health professionals 31, 33, 42, 113, 175, 198
    and communities 148
    and ethics 163
    and lay expertise 51, 55, 195
    and policy 87, 90
    and relationship with patients/clients 163, 194
health promotion research 18, 43, 149, 154, 159, 162–163, 205–206
Health and Social Care Act (2012) 192
health social movements (HSMs) 65–66
health trainers 53–54, 178, 188
health values 164–165
health visitors 177
health-institution 21–22
healthism 124, 129, 165
healthworlds concept 210–211
Healthy Cities initiative 25, 42, 66, 153, 178, 192
Heard, E. 200
heart disease 23, 45, 172
Helsinki Conference (WHO, 2013) 13, 75
Henderson, J. 195
Herzlich, C. 20, 23
HiAP (Health in All Policies) 13, **15**, 67, 75–82
    and complexity 77–78
    and health policy 80–82
    policy approaches 78, *78*
    principles/components of 76
    and social policy 79–80
Hilhorst, D. 170
Hillsden, M. 134, 135
HIV/AIDS 66, 163, 170, 196
    in Africa 16, 202, 204
    and health communication 108, 119, 120, 122
    and policy 87, 91, 96
Hogwood, B. 78–79, 89
holding frameworks 178
Holroyd, C. 175
Holtgrave, D.R. 66
homelessness 5, **78**, 153
homosexuality/homophobia 163, 200
Horsley, Katrice 64
hospitals 149, 151

housing 1, 6, 194, 203, 211
    and communities 51, 58
    and inequality/exclusion 27, 196, 202, 211
    policy 78, 80
HSMs (health social movements) 65–66
Hubley, J. 112
Hudson, J. 88, 90, 94
Hughner, R.S. 20
human rights 129–130, 171, 200, 221, 222
Human Rights, Universal Declaration of 1
humanistic approaches 25
Hunter, D.J. 152
hygiene 166–167
Hylton, K. 196

IBFAN (International Baby Food Action Network) 65
ICT (Information Communication Technology) *see* digital technology
ideologies 75, 84–86, **85**, 87, 96, 192
Ife, J. 32
immunization *see* vaccination
implementation of health promotion 149, 186, 187–192
    see also policy implementation
income 10, 27, 44, 211
India 164, 171, 177, 201, 213, 214, 215
indigenous peoples 16, 21, 32, 190, 214, 221
industrial diseases 23
infant/child mortality 8, 16, 53, 59, 81, 167, 204
infectious diseases 12, 16, 80, 83, 125, 203–204
infrastructure 7, 11, 12, 13, **15**, 32, 43, 49
Ingham, Harry 113
innovations 173
    diffusion of 118, 119
    policy 88
Innstrand, S.T. 225
interdisciplinary approach 53, 163
International Baby Food Action Network (IBFAN) 65
internet 122, 123, 124, 126, 126–127, 153, 207
    of Things (IoT) 107, 121, 127
interpersonal skills 107
intersectionality 200
intersectoral collaboration 12, 13, **15**, 75, 88, 94
intervention-driven approaches 43
    and intervention ladder 165, 166
Italy 190
IUHPE (International Union of Health Promotion and Education) 221

Jacobs, G. 29
Jakarta Conference/Declaration (WHO, 1997) 12–13, 75, 190
Janis, I.L. 166
Japan 4, 14, 16, 44
Jelsøe, E. 203

Joffe, M. 80
Johari window 113, 114
Johnson, A. 151
Johnston, R. 83
Jones, C.M. 187
Jones, M. 84
Jones, R. 190
Jordan 177
journals 160, 192, 213
Jovchelovitch, S. 58–59

Kamphuis, C.B.M. 46
Kane, S. 55–56
Karim, Q.A. 202
Kato, David 163
Katz, E. 118
Kawachi, I. 45
Kelly, G.P. 212–213
Kennedy, A. 128
Kenya 117–118, 168–169, 191
Keshavarz Mohammadi, N. 193–194, 195
Kharsany, A.B.M. 202
Khor, M. 201
Kickbusch, I. 190
Kiger, A. 107
Kim, C. 48
Kingdon, J.W. 90
Kingsley, J. 48
Kitzinger, C. 196
Kleine, S.S. 20, 24
Kleinman, A. 20, 51
Kloppers, R. 48
knowledge **9**, *64*, 108, 109–112, *110*, 116, 118, 138, 158, 163
    expert/professional 30–31, 110
    of grandmothers 50, 52
    lack of, as barrier to health 123, 126, 132
    lay 20–23, 24, 41, 50, 51, 53, 117
    local 32, 33, 47, 55
    and networks 156
    and peer education 119
    personal 45, 51
    renewal/exchange 179
    transfer 109–110, 112, 179, 208
    see also epistemology
Knowles, M. 111
Kobasa, S. 19
Kotter, John 155, 156
Kreuter, M.T. 116
Krieger, N. 84
Kubow, P. 168
Kumar, A. 213
Kuruvilla, S. 131–132
Kwok, C. 21
Kymlicka, W. 48, 168
Kyoto Protocol (2010) 76

Labonté, R. 14, 19, 94, 173, 175, 191, 202, 203
Lahtinen, E. 162, 205
Lalonde Report 10, 190, 192
Land, R. 7, 112
Landqvist, M. 195
Langer, A. 203
Langford, R. 128
Lapidos, A. 54
Larkin, F. 95
Larsen, E.L. 4, 6
Lasswell, H.D. 108
Latin America 16, 151, 201, 204
Latino communities 40, 53
Lave, J. 208
Laverack, G. 28, 29, 60, 61, 65, 94, 167, 173, 175
lay beliefs/knowledge 20–24, 33, 41, 50–56, 66, 189, 195, 211, 212
    and community health workers *see* CHWs
    and grandmothers 50, 52
    and health communication 117
    and health professionals 51, 55
lay epidemiology 195
Lazarfeld, P.F. 118
leadership 3, 32, 49, 59, *60*, 155, 178–179, 187
learning disability 199
Ledwith, M. 62
Lee, R.G. 107, 109, 110, 112
Leeds (UK) 87, 175, 209
Leeds Beckett University (UK) 16, 24, 88, 169, 205, 206, *208*
Lefebvre, R.C. 128
legislation 60, 80, 82, 91, 187
    Health Act (2007) 98
    Health and Social Care Act (2012) 192
    and lobby/interest groups *see* lobbying
    and top-down/bottom-up processes 89, 172
    and voluntary approach 88
    see also policy; taxation
Leninger, M. 116
Lesotho 120
leukaemia 117
Levitas, R. 201
LGBTQI+ communities 200
liberalism 85, 95, 111
libertarianism 88, 129, 165
libraries 64, 66
life expectancy 5, 14–16, 17, 81, 199, 221
life satisfaction 43, 44, 49, 213
lifestyles 10, 14, 91, 161, 210, 211
    and digital health promotion 123, 124
    and HiAP 76, 78
    and lay beliefs 21, 23
    and media 7
    and moralising/making 'right' choices 48, 165, 193
    unhealthy 7, 202, **211**, **217**
linear models 135, 136, 137, 212
    of communication 108, 215
    of policy 82, **83**

Linney, B. 120
Lipsky, M. 90
literacy 5, 27, 111, 116, 121
    health *see* health literacy
Liverpool (UK) 55
lobbying 86–87, 90, 92–93, 98
local government 42, 51, 58, 79, 125, 168–169, 192, 193
local knowledge 32, 33
loneliness *see* social isolation
Lowe, S. 88, 90
Luft, Joseph 113
Lundahl, B.W. 135
Lupton, D. 23–24, 126

Maass, R.B. 47
McCartney, G. 199
Macdonald, G. 24, 194, 195
McGregor, C. 221
McGuire, W. 108
Macintyre, S. 22
McKee, M. 84
Mackenzie, M. 23
McKinlay, J.B. 7, 8
McKnight, J.L. 42, 56, 58
Mackworth-Young, C.R.S. 66
McLuhan, Marshall 115
McNeill, D. 96
McQueen, D.V. 156, 194
Mad Management Virus 173
Mahoney, R. 32
Maio, G.R. 134
malaria 91, 120, 204
Malaysia 23
Mali 177
malnutrition 8, 11, 16, 96
Manderson, L. 4, 6
Manitoba Public Insurance campaigns (Canada) 92
Manji, F. 209
Manoff, Richard 127
Mantoura, R. 78
Maori people 32, 221
mapping *43*, 48, 58, *64*, 154, 168, 191, 206, 212
Marcano-Olivier, M.I. 129
Markel, H. 96
marketing 12, 24, 75, 194, 202
    social *see* social marketing
    see also advertising
Marks, D.F. 159
Marmot, Michael 2, 5, 78, 86, 193, 216
Marmot Review (2010) 5, 79, 190
Marotholi Travelling Theatre Company (Lesotho) 120
Marston, C. 66
Marteau, T.M. 129
Martell, L. 201
Marx, Karl 220
Marxism 47, 62

Mayall, Berry 198
Maycock, B. 93
Mayo, M. 41–42
Mda, Z. 120
MDGs (Millennium Development Goals) 96, 191
measles 2, 16
media 7, 23–24, 26, 86, 87, 92, 121, 194
    and health communication 115, 116, 117–118, 126
mediation 10, 11, **15**
medical model of health 9, **9**, 18, 76, 124, 151
    and health education 109
medical records 124, 125
Mendelsohn, H. 118
men's health 22, 189, 196
mental health 5, 52, 116, 119, 189, 195, 196, 204, 221
    and CHWs 53, 54
    and digital technology 122–123, 126
    and happiness/wellbeing/self-esteem 19, 133, 212, 213
    and policy 87, 90
    and social capital 44, 45
    and spiritual health 215
    and young people 121–122, 198
Mercer, H. 191
Merton, R.K. 118
Mexico Conference (WHO, 2000) 13, 75, 190
Meyer, J. 7, 112
Mezirow, J. 112
Michie, S. 138
Mill, John Stuart 165
Millennium Development Goals (MDGs) 96, 191
Miller, William 134
Milne, E. 192–193
Mindell, J. 80
Misan, G.M.H. 189
Mistry, Robinton 164
Mittelmark, M.B. 10, 175–176, 194
Mittelstadt, B.D. 125
mobile phones 115, 117, *120*, 121–122
Moghadam, V. 201
Mohan, M. 201–202
Monkman, K. 60
Montreal Declaration (2018) 127
Moore, S. 196
moral aspects 5, 21, 30, 48, 163, 164–165
    see also ethics
morbidity 9, 17, 162, 165, 202, 210
Morris, M. 200
Morrison, V. 78
mortality 7, 9, 14, 17, 44, 210
    infant/child 8, 16, 53, 59, 81, 167, 204
    maternal 120, 221
motivation 108, *109*, 118, 122, 133, 134, **217**
    three categories of 168
motivational interviewing 127, 133–135
    and brief behavioural counselling/health coaching 134–135
    critiques of 135
    principles of 134
    and step change theories/self-efficacy 135
Moyo, Dambisa 5
Muir Gray, J.M. 160, 162
Mullen, L. 21
Mullen, P.D. 152
Muller, R.F. 59
multi-disciplinary approach 24, 194, 205
multiculturalism 195, 196
Murray, M. 17
Musavengane, R. 48

Naidoo, J. 128, 176, 178
Nairobi Conference (WHO, 2009) 13, 191
Namibia 191
naming/shaming 167
'nanny state' 6, 78, 129, 187
Naples, N. 189
Narayan, D. 46
National Health Service *see* NHS
Navarro, Vincente 198–199
NCDs (non-communicable diseases) 7, 13, 189, 202, 204
    UN Resolution on Prevention/Control of (2011) 76
need assessment 59, 172, 209, **218**, **220**
neighbourhoods 7, 8, 41, 43, 49, 61, 193
Nelson, G. 194
neoliberalism 3, 25, 65, 79, 84, **85**, 86, 187, 190, 201, 202
Nepal 53, 167
Netherlands 124, 190
networks 13, 41, 46, 50, 52, 67, 148, 221
    bonding 45–46, 48
    bridging 46, 48, 49
    and leadership 148–149
    online 121, 122, 124, 127, 153
    and organizational change 156
    policy 88, 89, 94
    positive/negative effects of 46, 47
    and public health crises 50, 51
    and social capital 44, 45–46, 119
New Zealand 32, 203, 221
NGOs (non-governmental organizations) 148, 156, 167, 187, 201
    and bottom-up/top-down dilemma 149, 171
    criticisms of 170
    Hamara (Leeds, UK) 209
    and policy 87, 96, **97**
    Tostan (Senegal) 60, 61
NHS (National Health Service) 8, 56, 65, 79, 84, 121, 177, 199
    and digital technology 122, 125
    Five Year Forward View 65, 124–125, 193
    reorganization of 192–193
NICE (National Institute for Health and Clinical Excellence) 60, 158
Nigeria 21, 23, 77–78, 165, 191
non-communicable diseases *see* NCDs

non-governmental organizations *see* NGOs
non-maleficence 163, 164, **218**, **220**
non-verbal communication 115
Norman, C. 126
Norman, P. 138
Norman, W. 168
North Karelia Project 172
Norway 209
nudging 87, 166
Nuffield Ladder of Intervention 87–88
Nussbaum, M.C. 214
Nutbeam, D. 80, 130, 162
nutcracker effect 3, 43
nutrition *see* diet/nutrition

obesity 7, 8, 46, 76–77, 195
    in children 90, 164, 203
Obrist, H.U. 121
Occupy Movement 65–66, 168
O'Donnell, M.P. 214
Ofili, A.N. 94
O'Hara, L. 33, 164, 216, 219
older people 12, 22, 58, 123, 126, 190, 198
    projects with grandmothers 50, 52
Oliver, Jamie 115
Oliver, M. 199
Omonzejele, P.F. 21, 23
O'Neil, I. 127
oppression 25–26, 27
    challenging 26, 28–29, 111, 195–201
organizational change 149, 155–156, 173
    eight steps to 156
    five areas for development in 156
organizations 148, 152
    learning 155–156
Orton, L. 60
Osaghae, E.E. 171
Osgood–Schramm model of communication 108, *109*
O'Sullivan, T. 50
Ottawa Charter (WHO, 1986) 2, 13–14, 75, 127, 172, 192, 193, 205, 209
    and Bangkok Charter, compared 190
    empowerment in 24, 42, 135, 162
    environmental concerns in 202
    ethos/aims of 4, 10–11
    and reorienting health services 176, 177, 189
    and settings approach 150, 151, 154
    significance of 4, 187
Ottersen, O.P. 96
Outram, D. 211–212
Oxfam 96, **97**, 170

Pacific islands 151
Pakistan 177
Palmer, S. 134–135

pandemics 50, 51, 66
Panter-Brick, C. 20, 128
parents 79, 122, 175, 177, 195
Paris Agreement (2016) 76
Park, J.D. 6
Parry, G. 168
Parsons, W. 82, 92, 98
participation 31, 41, 52, 66–67, 123, **217**, **218**
    community *see* community participation
    and empowerment 29, 30, *30*, **219**
    in health promotion research 162–163, 205
    and top-down/bottom-up conundrum 172, *172*, 173, *174*
participatory budgeting (PB) 58–59, 66
partnerships 13, **15**, 32, 33, 127, 168, 191, 194
    and communities 55, 56, 66, 59.61.64
    and empowerment 29, *29*
    and policy 75, 94–96
    and universities 176, 207, 209
paternalism 5, 50, 56, **85**, 93, 110, 114, 129
patient-centred approach 51
Pawson, R. 59, 159
peace 3, 10, 32
Pearce, J. 170
Peckham, S. 193
Pedersen, A. 196
Pedler, M. 156
peer education/interventions 28, 54, 67, 118–119, 156, 207
Peerson, A. 130–131
People in Public Health Project (UK) 149
people-centred health promotion 31–32, 43, 54, 56, 148
People's Health Movement 3
Perkmann, M. 90
Perry, H.B. 52–53
personal development/skills 11
personal skills development 10, 11, **15**, 135, 188, **218**
Pescosolido, B.A. 189
Petterson, B. 187, 189
Petticrew, M. 159
pharmaceutical industry 92, 96, 167
PHC (primary health care) 14, 31, 94, **97**, 186, 187
    Alma-Ata Declaration on *see* Alma Ata Declaration
    and community health workers *see* CHWs
PHE (Public Health England) 56, 192
physical exercise 7, 8, 50, 123, 135
Pickett, K. 4–5
Pierret, J. 20, 21–22
Pill, R. 21, 22
Planned Behaviour Theory 132, 133, 136, 138
Platt, L. 80
Pleasant, A. 131–132
pluralism **83**, 93, 95, 115, 119
    medical 189
Pogge, Thomas 5
Poland 190
policy 7, 21–22, 75–99, 106, 119, 187
    and advocacy 75, 90–94
    and agenda setting 75

analysis 97–98
defined 79–80
entrepreneurs 90
evidence-based 161–162
health *see* health policy
Health in All *see* HiAP
ideological basis of 75, 84–86, **85**
and intersectoral collaboration 75, 88, 94
narratives 84
networks 88, 89
and nudging 87, 166
and Ottawa Charter 10, **15**
and partnerships 75, 94–95, 148
and power 78, **78**, 82, 86, 95, 98, 99
rationalist model of 82, **83**, 89
role of government in 87–88, 202
sectors 75
social 22, 79–80, 194
and social marketing 128
and social model of health 33, 81, 221
and social movements 65
and top-down/bottom-up processes 3, 172–173
see also HiAP
policy actors/stakeholders 79, 82, **83**, 84, 86–87, 94
three categories of 86
policy implementation 88–90
and advocacy 92
barriers to 89
bottom-up 89, 90
factors in 88–89
integrated 89
top-down 89–90
policy process 82–84
and advocacy 92
citizen participation in 95–96
eight steps of 82
and influencing factors 84
and policy-making theories 82, **83**
role of evidence in 82–83
wicked problems in 83
polio 16
political aspects of health promotion 1, 4, 14, 42, 123, 165, 192
see also democracy; global health policy; governments; ideologies
Pollock, A. 81
pollution 3, 7, 77, 77, 80, 125
Pols, J. 195
Polynesia 20, 21
Popay, J. 26, 210
population health 190
Porter, C. 190
Portman Group 92
Porto Alegre (Brazil) 58–59
positivism 158, 163, 211, **217**
Poskitt, E. 203
Potvin, L. 187

poverty 2, 3, 7, 8, 16, 96, 116, 191, 210–211, 222
child 5, 81
and globalization 201
Power for Health project (Oregon, USA) 53
power/powerlessness 25–27, 54, 67, 164, **172**, 199, **218**
citizen 56, 57
and digital technology 124, 125
and discourse analysis 189–190
and health education 110, 113
and health professionals 55, 163
and marketing 128
and policy 78, **78**, 82, 86, 95, 98, 99
and social capital 46
and transformational change 148
see also control; empowerment
Pratt, D.D. 109, 110, 112
praxis 62
precautionary principle 165–166
Prilleltensky, I. 194
Primary Care Trusts 192
primary health care *see* PHC
Prior, L. 195
prisons/prisoners 16, 30, 90, 119, 152, 154–155, 175
health-promoting 150, 151, 153, 154
private sector 148, 167, 170
privatization 85, **85**, 97
problem-solving approach 52, 63, 111, 121, 127, 155, 172
processes of health promotion 10, 11
professional development 175, 177, 206
professionalization 55, 175
propaganda 108, 117, 118
Protection Motivation Theory 132, 133, 136, 138, 166
psychology/psychoanalysis 106, 194, 195, 212, 213
public health 4, 110, 125, 193
decision-making model of 93
and health literacy 131, 132
and lobbying 93
Public Health Alliance 192
Public Health England (PHE) 56, 192
Public Health Skills and Career Framework 177–178
public spaces 48, 50
PubMed 160
Putnam, R.D. 45, 47, 48

quality of life 11, 18, 28, 132, 162, 165, 193, *200*, 201
and freedom 214

race/racism 44, 49, 66, 195–196
radio 115, 116, 117, 119, 121
Radley, A. 210
Raeburn, J.M. 25, 31–32
randomized controlled trials (RCTs) 59, 157, 159
Rao, H. 51
Raphael, D. 190
Ratcliffe, T. 2

Index 245

Ratima, M. 203
Rawls, J. 220
Raworth, K. 17
red lotus model 216, 219
redistributive justice 3
Redzuan, M. 30
refugees/asylum seekers 16, 122, 178
Reilly, R.G. 84
religion 5, 199, 214, 215, *216*
Renfrew, M.J. 161
reorienting health services 176, 177, 189, 203
reproductive health/rights 79, 120, 122, 196
resilience 41, 42, 48, 49, 50, 65, 81, 122, 137
    and health education 119
respiratory infections 2, 16, 204
Restrepo-Estrada, S. 113
Reynolds, A. 155
Rice, L. 125
Riddell, R.C. 6
Rifkin, S.B. 56, 57, 59
Riger, S. 30
rights-based approach 1
Rio+20 summit (2012) 96
Rio Declaration (2011) 76
risk-taking behaviour 14, 33, 46, 47, 122, 137, 198
Rissel, C. 25
road traffic accidents 58, 204
road-building 77–78, 80
Roberts, H. 159
Robertson, A. 210
Robertson, S. 22, 131, 189
Robinson, M. 131
Rocha Franco, S.H. 59
Roderick, P. 81
Rogers, Carl 111, 112, 173
Rogers, E.M. 118, 173
Rogers, R.W. 118
Rollnick, S. 134
Roma communities 16, 199–200
Rootman, I. 25, 31–32
Roseto, Pennsylvania (US) 44, 45
Rotorua Statement (2019) 221
Roy, M.J. 62
Russia 20, 21, 22
Rutten, A. 98
Rychetnik, L. 161

Salamon, L.M. 170
Salant, T. 195
salutogenesis 9–10, 17–18, 33, 50, 194, **219**
Sampson, U.K.A. 191
Sanders, D. 6, 127
Sanson-Fisher, R. 156–157
Sara, R. 125
Saudi Arabia 98
Saunders, M. 130–131

schools 149, 153, 155, 173, 175, 198
Schrecker, T. 3
Schwab, K. 216
Science Citation indices 160
Scotland 21, 22, 23, **85**, 95
Scott, K. 186
Scott-Samuel, A. 189–190, 192, 193
SDGs (Sustainable Development Goals) 3, 13, 17, 86, 96, 176, 203, 204
sedentary lifestyles 12, 80, 122, 165
Seedhouse, D. 17, 30, 93, 194
Seidler, Z.E. 189
self-efficacy 27, 111, 119, 122, 124, 126, 133, 134
self-esteem 27, 119, 122, 133, 154, 164
Sen, A. 24, 214
Sena, R. 42
Senegal 52, 60, 61
Senge, P.M. 155, 156
Serrat, O. 156
Serrata, J. 28
settings approach 149–155
    benefits of 150
    challenges with 152–153
    criticisms of 152, 153
    evaluation of effectiveness of 153–155
    limiting factors in 151
    and marginalized groups 153
    and range of/connections between settings 152
    terminology of 150–151
    and variability of practice 151, **152**
    and virtual settings 149, 153
settings for health 13
sexual health *see* reproductive health/rights
sexually transmitted diseases 16, 120
Sfard, A. 109–110, 111, 112
Shanghai conference (WHO, 2016) 13, 14, 42
Shannon-Weaver model of communication 108
Sharma, M. 135
Shepherd, J. 159
shock tactics 166
Shoemaker, F. 118
Shove, E. 137
Shuga (TV show) 117–118
Sierra Leone 167
Silva, K. 42
Simnett, I. 165
Sindall, C. 163
Small, N. 22–23
Smith, J. 2
Smith, K.E. 210–211
Smithies, J. 90–91
smoking *see* tobacco
Smyth, R.L. 161
social capital 41, 43–50, 57, 61, 65, 66, 119, 122, 188, 221
    and Covid-19 crisis 51
    and happiness/wellbeing 213, 214

and health promotion 47–48, 213
and healthy communities 49–50
and networks *see* networks
problems with 48–49
and trust 46–47, 48, 49
social care 2, 51, 196
social change 29, 61, 93, 111–112, 124, 148, 214, 222
social constructionism 158–159
social determinants of health (SDH) 1–4, *3*, 5, 32, 123, 189, 190, 193, 210, 221
and children/young people 198
and communities 41, 42, 43
and HiAP 76
and ICT 125
and individual empowerment 27
and policy 81, 161–162, 202
seven discourses in 190
and social change 125
WHO Commission for (CSDH, 2008) 2–3, 78, 176, 199
social exclusion 83, 95, 154, 193, *200*, 201
social isolation 47, 198, 214
social justice 1, 10, 14, 32, 171, 190, 191, 195, 200, 216, 221
and community development 60, 61, 65
as core value **15**, 31, 41, 106, 123
and social change 28
social marketing 106, 117, 127–130, 138
and advocacy 128
and behaviour change/choice 128, 129
downstream/upstream 128
and health promotion, compared 128
and nudging/choice architecture 128–130
social media 23, 87, 93, 115, 121, 122, 123, 125, 126, 153
social mobilization 65, 162
social model of health 8–9, **9**, 194
social movements 65–66, 93, 186
social policy 22, 79–80, 194
social relations 49
Social Science Citation Indices 160
social systems *see* settings approach
socialism 52, 57, 79, **85**
socio-economic aspects 8, 10, 14, 17
sociology 20, 24, 194, 195, 211
solid waste management 149, 168–169, *169*, 188
Solomon, B.B. 26
Soul City (TV show) 120
South Africa 16, 55, 120, 191, 210
South, J. 43, 55, 56, 60, 119, 162, 168, 205
Southby, K. 199
Spain 98
Sparks, M. 187
Spencer, G. 29
Spicker, P. 86
spiritual health 214–215
spirituality 17, 21, 32
Springett, J. 55, 189–190, 192, 193

Sri Lanka 14–16
Stainton-Rogers, W. 17
Standing, H. 52
Staples, L.H. 27
Staying Alive initiative 120
Stenning, A. 81
sterilization campaigns 164
Stiglitz, J. 201
storytelling 62, 64, 115, 116
Stott, N. 21, 22
stress 3, 122, 123, 124, 134, 189, 211
structural adjustment 57, 78
Stuckler, D. 81
subsidies 11
sugar 77, 80, 92
Sullivan, G. 21
Sundsval conference (WHO, 1991) 11, 12, 13–14
Sunstein, C.R. 129, 215
supportive environments 12, 13, 14, 188
sustainability 32, 33, 148, 202–203, 205, **218**, 221
and community development/participation 54, 56, 59, 60
and health communication 119, 120, 122, 123
and health literacy 130
and policy 80, **85**, 94, 95, 155
see also SDGs
Sustainable Development, 2030 Agenda for 1, 56
Sutton, R. 88–89
Sutton, S. 135
Svalastog, A.L. 17
Swami, V. 23
Swaziland 191
Sweden 14, 22, 124
Szreter, S. 49

Tanzania 52, 156, 168–169, 209
taxation 3, 11, 77, **78**, 81
Taylor, P. 50, 56, 66, 95
Taylor, R. 186
TB (tuberculosis) 54, 80, 91, 120
technology 41, 204, 212
digital *see* digital technology
Teixeira Assis, W.F. 59
telehealth/telecare platforms 123
telephone 121
see also mobile phones
television 115, 117–118, 120, 121
Thaler, R.H. 129, 215
Thatcher government 192
theatre/drama 62, 115, 116, 117, 120, 121
Thompson, S. 14
threat perception 133
threshold concepts 7–10, 24, 112
Thunberg, Greta 93
Tilford, S. 56
Tilley, N. 159

tobacco 7, 23, 80, 92
    anti-smoking campaigns 98, *116*, 117, 121, 122
    and communities 46, 47, 55
    Framework Convention on see FCTC
    and lobbying 91, 98
    marketing 12, *81*
    smoking bans 76, 98
Tobin, G. 50
Tod, A. 195
Tomlinson, M.W. 212–213
Tones, K. 56, 130
Tones, Keith 24
top-down processes 25, 57, 60, 89–90, **172**
    and bottom-up processes 3, 43, 55, 148, 149, 171, 172–175, *174*
    challenges to 65
    in health communication 106–107, 109–110, 112, 113, 114, 127, 128, 138
Tostan (Senegal) 60, 61
trade 12, 75, 78
traditional societies/practices 23, 120, 164, 196
training 51, 119, 124, 125, 175, 176, 177, 206–207
    of CHWs 52, 53, 54, 55
transactional analysis 113–114
transmission model 107, 108, 109, 112
transport 7, 10, 155, 194
    policies 76, 77–78, 80, *81*, 87
Transtheoretical Model 132, 133, 135, 138
Tribes (TV show) 120
Trinidad and Tobago 120
triple burden of disease 204
trust 44, 45, 46–47, 48, 49, 51, 115
tuberculosis (TB) 54, 80, 91, 120
Tuckett, D. 51
Twelvetrees, A. 62

Uganda 113, 163, 168–169
UKPHSKF (UK Public Health Skills and Knowledge Framework) 188–189, 206
Ukraine 20
United Nations (UN) 76, 87, **97**, 212
United States (USA) 4, 21, 26, 126, 168, 189
    CHWs in 53, 54
    empowerment in 28
    evidence-based practice in 158, 160
    health inequalities in 14
    indigenous people of 32
    lobbying in 86–87, 92, 93
    and WHO 97
universal basic income 7
universities 149, 150, 151, 176, 187, 192, 194, 195, 205, 206
    and communities 208–209
upstream thinking 7–8
urbanization 12, 203
utilitarianism 57, 65, 122, 167

vaccination 15, 23, 80, 177
Vader, J.P. 214, 215
Valdiserri, R.O. 66
values-based approach 30–33, 205, 216–219, **217–218**, 219, **220**
Vannucci, A. 122
Vass, C. 189
Veary, J. 191
VHAI (Voluntary Health Association of India) 171
victim blaming 14, 23, 48, 110, 127, 138
video games 123
Viens, A.M. 189
Villalonga-Olives, E. 45
violence 5, 13, 16, 17, 86, 123, 204
    domestic/gender-based 28, 196
voluntarism 164
volunteering 48, 51, 66, 67, 161
    see also CHWs

Wachter review (2016) 125
Waiora 32, 221
Wales 22
Walker, A. 95
Wallerstein, N. 28, 29, 65
Walt, G. 84, 98
Wang, S. 161
Ward, K. 210
Warwick-Booth, L. 80, 136, 162, 206
waste management 149, 168–169, *169*
water fluoridation/chlorination 164
water quality 80, 94, 204
Watson, J. 162
Weaver, A. 54
Webb, D. 154
Webb, T.L. 124
Webster, G. 90–91
welfare state 79
wellbeing 9, 18–20, *19*, 198, *200*, 211–214, **217**, **219**
    and communities 41, 42, 43, 46, 49
    and empowerment 27
    measurement of 59, 213, 222
    politics of 212
    relational 214
    and spiritual health 17, 215
Wells, J.S.G. 90
Wenger, E. 208
Werner, D. 127
What Works for Wellbeing (UK) 213
Whetton, Noreen 198
White, A. 196
White, S.C. 213–214
Whitehead, D. 162
Whitehead, M. 2, 5, 82, 125
Whitelaw, S. 151, **152**

WHO (World Health Organization) 2–3, 30, 33, 51, 87, 98
   and CHWs 53
   and communities 42, 53, 56
   definition of health by 17, 18, 212, 214, 215
   and evaluation 157
   and health impact assessments 96
   Healthy Cities programme 25, 42, 66, 153, 178, 192
   and HiAP 76, 79
   history of 10–14, **15**
   and networks 156
   and obesity 203
   and settings approach 150, 154
   and social determinants of health 176, 199
   and USA 92, 97
   values-based approach of 31
   see also specific conferences/charters/declarations
whole systems approach 155, 156, 173, 195, **217**, **219**
Wiggers, J. 156–157
Wilkinson, R. 4–5
Wilkinson, S. 196
Williams, E. 14
Williams, S. 210
Wills, J. 30–31, 128, 176
Wilson-Clay, B. 92
Wimbush, E. 162
windows of opportunity 90, 98
Wise, S. 28–29
Witte, K. 166
Wolf, M. 201

women 11, 16, 22, 28, 51, 169, 195–196, 198
   and community participation 59, *60*
   and globalization 201–202
   maternal health 13, 52, 59, 88
   and pregnancy 54, 196
   and sustainability 203
   see also feminism
Woodall, J. 25, 157, 205
Woodhead, D. 30–31
Woolcock, M. 49
workplaces 149, 152, 155, 156
World Bank 57, 78, 79, 96, **97**, 201
World Economic Forum 18
Wren-Lewis, S. 86
Wright, D. 154
Wrigley, T. 173

Yardley, L. 66
young people 78, 79, **91**
   and health communication 118, 119, 120, 122–123
   neglected in health promotion 196–198, *197*
YouTube 115, 117, 121, 153
Yurt, S. 119

Zambia 23, 88, 168–169, 209, 214
Zarcadoolas, C. 132
Zarychta, A. 46
Zimbabwe 52, 66
Zoller, H.M. 65